Vaccine Delivery Strategies

Edited by

Guido Dietrich
Berna Biotech AG, 3018 Berne, Switzerland

Werner Goebel
University of Würzburg, D-97074 Würzburg, Germany

Copyright © 2002
Horizon Scientific Press
P.O. Box 1
Wymondham
Norfolk NR18 0EH
England

www.horizonpress.com

Distributed exclusively in the United States, its dependent territories, Canada, Mexico, Central and South America, and the Caribbean by Springer-Verlag New York Inc, 175 Fifth Avenue, New York, USA, by arrangement with BIOS Scientific Publishers Ltd, 9 Newtec Place, Magdalen Road, Oxford OX4 1RE, UK. Distributed exclusively in the rest of the world by BIOS Scientific Publishers Ltd, 9 Newtec Place, Magdalen Road, Oxford OX4 1RE, UK.

British Library Cataloguing-in-Publication Data

A catalogue record for this book is available from the British Library

ISBN: 1-898486-48-4

Description or mention of instrumentation, software, or other products in this book does not imply endorsement by the author or publisher. The author and publisher do not assume responsibility for the validity of any products or procedures mentioned or described in this book or for the consequences of their use.

Printed and bound in Great Britain by Cromwell Press Ltd., Wiltshire BA14 0XB

Contents

Books of Related Interest

For further information on these books contact:

Horizon Scientific Press
P.O. Box 1, Wymondham
Norfolk
NR18 0EH England

Tel: +44(0)1953-601106
Fax: +44(0)1953-603068
Email: mail@horizonpress.com
Internet: www.horizonpress.com

Our Web site has details of all our books including full chapter abstracts, book reviews, and ordering information:

Contributors

Eileen Barry
Univ. Maryland School of Med.
Center for Vaccine Development
685 W. Baltimore St. - HSF 480
Baltimore
MD 21201
USA

Jozef Bizik
Cancer Research Institute
Slovak Academy of Sciences
Bratislava
Slovakia

Christof Berberich
Inst. Mol. Biol. Infectious Diseases
University of Würzburg
Germany

James E. Carter
Ctr. Mol. Biol. Gene Therapy
School of Medicine
Loma Linda University
Loma Linda
California 92350
USA

Trinad Chakraborty
Inst. Med. Microbiol.
Faculty of Medicine
Justus-Liebig University
Frankfurterstrasse 107
D-35392 Giessen
Germany

Ewald M.B. Denner
Inst. Microbiol. and Genetics
University of Vienna
Althanstraße 14
A-1090 Wien
Austria

Guido Dietrich
Berna Biotech AG
Bacterial Vaccine Research
Rehhagstr. 79
CH-3018 Berne
Switzerland
(guido.dietrich@bernabiotech.com)

Francis Eko
Dept. Microbiol.Biochem. Immunol.
Morehouse School of Medicine
720 Westview Drive
S.W.Atlanta
GA 30310-1495
USA

Diana Felnerova
Berna Biotech AG
Vaccine Research
Rehhagstr. 79
CH-3018 Berne
Switzerland

Sonja Friederichs
Bayer AG
Animal Health
Biological R&D
D-51368 Leverkusen
Germany

Matthias Frosch
Inst. of Hygiene and Microbiology
Josef-Schneider-Str. 2
97080 Würzburg
Germany
(mfrosch@hygiene.uni-wuerzburg.de)

James E. Galen
Univ. Maryland School of Medicine
Center for Vaccine Development
685 W. Baltimore St. - HSF 480
Baltimore
MD 21201
USA

Ivaylo Gentschev
Department of Microbiology
University of Würzburg
Biocenter
D-97074 Würzburg
Germany
(gentsch@biozentrum.uni-
wuerzburg.de)

Gregory M. Glenn
IOMAI Corporation
20 Firstfield Rd.
Gaithersburg
MD 20878
USA
(gglenn@iomai.com)

Werner Goebel
Department of Microbiology
University of Würzburg
Biocenter
D-97074 Würzburg
Germany

George R. Gunn, III
Department of Microbiology
University of Pennsylvania
Philadelphia
Pennsylvania 19104
USA

Wolfgang Haidinger
Inst. Microbiology and Genetics
University of Vienna
Althanstraße 14
A-1090 Wien
Austria

Christoph Haller
BIRD-C GmbH & CoKEG
Schoenborngasse 12
A-1080 Wien
Austria

Alexander Haslberger
Inst. Microbiology and Genetics
University of Vienna
Althanstraße 14
A-1090 Wien
Austria

Andreas Hensel
Inst. für Tierhygiene und Öffentliches
Veterinärwesen
Universität Leipzig
Semmelweißstr. 4
D-04103 Leipzig
Germany

Klaus Heeg
Institute of Medical Microbiology
Philipps University Marburg
Pilgrimstein 2
35037 Marburg
Germany
(heeg@med.uni-marburg.de)

Jürgen Hess
Department of Molecular Therapy
november AG
Ulrich-Schalk-Str. 3
91056 Erlangen
Germany
(hess@november.de)

Alexander Indra
Institute of Microbiology and Genetics
University of Vienna
Althanstraße 14
A-1090 Wien
Austria

Wolfgang Jechlinger
Institute of Microbiology and Genetics
University of Vienna
Althanstraße 14
A-1090 Wien
Austria

Gudrun Kohl
BIRD-C GmbH & CoKEG
Schoenborngasse 12
A-1080 Wien
Austria

Pavol Kudela
Cancer Research Institute
Slovak Academy of Sciences
Bratislava
Slovakia

Vladimir Kutyrev
Russian Anti-Plague Research Institute
"Microbe"
Universitetskaya St. 46
Saratov 410005
Russia

William H.R. Langridge
Center for Mol. Biol. Gene Therapy
School of Medicine
Loma Linda University
Loma Linda
California 92350
USA
(blangridge@som.llu.edu)

Myron M. Levine
Univ. Maryland School of Medicine
Center for Vaccine Development
685 W. Baltimore St. - HSF 480
Baltimore
MD 21201
USA
(mlevine@medicine.umaryland.edu)

Werner Lubitz
BIRD-C GmbH & CoKEG
Schoenborngasse 12
A-1080 Wien
Austria
(lubitz@bird-c.com)

Jürgen Marchart
Institute of Microbiology and Genetics
University of Vienna
Althanstraße 14
A-1090 Wien
Austria

Ulrike Mayr
BIRD-C GmbH & CoKEG
Schoenborngasse 12
A-1080 Wien
Austria

Peter Mayrhofer
Institute of Microbiology and Genetics
University of Vienna
Althanstraße 14
A-1090 Wien
Austria

Heidrun Moll
Institut für Molekulare
Infektionsbiologie
Röntgenring 11
D-97070 Würzburg
Germany
(heidrun.moll@mail.uni-
wuerzburg.de)

Elisabetta Monaci
IRIS
Chiron S.p.A.
Via Fiorentina, 1
53100 Siena
Italy
(elisabetta_monaci@chiron.it)

Derek O'Hagan
Chiron Corporation
Emeryville
USA
(derek_o'hagan@chiron.com)

Marcela F. Pasetti
Univ. Maryland School of Medicine
Center for Vaccine Development
685 W. Baltimore St. - HSF 480
Baltimore
MD 21201
USA

Susanne Paukner
Institute of Microbiology and Genetics
University of Vienna
Althanstraße 14
A-1090 Wien
Austria

Yvonne Paterson
University of Pennsylvania
323 Johnson Pavilion
36th Street and Hamilton Walk
Philadelphia
PA 19104-6076
USA
(yvonne@mail.med.upenn.edu)

Mariagrazia Pizza
IRIS
Chiron S.p.A.
Via Fiorentina, 1
53100 Siena
Italy
(mariagrazia_pizza@chiron.it)

Rino Rappuoli
IRIS
Chiron S.p.A.
Via Fiorentina, 1
53100 Siena
Italy
(rino_rappuoli@chiron.it)

Stephanie Resch
Apovia AG
Fraunhoferstraße 10
D-82152 Martinsried
Germany

Jörg Reimann
Institute for Medical Microbiology
University of Ulm
Helmholtzstr.8/1
D-89081 Ulm
Germany
(joerg.reimann@medizin.uni-ulm.de)

Eva Riedmann
Institute of Microbiology and Genetics
University of Vienna
Althanstraße 14
A-1090 Wien
Austria

Holger Rüssmann
Max von Pettenkofer-Institut für
Hygiene, Medizinische Mikrobiologie
Ludwig Maximilians Universität
München
Pettenkoferstrasse 9a
80336 München
Germany
(ruessmann@m3401.mpk.med.uni-
muenchen.de)

Reinhold Schirmbeck
Institute for Medical Microbiology
University of Ulm
Helmholtzstr.8/1
D-89081 Ulm
Germany

Tobias Schlapp
Bayer AG
Animal Health
Biological R&D
Building 6210/Monheim
D-51368 Leverkusen
Germany

Tatiana Schukovskaya
Russian Anti-Plague Res. Institute
"Microbe"
Universitetskaya St. 46
Saratov 410005
Russia

Wolfgang Strittmatter
Merck KgaA
Darmstadt
Germany

Michael Szostak
BIRD-C GmbH & CoKEG
Schoenborngasse 12
A-1080 Wien
Austria

Marcelo B. Sztein
Univ. Maryland School of Medicine
Center for Vaccine Development
685 W. Baltimore St. - HSF 480
Baltimore
MD 21201
USA

Carol O. Tacket
Univ. Maryland School of Medicine
Center for Vaccine Development
685 W. Baltimore St. - HSF 480
Baltimore
MD 21201
USA

Petra Walcher
Institute of Microbiology and Genetics
University of Vienna
Althanstraße 14
A-1090 Wien
Austria

Siegfried Weiss
Molecular Immunology
GBF - German Research Centre for
Biotechnology
Mascheroder Weg 1
D-38124 Braunschweig
Germany
(siw@gbf.d)

Jie Yu
Center for Mol. Biol. Gene Therapy
School of Medicine
Loma Linda University
Loma Linda
California 92350
USA

Stefan Zimmermann
Institute of Medical Microbiology
Philipps University Marburg
Pilgrimstein 2
35037 Marburg
Germany

Abba C. Zubair
Center for Hematologic Oncology
Department of Adult Oncology
Dana-Farber Cancer Institute
44 Binney St.
Boston
MA 02115
USA

Rinaldo Zurbriggen
Pevion Biotech Ltd.
Rehhagstrasse 79
CH-3018 Berne
Switzerland
(zurbriggen@pevion.com)

Preface

Infectious diseases and cancer continue to claim a deadly toll and are still the most important causes of death in mankind. The increasing cost of modern health care, that relies heavily on the direct treatment of on-going disease, stresses the need to reappraise current medical practice. Thus, it is highly desirable to place more emphasis on preventive medicine. Vaccination has proven to be the most efficient, cost-effective means for the prevention of a wide variety of infectious diseases. Concerted immunization programs have resulted in the eradication of smallpox, and the virtual eradication of polio from the Americas. The diligent use of measles, diphtheria, tetanus and pertussis vaccines has also been associated with a dramatic reduction in the incidence of these diseases worldwide. However, modern vaccinology faces two major challenges (i) prevention of the inadequate use of existing vaccines as well as (ii) the development of vaccines against diseases for which no protective vaccine exists to date. (i) Anti-vaccination movements expressing concerns over the safety of vaccines or the insufficient availability of vaccines in certain regions of the world can lead to rapid resurgance of diseases which were thought to be defeated. Similarly, failure to complete multi-dose vaccination regimens, especially in childhood, can severely affect the efficacy of routine vaccination programs. Indeed, in both developed and developing regions of the world a substantial number of infants fails to receive the number of recommended vaccine doses necessary to achieve optimal protection. (ii) the currently available vaccines are suitable for the elicitation of protective immunity against a variety of diseases. There are, however, novel diseases like AIDS caused by human immunodeficiency virus or hepatitis caused by hepatitis C virus for which the key to protective immunization has not been found yet. For other diseases, like tuberculosis caused by *Mycobacterium tuberculosis*, vaccines exist, but these are protective only against certain forms of disease or in certain populations or parts of the world. These diseases can only be prevented by novel approaches in vaccinology.

Approaches to solve both problems, the insufficient utilization of existing protective vaccines and the lack of efficacious vaccines against a variety of diseases, are therefore central to modern vaccine research. An important path that is followed by many vaccine researchers is the development of innovative vaccine delivery technologies. The delivery strategy represents a crucial determinant for the success of a vaccine. Novel vaccine delivery systems have many advantages: Delivery of vaccines via the oral route practised with vaccines against polio, cholera and typhoid fever or recent developments like transcutaneous or intranasal vaccination and edible vaccines offer an obvious practical advantage over parenteral administration which necessitates the presence of healthcare professionals and has all disadvantages connected with needle-injection. Vaccine delivery systems can enhance the immunogenicity of known protective antigens, which may allow the reduction of doses to be applied, ideally to a single dose that causes life-long protection. Alternatively, they can provide adjuvant functions which convert weakly immunogenic antigens like polysaccharides into vaccines that induce protective immunity and memory. Vaccine delivery systems can also induce arms of the immune system which can not be targeted with conventional vaccination approaches and achieve modulation of the immune response as desired. As prominent examples, induction of cellular and/or mucosal immunity may be the only key for protection against a wide range of pathogens and diseases. Finally, suitable delivery systems enable the prolonged release of antigens and their targeting to specific cells and organs.

This book aims at covering the most important and modern vaccine delivery systems available to date. The immunological principles upon which these systems are based, their potential applications and current clinical status are detailed. The choice of a delivery system aimed at developing a new vaccine should be based upon an understanding of both the disease and the type of immune response needed to confer protection. Each antigen must be considered carefully in terms of its delivery needs and the clinical performance specifications. It is thus extremely unlikely that any given delivery system will be suitable for all antigens, routes of administration and clinical applications. Each system will have its strengths and weaknesses and best applications. The very nature of available antigenic materials (in the form of whole inactivated pathogens, cell fractions, membrane proteins, surface carbohydrates, antigenic peptides, peptide-toxin constructs etc.) would suggest that different formulations and delivery systems may be equally successful or indeed necessary. The variety of systems covered in this volume is highlighted by the fact that some are still in the preclinical phase of research, others are already in clinical development and still others have already been licensed for many years and applied to millions of vaccinees. Nevertheless, the recent focus in vaccine research on delivery strategies has led to a breadth of approaches and information that can not be covered by a single book. To the investigators and advocates of technologies that have been missed, we apologize.

As this book is covering the most modern technologies and methods in vaccine delivery, it might be of interest to mention the first vaccine "delivery" in human history: In 1796, Edward Jenner discovered the protective efficacy of cowpox virus taken from human pustular lesions and inoculated into the skin of another person. The de Balmis expedition transported in 1803 to 1806 the vaccine to Spanish colonies in the Americas and Asia. Orphaned children were carried along and the vaccine was transferred from arm-to-arm in these children to deliver it in an active form to the expedition's destinations. This mode of delivery ensured that Jenner's vaccine was transported to countries throughout the world within a decade of its discovery.

We would like to thank the contributors of this book for their excellent chapters and their time and effort invested.

July 2002,

Guido Dietrich, Berne
Werner Goebel, Würzburg

From: *Vaccine Delivery Strategies*
Edited by: Guido Dietrich and Werner Goebel

Chapter 1

Bacterial Polysaccharide Conjugate Vaccines

Matthias Frosch

ABSTRACT

Bacterial polysaccharide conjugate vaccines are defined as delivery systems composed of bacterial capsular polysaccharide or lipopolysaccharide antigens, which are coupled to protein carrier molecules. The application of isolated polysaccharides results in a T-cell independent immune response, which is not boostable and elicits low-affinity IgM antibodies. Due to the immature immune system of infants, plain polysaccharides are non-immunogenic below the age of 18 months. However, by conjugation to a T-cell dependent protein carrier molecule, the polysaccharides become T-cell dependent and boostable, and protective antibody responses are elicited even in infants. This strategy was most successfully applied for the design of a vaccine against *Haemophilus influenzae* type b infections. Since the introduction of this vaccine, severe and invasive infections caused by this pathogen almost completely disappeared in those countries that included the vaccine in their national vaccination programmes. The prinicple of conjugate vaccines is currently propagated especially for the prevention against infections caused by *Streptococcus pneumoniae* and *Neisseria meningitidis*.

INTRODUCTION

Many bacterial pathogens causing respiratory tract infections, sepsis and meningitis express capsules which are composed of acidic polysaccharides. Especially, infections with *Streptococcus pneumoniae* (the pneumococcus), *Neisseria meningitidis* (the meningococcus) and *Haemophilus influenzae* cause a major disease burden. Pneumococci are the leading cause of community-acquired pneumonia, otitis media and sinusitis. In addition, the pneumococcus is among the most common pathogens causing acute bacterial meningitis in Europe and North America (Schuchat *et al.*, 1997). Invasive pneumococcal disease in all age groups reaches incidence rates of up to 72/100,000 (Zangwill *et al.*, 1996) and it has been calculated that pneumococci kill more than 1 million children each year world wide (Stansfield, 1987). The emergence of pneumococcal strains resistent against penicillin, chloramphenicol, macrolides and third-generation cephalosporines, which account for more than 30% of clinical isolates in the United States and several European countries, is alarming and underlines the need for effective preventive measures (Hoban *et al.*, 2001; Sahm *et al.*, 2000).

The leading cause of bacterial meningitis is the meningococcus with incidence peaks in young children at the age of 6 months to five years and in teenagers. World-wide, about 500,000 to 1 million cases of invasive meningococcal disease occur every year. The incidence of meningococcal sepsis and meningitis varies from 1-5 per 100,000 in most industrialized countries to up to 2% in developing countries during epidemics (Connolly and Noah, 1999). *H. influenzae* is a further important pathogen causing infections of the respiratory tract, meningitis, septicemia and septic arthritis, but its significance in invasive disease has dramatically dropped since the introduction of a conjugate vaccine against *H. influenzae* type b in 1990 (Peltola, 2000).

Based on the chemical composition and the immunological characteristics of the capsular polysaccharides, pneumococci, meningococci and *H. influenzae* are classified in serogroups or serotypes. In pneumococci, 90 capsular serotypes are known, which differ in their geographical distribution (Butler, *et al.*, 1995; von Kries *et al.*, 2000). In *H. influenzae*, six capsular polysaccharide serotypes, i.e. a, b, c, d, e and f, have been described, but most (ca. 95%) of the isolates from invasive disease were of serotype b (Pittman, 1931). Among the 13 capsular serogroups of meningococci, five of them, i.e. A, B, C, W135 and Y, are associated with invasive disease. Serogroup A meningococci cause epidemics in the African meningitis belt

Table 1. Structures of the capsular polysacharides of *H. influenzae* and *N. meningitidis* (Bundle *et al.*, 1974; Bhattacharjee *et al.*, 1975a and 1975b; Crisel *et al.*, 1975)

		Repeat structure	Linkage
H. influenzae	type b	D-ribofuranosyl-D-ribitolphosphate-	$\beta\ 5{\rightarrow}3$
N. meningitidis	serogroup A	N-acetyl-D-mannosamine-1-phosphate	$\alpha\ 1{\rightarrow}6$
	serogroup B	N-acetylneuraminic acid	$\alpha\ 2{\rightarrow}8$
	serogroup C	N-acetylneuraminic acid	$\alpha\ 2{\rightarrow}9$
	serogroup	W1354-O-α-D-galactopyranosyl- N-acetylneuraminic acid	$\alpha\ 2{\rightarrow}6$
	serogroup Y	4-O-α-D-glucopyranosyl- N-acetylneuraminic acid	$\alpha\ 2{\rightarrow}6$

and are also important in China and Russia (Achtman, 1995), whereas sporadic cases and outbreaks in Europe and Northern America are usually due to meningococci of the serogroups B and C with a predominance of 65% for serogroup B in Europe (Connolly and Noah, 1999). Recently, an increase of serogroup Y meningococcal disease has been reported in the US (Rosenstein *et al.*, 1999). The most common meningococcal and *H. influenzae* serogroups/serotypes and the chemistry of their capsular polysaccharides are summerized in Table 1.

Work in many laboratories over the last decades provided clear evidence that expression of the capsular polysaccharides is essential for the virulence of these pathogenic bacterial species, as the capsules interfere with complement activation, complement mediated bacteriolysis and opsonophagocytosis (Lee *et al.*, 1991; Vogel and Frosch, 1999; Roche and Moxon, 1995). However, these virulence attributes can be overcome by antibodies that bind to the capsule, leading to the clearance of the microorganisms by opsonin-dependent phagocytosis. This capsule-based immunity is serotype specific. The observation that capsule specific antibodies provide immunity to infection made the capsular polysaccharides an attractive target for the development of vaccines against disease caused by pneumococci, meningococci and *H. influenzae*. Remarkably, the capsular polysaccharide of serogroup B meningococci is non-immunogenic due to its identity to the carbohydrate modification of the eukaryotic neural cell adhesion molecule (N-CAM). Especially, the embryonic N-CAM is modified by long-chain polysialic molecules, which contain the epitopes common to the group B meningococcal capsular polysaccharide (Troy, 1992; Frosch *et al.*, 1985). Thus, antigenic mimicry may have contributed to the dominance of serogroup B strains in invasive meningococcal disease.

VACCINES COMPOSED OF PURIFIED CAPSULAR POLYSACCHARIDES

In the 1970ies, vaccines based on the group A and C meningococcal polysaccharide (Gold *et al.*, 1975) and the *H. influenzae* type b capular antigen were evaluated. High-molecular weight antigen preparations of the group A and C antigens were shown to elicit bactericidal antibodies (Gotschlich *et al.*, 1969). In U.S. Army recruits, the group C polysaccharide vaccine was safe and effective (Artenstein *et al.*, 1970) and field trials in Brazil indicated that this vaccine provides protection against disease in children above 2 years of age (Taunay *et al.*, 1974). Similarly, high levels of protection were achieved in children between 18 months and 5 years. However, in infants below 18 months, i.e. the age group with the highest attack rates of invasive disease caused by meningococci and *H. influenzae*, plain polysaccharide vaccines did not elicit significant and protective polysaccharide specific antibody titers (Gold *et al.*, 1975; Peltola *et al.*, 1984). Consequently, with the exception of the United States and Canada the *H. influenzae* type b vaccine was not recommended for general use in any other part of the world.

For the protection against meningococcal disease, two preparations are available consisting either of the group A and C polysaccharide or of the capsular antigens of group A, C, W135 and Y meningococci. The application of these vaccines is limited by the lack of protection against the group B meningococci, which predominate by far in Europe and America, and by their inability to elicit protective antibody titers in infants. Thus, the application of the meningococcal polysaccharide vaccines is restricted (i) to inhabitants of and travellers to regions with high incidence rates and epidemics due to group A, C, W135 and Y meningococci, (ii) to the control of outbreaks with meningococcal serogroups covered by the vaccine and (iii) to laboratory workers (Peltola, 1998).

Since 1983, a vaccine containing 23 purified capsular polysaccharides of the most prevalent pneumococcal serotypes is available, which covers more than 90% of the isolates responsible for invasive pneumococcal disease. This vaccine is recommended for the elderly and patients with predesposing conditions, like asplenia, diabetes, alcoholism, heart, lung and kidney disease and immunosuppression, particularly AIDS (Breiman *et al.*, 1990). While the efficacy of the vaccine is good in immunocompetent adults (Fine *et al.*, 1994; Christenson *et al.*, 2001), its application in patients with immunodeficiencies and hematologic malignancies is a matter of debate (Butler *et al.*, 1993). Furthermore, like the *H. influenzae* polysaccharide, the 23-valent pneumococcal polysaccharide vaccine is not immunogenic in the age group of infants below 18 months, in which the disease rates are especially high.

The failure in eliciting antibody responses in infants is a general property of polysaccharide molecules, since the immune response against these antigens does not involve T-cells. Thus, mostly low-affinity IgM antibodies are elicited, an immunological memory is not established and any booster effect against polysaccharide antigens is principally lacking (Stein, 1992). Repeated vaccination with group A and C meningococcal polysaccharides even induced hyporesponsiveness and lower bactericidal antibody titers after revaccination (MacLennan *et al.*, 1999). These limitations in the use of bacterial polysaccharide antigens for vaccines can be overcome by linkage of the T-independent polysaccharide antigen to a T-dependent protein carrier molecule. The polysaccharide-protein conjugate is processed and presented to T cells that bear receptors with specificity for the polysaccharide-protein complex. As a result, polysaccharide specific B-cells vigorously proliferate and mature to B-memory cells. Most important, this enhanced immune response against the conjugated polysaccharides also occurs in infants below the age of 18 months, thus eliciting high-titer and boostable protective antibody titers even in this age group.

CHEMICAL COUPLING OF POLYSACCHARIDE ANTIGENS TO CARRIER PROTEINS

Basically, two protocols for the covalent linkage of the polysaccharides to the protein carriers have been described. Jennings and Lugowski (1981) linked meningococcal group A, B, and C capsular polysaccharides to tetanus toxoid by limited periodate oxidation and, thus, introduction of aldehyde groups at the non-reducing terminus of the carbohydrates. This derivate was bound to the protein by reductive amination. Preparation of a conjugate vaccine by this approach induced high-titer and boostable bactericidal antibodies against the group A and C polysaccharides, but due to immunotolerance not against the group B antigen.

Schneerson *et al.* (1980) described a method for covalent coupling of the *H. influenzae* type b polysaccharide to carrier proteins by the introduction of adipic acid hydrazide as a six carbon spacer molecule. Several protein carriers, e.g. bovine and human serum albumine, diphtheria toxoid and horseshoe crab hemocyanin, were used, which first were derivatized with adipic acid hydrazide before reacting with 1-ethyl-3-(3-dimethylaminopropyl) carbodiimide. Conjugation was achieved after CNBr-activation of the type b polysaccharide. In these preparations the ratio of polysaccharide to protein varied from 0.5:1 to 1.5:1. These conjugates strongly induced bactericidal antibodies.

THE *HAEMOPHILUS INFLUENZAE* CONJUGATE VACCINES

The licencing of the *H. influenzae* type b conjugate vaccine in the late 80ies and its introduction in almost all developed countries until the early 90ies of the 20th century was a milestone in the history of vaccination as there are only a few vaccines against bacterial pathogens that led to such a dramatic decline in the incidence of a widely distributed infectious disease. Currently, four vaccine formulations have been licensed and are commercially available, i.e. a diphtheria toxoid conjugate (ProHIBiT), a mutant diphtheria toxin (CRM) conjugate (HibTITER), a meningococcal outer membrane protein conjugate (PedvaxHIB) and a tetanus toxoid conjugate (ActHIB, OmniHIB; Hiberix). In a recent excellent review, Peltola (2000) summarized the impact of large-scale vaccination on *H. influenzae* type b disease. In those countries, like the United States and most European countries which have introduced routine immunization in infants, a 90-98% reduction was seen and *Haemophilus* meningitis, septicemia and septic arthritis almost completely disappeared. Furthermore, the conjugate vaccine induces a *Haemophilus influenzae* type b specific mucosal immunity. The generation of mucosal IgA antibodies reduces nasopharyngeal colonization with *H. influenzae* type b and the decreased carriage rates presumably led also to an almost complete disappearance of *Haemophilus* epiglottitis and pneumoniae (Mohle-Boetani *et al.*, 1993).

However, from a global point of view the prevalence of invasive *Haemophilus* disease is still alarming. World-wide only 2% of all cases of invasive *H. influenzae* type b disease are prevented annually, since some

Table 2. Pneumococcal serotypes included in conjugate vaccines

7-valent conjugate vaccine	4, 6B, 9V, 14, 18C, 19F, 23F
11-valent conjugate vaccine	1, 3, 4, 5, 6B, 7F, 9V, 14, 18C, 19F, 23F

80% of all countries do not use the *H. influenzae* type b conjugate vaccine. Currently, The Gambia and South Africa are the only African countries which introduced the vaccine as part of their national vaccination programmes. Consequently, only in these developing countries *H. influenzae* type b disease is strongly declining (Adegbola *et al.*, 1999).

PROSPECTS AND LIMITATIONS OF NOVEL CONJUGATE VACCINES

Pneumococcal Conjugate Vaccines

The enormous success of the *H. influenzae* type b conjugate vaccine initiated efforts for the prevention against pneumococcal disease by a similar approach. Seven pneumococcal capsular polysaccharides from serotypes most prevalent in the United States (Table 2) were chosen and covalently linked to the same carrier proteins, which had previously been used for the preparation of the *H. influenzae* conjugate vaccine. On the basis of epidemiological data, these conjugates were expected to prevent 86% of the cases of septicemia and 83% of the cases of meningitis in children below the age of 6 years (Butler *et al.*, 1995; Yu *et al.*, 1999).

As with the *H. influenzae* type b vaccine, the pneumococcal conjugate vaccines are safe with only local reactions at the injection site, which were even less frequent and severe than the diphtheria-tetanus-whole cell pertussis vaccine, that was simultanously administered at different sites (Eskola *et al.* 2001; Black *et al.*, 2000). The immunogenicity of the vaccine in infants has been demonstrated in numerous studies (Yu *et al.*, 1999; Eskola *et al.*, 2001; Black *et al.*, 2000; Eskola and Antilla, 1999) and the opsonophagocytic activity of the vaccine-induced antibodies characterized (Yu *et al.*, 1999). The induction of IgA antibodies that are found in mucosal secretions resulted in a decreased pneumococcal carriage rate in the nasopharynx (Dagan *et al.*, 1996).

The efficacy of the 7-valent pneumococcal conjugate vaccine was clearly demonstrated at the Northern California Kaiser Permanente study site. In a recently finished study (Black *et al.*, 2000) 37,868 infants were included and immunized at the age of 2, 4, 6, and 12-15 months. After application of three vaccine dosages, an efficacy of 97.4% for the prevention of invasive pneumococcal disease for serotypes included in the vaccine was achieved. The serotype-specific efficacy ranged from 87% for serotype 19F to 100% for the serotypes 14, 18C and 23F, reflecting the different immunogenicity of each of the polysaccharides. Including cases of invasive pneumococcal disease by serotypes not covered by the vaccine the efficacy of 92.9% was roughly identical. The impact of vaccination for prevention of pneumonia (as a clinical diagnosis including abnormous chest-ray, but without microbiological examination and isolation of the causative organism) was also evaluated. The efficacy was 33% and was thus in the range of the expected cases of pneumococcal pneumonia among all cases of bacterial pneumonia (Heiskanen-Kosma *et al.*, 1998).

The efficacy to prevent otitis media was less evident. In a recent Finish study in children (Eskola *et al.*, 2001), the vaccine reduced the number of otitis media episodes independent of the causative organism only by 6%. However, cases of otitis media caused by pneumococci were reduced by 34% and episodes of pneumococcal otitis media caused by the serotypes covered by the vaccine were reduced by 57%. Interestingly, the number of cases of otitis media caused by pneumococcal serotypes not covered by the vaccine increased by 33%.

Although different clinical presentations and age groups were analysed at the Northern California Kaiser Permanente study site and in the Finish otitis media study, the discrepency in the efficacy to prevent pneumococcal disease independent of the serotypes included in the conjugate vaccine is remarkable and at least partially reflects the different epidemiology and distribution of pneumococcal serotypes in the United States and European countries. The 7-valent conjugate vaccine was designed according to the most prevalent pneumococcal serotypes in the United States (Butler *et al.*, 1995). However, in Germany these serotypes cover only 52% of strains responsible for systemic pneumococcal disease in children below 16 years of age (von Kries *et al.*, 2000), but differences in the age-related serotype distribution have been observed with higher coverage rates in the 1-5 years old (R. Reinert, pers. communication).

Currently, in contrast to the United States, where the licenced pneumococcal conjugate vaccine was recommended for general use on the basis of the results from the Kaiser Permanente study and calculation of the cost-effectiveness (Lieu *et al.*, 2000), no general recommendation is yet given in

European countries. The discussion about the recommendation of the pneumococcal conjugate vaccine compromises several aspects:

- The population to be vaccinated needs a revised definition. The immunogenicity in infants opens new horizons for vaccine application extending earlier recommendations for groups at risk, especially elderly and immunocompromised patients. The burden of severe pneumococcal disease in children justifies the general recommendation, if the coverage of a vaccine is broad enough to achieve a significant decrease especially of severe and systemic pneumococcal disease. Therefore, large-scale vaccination and efficacy trials are urgently needed for Europe using conjugate vaccines, including vaccine fomulations with an enhanced spectrum of epidemiological relevant serotypes, like the 11-valent conjugate vaccine (Table 2). Cost-benefit calculations are to be performed on the basis of epidemiological data and age-dependend distribution of the serotypes included in vaccines.

- If – on the basis of current epidemiological data and valid cost-benefit analyses – the pneumococcal conjugate vaccine will be introduced, carefully performed epidemiological surveys are urgently required for the next years to address concerns about serotype switching and replacement. The Finish otitis media study demonstrated a significant increase after vaccination of disease causing pneumococcal serotypes which were not covered by the vaccine. This short-term effect indicates that the nasopharyngeal niche from which a limited number of pneumococcal serotypes have been eliminated by vaccination will be filled up again by other important pneumococcal serotypes with pathogenic potential. As an alternative to this scenario the same currently most prevalent disease associated clonal lineages remain within the population after they have undergone genetic recombination and exchange of capsule biosynthesis genes. The frequency of allelic exchange may be enhanced by immune selection after vaccination (Enright and Spratt, 1999).

- Multi-drug resistant pneumococci are limited to only a few clonal lineages. These express serotypes covered by the 7-valent conjugate vaccine (Enright and Spratt, 1999). Therefore, vaccination might eliminate the spread of antibiotic resistant pneumococci. In fact, this aim could potentially be achieved by the reduction of the carriage with resistant strains and by decreased usage of antibiotics, when the incidence of pneumococcal disease declines.

Meningococcal Conjugate Vaccines

A meningococcal vaccine protecting against all cases of meningococcal disease, which is based on conjugated capsular polysaccharides, faces major difficulties. One limitation of a meningococcal conjugate vaccine is the lack of immunogenicity of the serogroup B specific capsular polysaccharide, which is composed of α-2,8 linked poly-neuraminic acid (polysialic acid) and expressed by some 65% of disease isolates in Europe and North America (Connolly and Noah, 1999). The lack of immunogenicity, which is observed in all age groups, is due to immunotolerance, since an identical carbohydrate is part of carbohydrate modifications of the neural cell adhesion molecule and is expressed in embryonic neural tissue, on natural killer cells and regenerating nerves (Finne, 1982; Husmann *et al.*, 1989; Zhang *et al.*, 1995).

An interesting approach to overcome the lacking immunogenicity came from the group of Jennings, who chemically modified the α-2,8 linked *N*-acetyl-neuraminic acid of the group B capsular antigen by replacement of the *N*-acetyl groups by *N*-propionyl groups. After conjugation to tetanus toxoid the modified group B meningococcal polysaccharide was highly immunogenic and elicited bactericidal antibodies against group B meningococci in mice, which conferred protection in animal studies (Jennings *et al.*, 1986, 1987; Ashton *et al.*, 1989). Thus, the modified group B meningococcal capsular antigen was able to break immunotolerance. However, there is strong concern, that antibodies elicited by immunization with the *N*-propionylated group B meningococcal polysaccharide may induce autoimmune inflammatory disease or adversely affect the neural development of the fetus, when IgG antibodies cross the placenta.

Jennings *et al.* proposed that the bactericidal epitope that is mimicked by the *N*-propionylated polysialic acid has a restricted occurrence in the high molecular weight fraction of the meningococcal group B polysaccharide as a part of polysaccharide aggregates (Pon *et al.*, 1997). This interesting observation could lead to the conclusion that a broad cross-reactivity of antibodies elicited by this vaccination strategy with host tissue is not necessarily expected, since the N-CAM modification of host cells comprises α-2,8 linked poly-neuraminic acid chains of less than 50 residues in length (Troy, 1992). However, several monoclonal antibodies have been generated by immunization with *N*-propionylated poly-neuraminic acid that show bactericidal acitivity as well as a strong cross-reactivity with human polysialylated cells (Granoff *et al.*, 1998; Häyrinen *et al.* 1995). These data are in accordance with earlier observations, which suggested that patients suffering from systemic meningococcal B disease develop capsule specific

IgM antibodies that cross-react with polysialylated N-CAM and lyse N-CAM expressing eukaryotic cells in a complement-dependent manner (Nedelec *et al.*, 1990). Therefore, despite promising preclinical studies with a meningococcal *N*-propionylated group B conjugate vaccine (Zollinger *et al.*, 1997; Fusco *et al.*, 1997; Devi *et al.*, 1997) any attempt to apply such a vaccine in clinical studies and recommend it for general human use should be met with reserve for safety and ethical reasons. Possible long-term effects on the development of autoimmune disorders, which may not be recognized in the short-term observation period of clinical studies with only limited numbers of individuals, and the potentially severe damage of the fetal neural tissue following vaccination should rule out the application of a serogroup B meningococcal vaccine based on a modified polysaccharide antigen that overcomes immunotolerance.

Conjugate vaccines against group C meningococci have been licenced and conjugates with the group A, W135 and Y capsular antigens are currently under development or clinical evaluation. On the basis of safety and immunogenicity data (Richmond *et al.*, 1999 and 2000; MacLennan *et al.*, 2000), but without prior performance of efficacy studies, the United Kingdom was the first country to introduce the meningococcal C conjugate vaccine into the routine infant vaccination schedule since November 1999. The vaccine was also offered to all children younger than 18 years. The results from the first 9 months of the vaccination programme were promising. In the adolescent target group, the efficacy of the vaccine was 97% and 92% in toddlers (Ramsay *et al.*, 2001). Thus, it seems realistic that meningococcal disease due to serogroup C meningococci can be eradicated. This is an encouraging prospect, since disease caused by serogroup C organisms tends to be severe and associated with high mortality rates.

The introduction of the group C conjugate vaccine had a significant impact on the epidemiology of meningococcal disease in the UK. In the second half of the year 2000, a 49% reduction of cases of group C meningococcal disease was observed (as compared to the number of cases in 1999). In the age-group of the under 20 years old the decline was even more apparent and a reduction in the number of cases by 72% observed (CDR Weekly, 2001). It has been estimated that in the first year of the introduction of the vaccine, a total of 500 cases and 50 deaths have been prevented in the UK. Interestingly, in the same period a significant increase of confirmed cases of meningococcal disease due to serogroup B strains was observed. Presently, it is not clear whether this change in the prevalence of disease causing meningococcal serogroups was induced by the vaccination campaign, or whether it is in line with the increase of group B cases observed already before the vaccination campaign started. As with the pneumococcal conjugate vaccine (Eskola *et al.*, 2001), meningococcal serogroups not covered by the vaccine may occupy the vacant niches. Of particular concern is the capability of the meningococcus to alter antigenic determinants by horizontal DNA transfer. Likewise, it has been shown, that by transformation with DNA fragments harbouring genes of the capsule locus, a serogroup switch can be induced (Vogel *et al.*, 2000). As a consequence of the immunity against serogroup C meningococci within a population, capsular variants expressing the serogroups B, W135 or Y may spread in the vaccinated population. Currently, the effect of the vaccination campaign, that targets only one among several disease causing serogroups, on the serogroup-independent overall incidence rates of meningococcal disease cannot be predicted and possible changes in the disease rates, the epidemiology and the population biology of the meningococcus will only be known in the next months and years. Carefully performed epidemiological surveys and analysis of alterations in the meningococcal population structure are in progress, which will shed light on these urgent questions (Maiden and Spratt, 1999). The results from these studies will contribute to decisions of vaccination advisory committees on the future application of meningococcal conjugate vaccines.

POLYSACCHARIDE VACCINES AGAINST OTHER BACTERIAL PATHOGENS

In addition to the conjugate vaccines discussed in this contribution the approach of conjugating capsular polysaccharides and lipopolysaccharide antigens to carrier proteins has also been applied for the prevention of infectious diseases caused by *Staphylococcus aureus* (Tollersrud *et al.*, 2001), group B streptococci (Baker *et al.*, 1999) and a number of pathogens of the gastrointestinal tract (Gupta *et al.*, 1998; Konadu *et al.*, 1999; Pozsgay *et al.*, 1999; Singh *et al.*, 1999). Furthermore, a *Pseudomonas aeruginosa* O-polysaccharide toxin A conjugate vaccine has been developed for patients suffering from cystic fibrosis (Cryz *et al.*, 1987). First clinical studies showed promising results (Schaad, *et al.*, 1991).

CONCLUSIONS

The optimism on bacterial conjugate vaccines derived from the success of the *H. influenzae* conjugate vaccine. However, in contrast to pneumococci and meningococci, only a single *H. influenzae* serotype, i.e. type b, is associated with invasive disease, which made the objective for vaccine design clear-cut and straightforward. The complex epidemiology and population biology of pneumococcal serotypes and meningococcal serogroups together with the lack of immunogenicity of the most common meningococcal serogroup B capsule raises concerns, whether pneumococcal and meningococcal conjugate vaccines will have the same potential as the *H. influenzae* conjugate vaccine in prevention and elimination of all cases of invasive pneumococcal and meningococcal disease. Even if the demonstrated obstacles can be overcome, the costs of these kinds of vaccines will prevent their global distribution and application. As with the *H. influenzae* conjugate vaccine, for economical reasons the pneumococcal and meningococcal conjugate vaccines will probably never enter the developing countries, where most cases of disease and death are registered. Thus, conjugate vaccines are of potential use for a transitional period in developed countries until broadly effective and much cheaper vaccines against these important bacterial pathogens become available.

REFERENCES

Achtman, M. 1995. Global epidemiology of meningococcal disease. In: Meningococcal Disease. K. Cartwright, ed. John Wiley & Sons, Ltd. Chichester, England. p. 159-175.

Adegbola, R.A., Usen, S.O., Weber, M., Lloyd-Evans, N., Jobe, K., Mulholland, K., McAdam, K.P.W.J., Greenwood, B.M., and Milligan, P.J.M. 1999. *Haemophilus influenzae* type b meningitis in The Gambia after introduction of a conjugate vaccine. Lancet 354: 1091-1092.

Artenstein, M.S., Gold, R., Zimmerly, J.G., Wyle, F.A., Schneider, H., and Harkins, C. 1970. Prevention of meningococcal disease by group C polysaccharide vaccine. N. Engl. J. Med. 282: 417-420.

Ashton, F.E., Ryan, J.A., Michon, F., and Jennings, H.J. 1989. Protective efficacy of mouse serum to the *N*-propionyl derivative of meningococcal group B polysaccharide. Microb. Pathogen. 6: 455-458.

Baker, C.J., Paoletti, L.C., Wessels, M.R., Guttormsen, H.K., Rench, M.A., Hickman, M.E., and Kasper, D.L. 1999. Safety and immunogenicity of capsular polysaccharide-tetanus conjugate vaccines for group B streptococcal types Ia and Ib. J. Infect. Dis. 179: 142-150.

Bhattacharjee, A.K., Jennings, H.J., Kenny, C.P., Martin, A., and Smith, I.C.P. 1975a. Structural determination of the sialic acid polysaccharide antigens of *Neisseria meningitidis* serogroup B and serogroup C with carbon 13 nuclear magnetic resonance. J. Biol. Chem. 250: 1926-1932.

Bhattacharjee, A.K., Jennings, H.J., Martin, A., and Smith, I.C.P. 1975b. Structural determination of the polysaccharide antigens of *Neisseria meningitidis* serogroups Y, W-135, and BO. Can. J. Biochem. 54: 1-8.

Black, S., Shinefield, H., Fireman, B., Lewis, E., Ray, P., Hansen, J.R., Elvin, L., Ensor, K.M., Hackell, J., Siber, G., Malinoski, F., Madore, D., Chang, I., Kohberger, R., Watson, W., Austrian, R., and Edwards, K. 2000. Efficacy, safety and immunogenicity of heptavalent pneumococcal conjugate vaccine in children. Pediatr. Infect. Dis. J. 19: 187-195.

Breiman, R.F., Spika, J.S., Navarro, V.J., Darden, P.M., and Darby, C.P. 1990. Pneumococcal bacteremia in Charlston County, South Carolina. A decade later. Arch. Intern. Med. 150: 1401-1405.

Bundle, D.R., Smith, I.C.P., and Jennings, H.J. 1974. Determination of the structure and confirmation of bacterial polysaccharides by carbon-13 nuclear magnetic resonance. J. Biol. Chem. 249: 2275-2281.

Butler, J.C. Breiman, R.F., Campbell, J.F., Lipman, H.B., Broome, C.V., and Facklam, R.R. 1993. Pneumococcal polysaccharide vaccine efficacy. An evaluation of current recommendations. JAMA 270: 1826-1831.

Butler, J.C., Breiman, R.F., Lipman, H.B., Hofmann, J., and Facklam, R.R. 1995. Serotype distribution of *Streptococcus pneumoniae* infections among preschool children in the United States, 1978-1994: implication for development of a conjugate vaccine. J. Infect. Dis. 171: 85-889.

CDR Weekly. 2001. The impact of conjugate group C meningococcal vaccination. Vol. 11: No. 2.

Connolly, M., and Noah, N. 1999. Is group C meningococcal disease increasing in Europe? A report of surveillance of meningococcal infection in Europe 1993-1996. Epidemiol. Infect. 122: 41-49.

Christenson, B., Lundbergh, P., Hedlund, J., and Örtquist, A. 2001. Effects of a large-scale intervention with influenza and 23-valent pneumococcal vaccines in adults aged 65 years and older: a prospective study. Lancet 357: 1008-1011.

Crisel, R.M., Baker, R.S., and Dorman, D.E. 1975. Capsular polymer of *Haemophilus influenzae* type b. Part 1. Structural characterization of the capsular polymer of strain Eagan. J. Biol. Chem. 250: 4926-4930.

Cryz, S.J., Fürer, E., Cross, A.S., Wegmann, A., Germanier, R., and Sadoff, J.C. 1987. Safety and immunogenicity of a *Pseudomonas aeruginosa* O-polysaccharide toxin A conjugate vaccine in humans. J. Clin. Invest. 80: 51-56.

Dagan, R., Melamed, R., Muallem, M., Piglansky, L., Greenberg, D., Abramson, O., Mendelman, P.M., Bohidar, N., and Yagupsky, P. 1996. Reduction of nasopharyngeal carriage of pneumococci during the second year of life by a heptavalent conjugate pneumococcal vaccine. J. Infect. Dis. 174: 1271-1278.

Devi, S.J.N., Zollinger, W.D., Snoy, P.J., Tai, J.Y., Constantini, P., Norelli, F., Rappuoli, R., and Frasch, C.E. 1997. Preclinical evaluation of group B *Neisseria meningitidis* and *Escherichia coli* K92 capsular polysaccharide-protein conjugate vaccines in juvenile rhesus moneys. Infect. Immun. 65: 1045-1052.

Enright, M.C. and Spratt, B.G. 1999. Multilocus sequence typing. Trends Microbiol. 7: 482-487.

Eskola, J., and Antilla, M. 1999. Pneumococcal conjugate vaccines. Pediatr. Infect. Dis. J. 18: 543-551.

Eskola, J., Kilpi, T., Palmu, A., Jokinen, J., Haapakosi, J., Herva, E., Takala, A., Käyhty, H., Karma, P., Kohberger, R., Siber, G., and Mäkelä, P.H. 2001. Efficacy of a pneumococcal conjugate vaccine against otitis media. N. Engl. J. Med. 344: 403-409.

Fine, M.J., Smith, M.A., Carson, C.A., Meffe, F., Sankey, S.S., Weissfeld, L.A., Detsky, S., and Kapoor, W.N. 1994. Efficacy of pneumococcal vaccination in adults. A meta-analysis of randomized controlled trials. Arch. Intern. Med. 154: 2666-2677.

Finne, J. 1982. Occurrence of unique polysialosyl carbohydrate units in glycoproteins of developing brain. J. Biol. Chem. 257: 11966-11970.

Frosch, M., Görgen, I., Boulnois, G.J., Timmis, K.N., and Bitter-Suermann, D. 1985. NZB-mouse system for production of monoclonal antibodies to weak bacterial antigens: isolation of an IgG antibody to the polysaccharide capsules of *Escherichia coli* K1 and group B meningococci. Proc. Natl. Acad. Sci. USA. 82: 1194-1198.

Fusco, P.C., Michon, F., Tai, J.Y., and Blake, M.S. 1997. Preclinical evaluation of a novel group B meningococcal conjugate vaccine that elicits bactericidal activity in both mice and nonhuman primates. J. Infect. Dis. 175: 364-372.

Gold, R., Lepow, M.L., Goldschneider, I., Draper, T.L., and Gotschlich, E.C. 1975. Clinical evaluation of group A and group C meningococcal polysaccharide vaccines in infants. J. Clin. Invest. 56: 1536-1547.

Gotschlich, E.C., Goldschneider, I., and Artenstein, M.S. 1969. Human immunity to the meningococcus. IV. Immunogenicity of group A and group C meningococcal polysaccharides in human volunteers. J. Exp. Med. 129: 1367-1384.

Granoff, D.M., Bartoloni, A., Ricci, S., Gallo, E., Rosa, D., Ravenscroft, N., Guarnieri, V., Seid, R.C., Shan, A., Usinger, W.R., Tan, S., McHugh, Y.E., and Moe, G.R. 1998. Bactericidal monoclonal antibodies that define unique meningococcal B polysaccharide epitopes, that do not cross-react with human polysialic acid. J. Immunol. 160: 5028-5036.

Gupta, R.K., Taylor, D.N., Bryla, D.A., Robbins, J.B., and Szu, S.C. 1998. Phase 1 evaluation of *Vibrio cholerae* O1, serotype Inaba, polysaccharide-cholera toxin conjugates in adult volunteers. Infect. Immun. 66: 3095-3099.

Häyrinen, J., Jennings, H., Raff, H.V., Rougon, G., Hanai, N., Gerardy-Schahn, R., and Finne, J. 1995: Antibodies to polysialic acid and its N-propyl derivate: binding properties and interaction with human embryonal brain glycopeptides. J. Infect. Dis. 171: 1481-1490.

Heiskanen-Kosma, T., Korppi, M., Jokinen, C., Kurki, S., Heiskanen, L., Juvonen, H., Kallinen, S., Sten, M., Tarkiainen, A., Ronnberg, P.R., Kleemola, M., Mäkelä, P.H., and Leinonen, M. 1998. Etiology of childhood pneumonia: serologic results of a prospective, population-based study. Pediatr. Infect. Dis. J. 17: 986-991.

Hoban, D.J., Doern, G.V., Fluit, A.C., Roussel-Delvallez, M., and Jones, R.N. 2001. Worldwide prevalence of antimicrobial resistance in *Streptococcus pneumoniae, Haemophilus influenzae*, and *Moraxella catarrhalis* in the SENTRY Antimicrobial Surveillance Program, 1997-1999. Clin. Infect. Dis. 32: S81- S93.

Husmann, M., Pietsch, T., Fleischer, B., Weisgerber, C., and Bitter-Suermann, D. 1989. Embryonic neural cell adhesion molecules on human natural killer cells. Eur. J. Immunol. 19: 1761-1763.

Jennings, H.J., and Lugowski, C. 1981. Immunochemistry of groups A, B and C meningococcal polysaccharide-tetanus toxoid conjugates. J. Immunol. 127: 104-108.

Jennings, H.J., Roy, R., and Gamian, A. 1986. Induction of meningococcal group B polysaccharide-specific IgG antibodies in mice by using an *N*-propionylated B polysaccharide-tetanus toxoid conjugate vaccine. J. Immunol. 137: 1708-1713.

Jennings, H.J., Gamian, A., and Ashton, F.A. 1987. *N*-propionylated group B meningococcal polysaccharide mimics a unique epitope on group B *Neisseria meningitidis*. J. Exp. Med. 165: 1207-1211.

Konadu., E., Donohue-Rolfe, A., Calderwood, S.B., Pozsgay, V., Shiloah, J., Robbins, J.B., and Szu, S.C. 1999. Syntheses and immunologic properties of *Escherichia coli* O157 O-specific polysaccharide and Shiga toxin 1 B subunit conjugates in mice. Infect. Immun. 67:6191-6193.

Lee, C.J., Banks, S.D., and Li, J.P. 1991. Virulence, immunity, and vaccine related to *Streptococcus pneumoniae*. Crit. Rev. Microbiol. 18: 89-114.

Lieu, T.A., Ray, G.T., Black, S.B., Butler, J.C., Klein, J.O., Breiman, R.F., Miller, M.A., and Shinefield, H.R. 2000. Projected cost-effectiveness of pneumococcal conjugate vaccination of healthy infants and young children. JAMA 283: 1460-1468.

MacLennan, J., Obaro, S., Deeks, J., Williams, D., Pais, L., Carlone, G., Moxon, R., and Greenwoord, B. 1999. Immune response to revaccination with meningococcal A and C polysaccharides in Gambian children following repeated immunisation during early childhood. Vaccine 17: 3086-3093.

MacLennan, J.M., Shackley, F., Heath, P.T., Deeks, J.J., Flamank, C., Herbert, M., Griffiths, H., Hatzmann, E., Goilav, C., and Moxon, E.R. 2000. Safety, immunogenicity, and induction of immunologic memory by a serogroup C meningococcal conjugate vaccine in infants. A randomized controlled trial. JAMA 283: 2795-2801.

Maiden, M.J.C., and Spratt, B.G. 1999. Meningococcal conjugate vaccines: new opportunities and new challenges. Lancet 354: 615-616.

Mohle-Boetani, J.C., Ajello, G., Breneman, E., Deaver, K.A., Harvey, C., Plikaytis, B.D., Farley, M.M., Stephens, and D.S., Wenger, J.D. 1993. Carriage of *Haemophilus influenzae* type b in children after widespread vaccination with conjugate *Haemophilus influenzae* type b vaccines. Pediatr. Infect. Dis. J. 12: 589-593.

Nedelec, J., Boucraut, J., Garnier, J.M., Bernard, D., and Rougon, G. 1990. Evidence for autoimmune antibodies directed against embryonic neural cell adhesion molecules (N-CAM) in patients with group B meningitis. J. Neuroimmunol. 29: 49-56.

Peltola, H., Käyhty, H., Virtanen, M., and Mäkelä, P.H. 1984. Prevention of *Haemophilus influenzae* type b bacteremic infections with the capsular polysaccharide vaccine. N. Engl. J. Med. 310: 1561-1566.

Peltola, H. 1998. Meningococcal vaccines. Current status and future possibilties. Drugs 55: 347-366.

Peltola, H. 2000. Worldwide *Haemophilus influenzae* type b disease at the beginning of the 21st century: global analysis of the disease burden 25 years after the use of the polysaccharide vaccine and a decade after the advent of conjugates. Clin. Microbiol. Rev. 13: 302-317.

Pittman, M.1931. Variation and type specificity in the bacterial species *Haemophilus influenzae*. J. Exp. Med. 53: 471-495.

Pon, R.A., Lussier, M., Yang, Q.-L., and Jennings, H.J. 1997. *N*-propionylated group B meningococcal polysaccharide mimics a unique bactericidal capsular epitope in group B *Neisseria meningitidis*. J. Exp. Med. 185: 1929-1938.

Pozsgay, V., Chu, C., Pananell, L., Wolfe, J., Robbins, J.B., and Schneerson, R. 1999. Protein conjugates of synthetic saccharides elicit higher levels of serum IgG lipopolysaccharide antibodies in mice than do those of the O-specific polysaccharide from *Shigella dysenteriae* type 1. Proc. Natl. Acad. Sci. U.S.A. 96: 5194-5197.

Ramsay, M.E., Andrews, N., Kaczmarski, E.B., and Miller, E. 2001. Efficacy of meningococcal serogroup C conjugate vaccine in teenagers and toddlers in England. Lancet 357: 195-196.

Richmond, P., Borrow, R., Miller, E., Clark, S., Sadler, F., Fox, A., Begg, N., Morris, R., and Cartwright, K. 1999. Meningococcal serogroup C conjugate vaccine is immunogenic in infancy and primes for memory. J. Infect. Dis. 179: 1569-1572.

Richmond, P., Goldblatt, D., Fusco, P.C., Fusco, J.D.S., Heron, I., Clark, S., Borrow, R., and Michon, F. 2000. Safety and immunogenicity of a new *Neisseria meningitidis* serogroup C-tetanus toxoid conjugate vaccine in healthy adults. Vaccine 18: 641-646.

Roche, R.J., and Moxon, E.R. 1995. Phenotypic variation of carbohydrate surface antigens and the pathogenesis of *Haemophilus influenzae* infections. Trends Microbiol. 3: 304-309.

Rosenstein, N.E., Perkins, B.A., Stephens, D.S., Lefkowitz, L., Cartter, M.L., Danila, R., Cieslak, P., Shutt, K.A., Popovic, T., Schuchat, A., Harrison, L.H., and Reingold, A.L. 1999. The changing epidemiology of meningococcal disease in the United States, 1992-1996. J. Infect. Dis. 180: 1894-1901.

Sahm, D.F., Jones, M.E., Hickey, M.L., Diakun, D.R., Mani, S.V., and Thornsberry, C. 2000. Resistance surveillance of *Streptococcus pneumoniae, Haemophilus influenzae* and *Moraxella catarrhalis* isolated in Asia and Europe, 1997-1998. J. Antimicrob. Chemother. 45: 457-466.

Schaad, U.B., Lang, A.B., Wedgwood, J., Ruedeberg, A., Que, J.U., F‚rer, E., and Cryz, S.J. 1991. Safety and immunogenicity of *Pseudomonas aeruginosa* conjugate A vaccine in cystic fibrosis. Lancet 338: 1236.

Schneerson, R., Barrera, C., Sutton, A., and Robbins, J.B. 1980. Preparation, characterization and immunochemistry of *Haemophilus influenzae* type b polysaccharide-protein conjugates. J. Exp. Med. 152: 361-375.

Schuchat, A., Robinson, K., Wenger, J.D., Harrison, L.H., Farley, M., Reingold, A.L., Lefkowitz, L., and Perkins, B.A. 1997. Bacterial meningitis in the United States in 1995. N. Engl. J. Med. 337: 970-976.

Singh, M., Ganguly, N.K., Kumar, L., and Vohra, H. 1999. Protective efficacy and immunogenicity of Vi-porin conjugate against *Salmonella typhi*. Microbiol. Immunol. 43: 535-542.

Stansfield, S.K. 1987. Acute respiratory infections in the developing world: strategies for prevention, treatment and control. Pediatr. Infect. Dis. 6: 622-629.

Stein, K.E. 1992. Thymus-independent and thymus-dependent responses to polysaccharide antigens. J. Infect. Dis. 165: S49-52.

Taunay, A., Galvao, P.A., de Morais, J.S., Gotschlich, E.C., and Feldman, R.A. 1974. Disease prevention by meningococcal serogroup C polysaccharide vaccine in preschool children: results after eleven months of vaccination. Pediatr. Res. 8: 429.

Tollersrud, T., Zernichow, L., Andersen S.R., Kenny, K., and Lund, A. 2001. *Staphylococcus aureus* capsular polysaccharide type 5 conjugate and whole cell vaccines stimulate antibody responses in cattle. Vaccine 16: 3896-3903.

Troy, F.A. 1992. Polysialylation: from bacteria to brains. Glycobiol. 2: 5-23.

Vogel, U., and Frosch, M. 1999. Mechanisms of neisserial serum resistance. Mol. Microbiol. 32: 1133-1139.

Vogel, U., Claus, H., and Frosch, M. 2000. The velocity of natural serogroup switching in *Neisseria meningitidis*. New Engl. J. Med. 342: 219-220.

von Kries, R., Siedler, A., Schmitt, H.J., and Reinert, R.R. 2000. Proportion of invasive pneumococcal infections in German children preventable by pneumococcal conjugate vaccines. Clin. Infect. Dis. 31: 482-487.

Yu, X., Gray, B., Chang, S., Ward, J.I., Edwards, K.M., and Nahm, M.H. 1999. Immunity to cross-reactive serotypes induced by pneumococcal conjugate vaccines in infants. J. Infect. Dis. 180: 1569-1576.

Zangwill, K.M., Vadheim, C.M., Vannier, A.M., Hemenway, L.S., Greenberg, D.P., and Ward, J.I. 1996. Epidemiology of invasive pneumococcal disease in southern California: implication for the design and conduct of a pneumococcal conjugate vaccine efficacy trial. J. Infect. Dis. 174: 752-759.

Zhang, Y., Campbell, G., Anderson, P.N., Martini, R., Schachner, M., and Lieberman, A.R. 1995. Molecular basis of interactions between regenerating adult rat thalamic axons and Schwann cells in peripheral nerve grafts I. Neural cell adhesion molecules. J. Comp. Neurol. 361: 193-209.

Zollinger, W.D., Moran, E.E., Devi, S.J.N., and Frasch, C.E. 1997. Bactericidal antibody responses of juvenile rhesus monkeys immunized with group B *Neisseria meningitidis* capsular polysaccharide-protein conjugate vaccines. Infect. Immun. 65: 1053-1060.

From: *Vaccine Delivery Strategies*
Edited by: Guido Dietrich and Werner Goebel

Chapter 2

Novel Adjuvants

Mariagrazia Pizza, Elisabetta Monaci,
Derek O'Hagan and Rino Rappuoli

ABSTRACT

The ideal vaccine has to be safe and able to induce an immune response that is strong and effective. Most of the vaccines currently available were generated a long time ago and are based on killed or live-attenuated microorganisms, or on purified antigens derived from these microorganisms. These vaccines are highly protective, but sometimes they are reactogenic. New generation vaccines, mainly based on highly purified material are safer than traditional vaccines, but are often poorly immunogenic. Therefore, the use of an adjuvant is crucial in rendering the vaccine able to induce an immune response. In the last years considerable efforts have been directed toward the development of new and improved vaccine adjuvants. Many new molecules have been proposed and some of them have been evaluated in clinical trials. In this chapter we will describe the properties of some of the novel adjuvants that are promising for the development of new vaccines. These include immunostimulatory adjuvants such as LPS derivatives, saponins, CpG oligonucleotides, cytokines, and vaccine delivery systems such as emulsions, iscoms, liposomes, and microparticles. Particular emphasis will be given to mucosal adjuvants such as genetically detoxified derivatives of cholera and heat-labile enterotoxins that have significant potential for the future development of mucosally delivered vaccines.

INTRODUCTION

The knowledge of the pathogenesis of many microorganisms, the identification of the main virulence factors and characterization of the immune response induced following infection has been crucial for the design of novel vaccines. The new vaccines proposed are mainly based on highly purified components such as recombinant antigens, synthetic peptides, protein polysaccharide conjugates or DNA. Although these vaccines are expected to be very effective, their immunogenicity is often very low. Therefore, their formulation with an adjuvant is crucial to render them immunogenic.

The induction of an immune response is a multifactor event, which initiates when the microorganism or the antigen are picked up by antigen-presenting cells (APC) (e.g. dendritic cells, macrophages, B lymphocytes) that are able to process the antigen and migrate to draining lymphnodes. The pathway of antigen processing, cytoplasmic for intracellularly produced bacterial or viral antigens and endosomal for exogenous antigens, drives the class I or class II MHC presentation, and the type of T cell precursor, CD8+ or CD4+ (Germain, 1994). Activation of the appropriate T-cell population is the key point for the induction of effector immune functions. CD8+ T cells mediate their function through the production of interferon-γ (IFN-γ) and TNF-α, and through a selective cytolytic activity of pathogen-infected cells expressing on their surface MHC class I molecules (Kagi *et al.*, 1996). CD4+ T cells have a helper function, since following activation and proliferation they produce cytokines that stimulate B-lymphocytes to differentiate into antibody secreting cells (Fearon and Locksley, 1996). CD4+ T cells differentiate into Th1, Th2 cells (T helper 1 and 2). The division into these subsets is mainly based on their secretion of different cytokines (Cherwinsky *et al.*, 1987, Romagnani, 1994; Mosmann and Sad, 1996). Th1 responses are typically characterized by secretion of IFN-γ. The secretion of IL-4, IL-5, IL-6 and IL-10 characterizes Th2 responses. The fine balance of the particular CD4+ T cells subset activated can influence the outcome of the infection. Protection against many bacterial infections has been associated to the induction of a Th1 response, as in the case of *Chlamydia* (Rank *et al.*, 1992), *Bordetella pertussis* (Mills *et al.*, 1993) and *Listeria monocytogenes* (Hsieh *et al.*, 1993), or of a Th2 response as in the case of *Leishmania major* (Milon *et al.*, 1995; Reiner and Locksley, 1995). Obviously, the knowledge of the type of response induced is fundamental for the design, development and testing of an effective vaccine. Although different adjuvants may induce comparable levels of functional antibodies, the cytokine and antibody profiles generated can be different. The most appropriate adjuvant to use will depend to a large extent on the type of immune response that is required for protective immunity. Therefore, the knowledge and critical evaluation of the immune response induced following infection can help in the adjuvant selection and in the rational design of new vaccines.

Adjuvants able to induce an immune response were first described by Ramon (Ramon, 1924) as substances that, when used in combination with a specific antigen, were able to induce a stronger immune response than the antigen alone. Although a large number of adjuvants have been proposed and tested for several decades, the only widely used adjuvant for human vaccines are aluminum salts whose mechanism of action remains poorly defined (Cox and Coulter, 1997). Experiments with radiolabeled antigens have shown that alum is not able to increase the persistence of antigen at the injection site, as originally thought (Gupta *et al.*, 1996). *In vitro,* alum is able to upregulate co-stimulatory signals on human monocytes and to promote the release of IL-4 (Ulanova *et al.*, 2001). In mice, antigen administration with alum tends to favor the polarization of CD4+ T cells toward a Th2 phenotype. Alum is a safe adjuvant, however, it is not devoid of possible side-effects; its ability to induce IgE antibody responses has been associated with allergic reactions in some subjects (Gupta, 1998; Relyveld *et al.*, 1998).

More recently, a number of new adjuvants for systemic or mucosal administrations have been proposed and are actually under investigation. Here we will describe some of them on the basis of their ability to directly activate an immune response (e.g. driving the activation of the appropriate T cell population) to act as delivery systems (e.g. facilitating antigen-uptake, transport or presentation to antigen presenting cells) or to act as mucosal adjuvants (e.g. inducing a systemic and mucosal response following mucosal immunization).

IMMUNOSTIMULATORY ADJUVANTS

Many of the adjuvants belonging to this family are directly derived from pathogens (e.g. bacterial cell wall components, CpG DNA etc.) and may represent a "danger signal" for the immune system, indicating a possible infection of the host. These antigens represent pathogen-associated molecular patterns (PAMP'S) that, interacting with a pattern recognition receptor (PRR), activate cells of the innate immune system. These cells not only phagocytose and kill pathogens but also drive the activation of the immune response by secreting a wide-range of inflammatory mediators and cytokines (Medzitov and Janeway, 1998; Aderem and Ulevitch 2000). Although not all the features that make pathogens immunogenic are known, some components, including PAMPS, have the ability to activate APC and initiate an immune response.

Monophosphoryl Lipid A (MPL)

Monophosphoryl Lipid A (MPL) is an adjuvant derived from LPS of *Salmonella minnesota*, able to induce CD4+ T cell response, the synthesis and release of cytokines, particularly IL-2 and IFN-γ, (generation of Th1 response) (Gustafson and Rhodes, 1992; Ulrich and Myers, 1995) and the maturation of DC (De Becker *et al.*, 2000). MPL has been extensively evaluated in the clinic in more than 10,000 subjects for cancer (melanoma and breast), infectious disease (genital herpes, HBV, malaria and HPV), and allergy vaccines. MPL maintains an adjuvant effect when used in combination with alum (Thoelen *et al.*, 1998) and has been also proposed as adjuvant for DNA vaccines (Sasaki *et al.*, 1997) and for mucosal delivery (Childers *et al.*, 2000).

Structure-function studies of MPL have allowed the identification of a new generation of synthetic adjuvants called AGPs (Johnson *et al.*, 1999), one of which, the Ribi.529, is currently being evaluated in a phase III trial for HBV.

C$_P$G

Bacterial DNA, but not vertebrate DNA, has immunostimulatory effects on immune cells *in vitro* (Messina *et al.*, 1991; Tokunaga *et al.*, 1984). This effect seems to be mediated by the unmethylated CpG dinucleotides (Krieg *et al.*, 1995), which are under-represented and methylated in vertebrate DNA. Unmethylated CpGs have probably the role to be recognized by cells of the immune system to allow discrimination of pathogen-derived DNA from self-DNA (Bird, 1986).

CpG motifs are able to induce a Th1 response, mainly through stimulation of TNFα, IL-1, IL-6 and IL-12, and expression of co-stimulatory molecules (Davis *et al.*, 1998; Sun *et al.*, 1998). The adjuvant effect of CpG increases following conjugation to protein antigens (Klinman *et al.*, 1999). Although CpG oligos have been mainly evaluated in mice, sequences active in humans have been recently described (Hartmann *et al.*, 2000) and human clinical trials are ongoing to evaluate the adjuvant effect.

Saponins

Saponins or triterpenoid glycosides are derived from the bark of a Chilean tree, *Quillaja saponaria*, and function as adjuvants mainly through the induction of cytokines (Kensil, 1996). Saponins have been shown to intercalate into cell membranes, through interaction with cholesterol, forming 'holes' or pores. Although it is unknown if the adjuvant effect of saponins is related to pore-formation, this may allow antigens to gain access to the endogenous pathway of antigen presentation. QS21, a member of this family is a potent adjuvant for CTL induction and induces Th1 cytokines (IL-2 and IFN-γ) and IgG2a antibodies (Soltysik *et al.*, 1995; Kensil *et al.*, 1996). A number of clinical trials on more than 1600 volunteers have been performed, using QS21 as an adjuvant, initially for cancer vaccines (melanoma, breast and prostate), and subsequently for infectious diseases, including HIV, influenza, herpes, malaria and hepatitis B (Waite *et al.*, 2001). The results show that the critical aspect for this adjuvant is to establish the effective adjuvant dose tolerable in humans (Keefer *et al.*, 1997; Waite *et al.*, 2001). QS21 has been also proposed as an adjuvant for DNA vaccines, following both systemic and mucosal administration (Sasaki *et al.*, 1998).

Cytokines

Most cytokines have the ability to modify and re-direct the immune response. The cytokines that have been evaluated most extensively as adjuvants include IL-1, IL-2, IFN-γ, IL-12, and GM-CSF (Heath, 1995). However, the dose-related toxicity, the low stability, and the high costs render their use in routine vaccination difficult.

DELIVERY SYSTEMS

The use of antigen delivery system as alternative to immunostimulatory adjuvants has been widely investigated. The particulate adjuvants (emulsion, liposomes, iscoms, virosomes and microparticles) have similar dimensions to pathogens and are able to target the associate antigens to macrophages and dendritic cells, facilitating antigen uptake, transport or presentation. As later shown, in some studies the delivery system and the immunostimulatory adjuvants have been combined to enhance the immune response or to direct the immune response through the desired pathway (e.g. Th1 or Th2).

Oil in Water Adjuvants

The most potent water in mineral oil adjuvant is the Freund's adjuvant, but it is too toxic to be used in humans. New members of this family have been proposed to substitute the Freund's for human use. One of them, the syntex adjuvant formulation, SAF (Allison and Byar, 1986), was developed in the 1980s using a biodegradable oil (squalen), but it resulted to be too toxic for human use (Quan *et al.* 1997).

More recently, a novel o/w emulsion, derived from squalene has been developed and named MF59 (Van Nest *et al*, 1992; Ott *et al.*, 1995). The adjuvant properties of MF59 have been demonstrated not only in different animal models but also in human clinical trials. More than 18,000 subjects have been immunized with MF59 in combination with HIV, HSV, CMV, HBV, and influenza, to evaluate the safety and potency of MF59. The results have shown that MF59 is safe and effective in promoting the induction of potent antibody responses (Kahn *et al.* 1994; Langenberg *et al.*, 1995; Pass *et al.*, 1999; Nitayaphan *et al.* 2000). MF59 has been recently licensed for use in humans in association with influenza vaccine (Minutello *et al.*, 1999; De Donato *et al.*, 1999; Menegon *et al.*, 1999). In addition, MF59 has also been shown to be an effective adjuvant for a protein/polysaccharide conjugate in infant baboons (Granoff *et al.*, 1997). The size of the MF59 particles is about 200nm and studies with labelled MF59 have shown that it is taken up by macrophages and DC, both at the site of injection and in local lymphnodes (Dupuis *et al.*, 1998).

Liposomes

Liposomes are phospholipid vesicles with a diameter ranging from 50nm to 10μm that have been evaluated both as adjuvants and as delivery systems for antigens and adjuvants (Gregoriadis, 1990; Alving, 1992). Liposomal vaccines based on viral membrane proteins (virosomes) have been extensively evaluated in the clinic and are approved as products in Europe for hepatitis A and influenza (Ambrosch *et al.*, 1997). Liposomes as well as virosomes are described in more detail in Chapter 4 by R. Zurbriggen.

Iscoms

Iscoms are complexes with a diameter of 40nm formed by cholesterol, phospholipids, cell membrane antigens, and saponins derived from *Q. saponaria* (Quil A) (Cox *et al.*, 1998). Iscoms are known to promote antibody responses and induce T cell help in a variety of animal models. They are generally considered to be the most potent adjuvant for the induction of CTL responses with recombinant proteins in pre-clinical models. A recent study has indicated that the induction of IL-12 is key to the adjuvant effect of iscoms (Smith *et al.*, 1999). An influenza iscom vaccine has shown to be more immunogenic and protective than a classical subunit vaccine in macaques (Rimmelzwaan *et al.*, 1997) and to induce CTL responses in human clinical trials (Ennis *et al.*, 1999). Potent T cell proliferative responses have been shown in primates immunized with iscom vaccines containing CMV, flu, HIV and EBV antigens (Cox *et al.*, 1998; Sjolander *et al.*, 2001). However, the efficacy for CTL induction, and the safety profile of iscoms needs to be further established in humans, although preliminary studies are encouraging (Bates *et al.*, 1996). A potential problem with iscoms is that inclusion of antigens into the adjuvant is often difficult and may require extensive antigen modification (Lovgren-Bengtsson and Morein, 2000); however, novel ways to associate antigens to iscoms, without significant formulation difficulties have been recently described (Polakos *et al.*, 2001). In this study, the immunization of rhesus macaques with the core of hepatitis C virus adsorbed to iscoms has been shown to induce a potent long-lasting CTL response.

Microparticles

Polylactide-co-glycolides (PLG) have been used in humans for many years as suture material and as controlled release drug delivery systems (Okada and Toguchi, 1995; Putney and Burke, 1998) and are actually the primary candidates for the development of microparticles as adjuvants. The adjuvant effect of PLG microparticles has been shown only recently (Eldridge *et al.*, 1991; O'Hagan, *et al.*, 1991a, 1991b, and 1993) and is mediated by the uptake into DC, macrophages and local lymphnodes. Microparticles have a diameter ranging from 100nm to 10μm, can be positively or negatively charged and be effective for the absorption of protein antigens and DNA vaccines (Hedley *et al.*, 1998; Gupta *et al.*, 1998; Singh *et al.*, 2000; O'Hagan, 2001). A particularly attractive feature of microparticles is their ability to control the rate of release of entrapped antigens (Singh *et al.*, 1997). Cationic microparticles with adsorbed DNA are able to enhance both antibody and CTL responses in a range of animal models (Singh *et al.*, 2000). Anionic microparticles with adsorbed proteins are effective for CTL induction in mice (Kazzaz *et al.*, 2000). In a recent study with HIV vaccines, the potency of microparticles as an adjuvant has been shown to increase significantly following formulation into MF59 emulsion (O'Hagan *et al.*, 2000).

MUCOSAL DELIVERY OF VACCINES

Most of the vaccines available are administered by subcutaneous or intramuscular routes. Nevertheless, mucosae represent ideal sites to deliver vaccines against those pathogens that infect hosts through mucosal surfaces. Mucosal surfaces provide a physical barrier between the external environment and the body being constantly exposed to thousands of foreign substances that are acquired through eating, breathing, touching, etc. It would be wasteful and potentially dangerous to mount inappropriate immune responses against these environmental antigens. They are in fact substantially ignored by the healthy immune system that induces an immunological tolerance to them (Strober *et al.* 1988). As a consequence, only few molecules have the unique property to act as immunogens when they contact mucosal surfaces.

Several approaches to deliver vaccines at mucosal surfaces have been described and many others are currently under investigation. Many of these approaches as the use of live-attenuated bacteria as delivery system for heterologous antigens or the use of plants, such as bananas or potato tubers, as expression system for viral and bacterial antigens will be extensively described in the following chapters of this book. Here we will focus on those molecules that behave as strong adjuvants when given in combination with soluble antigens.

The most attractive route for mucosal immunization is the oral route. Unfortunately, oral immunization is difficult with non-living antigens, since they are exposed to the low pH of the stomach and to digestive enzymes present in the intestine. A number of different delivery systems has been evaluated for their ability to act as adjuvants following oral immunization (O'Hagan, 1998). Among them, microparticles have been shown to be effective adjuvants following oral immunization, probably as a consequence of their uptake into specialized sites of mucosal immune response induction (e.g. mucosal associated lymphoid tissues or MALT) (O'Hagan, 1996). Alternative routes of mucosal immunization including nasal, pulmonary, intra-vaginal and intra-rectal have been extensively evaluated. Of these, the intranasal route is the most promising and the most convenient since small amounts of antigen and adjuvant can induce strong immunogenicity and adjuvanticity.

The most powerful mucosal immunogens and adjuvants recognized to date are cholera toxin (CT) and *Escherichia coli* heat-labile enterotoxin (LT), responsible for the watery secretions typical of cholera and traveller's diarrhoea, respectively (Mekalanos *et al.*, 1983; Spangler, 1992). Although LT and CT have been extensively investigated as mucosal immunogens and adjuvants in animal models, their use in humans has been prohibited by their toxicity. Knowledge of the molecular structure of LT and CT has allowed a rational design of LT and CT derivatives, which are non-toxic but still active as mucosal immunogens and adjuvants as will be later described.

CT and LT Structure and Activity

CT and LT are 80% identical in their amino acid sequence (Dallas and Falkow, 1980; Spicer *et al.*, 1981) and have an identical tertiary structure (Sixma *et al.*, 1991). They are composed of two subunits A and B, organized in an AB5 structure. The A subunit is an enzyme with ADP-ribosylating activity that is responsible for the toxicity, whereas the B subunit is a pentameric oligomer that binds the receptor located on the surfaces of eukaryotic cells. The A subunit is composed of two domains: the enzymatically active A1 and the A2, which is formed by a long α-helix that enters into the central cavity of the B oligomer. The two domains are linked by a trypsin-sensitive loop and by a disulphide bridge between the A1-cys 187 and the A2-cys 199. In order to generate the enzymatic activity, the loop has to be cleaved and the disulphide bridge reduced (Gill and Rappaport, 1979). CT is secreted by *Vibrio cholerae* already in the active form since the bacterium produces a specific haemagglutinin protease that processes the A subunit (Booth *et al.*, 1984), whereas LT is activated by non-specific enzymes produced by the host.

The A1 subunit binds nicotinamide adenine dinucleotide (NAD) and transfers the ADP-ribose group to the α subunit of G_s, a GTP-binding protein which regulates the activity of adenylate cyclase causing its permanent activation and abnormal intracellular accumulation of cAMP (Holmgren, 1981; Moss and Vaughan, 1984; Field *et al.*, 1989; Gill and Woolkalis, 1991; Pizza *et al.*, 1999).

The B subunit is formed by five monomers that are arranged in a ring-like structure with a central pore containing five symmetrical cavities responsible for binding to the eukaryotic cell receptor (Sixma *et al.*, 1993a, and 1993b). The receptor-binding site is specific for a variety of galactose-containing molecules and shows a different fine specificity between LT and CT. CT binds mostly to the ganglioside GM1 that is believed to be the major toxin receptor (Holmgren *et al.*, 1973), while LT binds not only to GM1 (Sugii, 1989) but also to other glycosphingolipids (Tenenberg *et al.*, 1994), to glycoprotein receptors present in the intestine of rabbits and humans (Holmgren *et al.*, 1982, and 1985; Griffiths *et al.*, 1986), to polyglycosilceramides (PCGs) (Karlsson *et al.*, 1996), and to paragloboside (Tenenberg *et al.*, 1994).

After the binding of the B subunit to the receptor, the toxin is transported to the Golgi compartment and undergoes retrograde transport from the Golgi to the endoplasmic reticulm (ER). The A subunit (or the A1) is then translocated, by an unknown mechanism, from the ER to the cytosol (Bastiaens *et al.*, 1996; Majoul *et al.*, 1996) where it can interact with ADP-ribosylation factors (ARFs), a family of 20 kDa proteins with a role in vesicular membrane trafficking and able to enhance the CT or LT enzymatic activity (Tsai *et al.*, 1988). Once activated, the A1 peptide ADP-ribosylates the α subunit of G_s and possibly other G proteins located on the plasma membrane.

To better characterize the role of the CT and LT and of their A and B subunits in mucosal immunogenicity as well as to define molecules that are nontoxic but still active as mucosal adjuvants and immunogens, more than fifty different site-directed mutants have been produced (Giuliani *et al.*, 1998; Lycke *et al.*, 1992; Pizza *et al.*, 1994a; 1994b; Fontana *et al.*, 1995; Dickinson and Clements 1995; Douce *et al.*, 1995; De Haan *et al.*, 1996; Douce *et al.*, 1997; Yamamoto *et al.*, 1997; De Haan *et al.*, 1998; Douce *et al.*, 1998). Here we will not describe all of them but we will focus only on those that have been best characterized and are relevant for this chapter.

Mutations in the B Subunit

The B subunits of LT and CT (LTB and CTB) were the first non-toxic derivatives of CT and LT produced. Initial commercial preparations of CTB, in which the B subunit was purified from the active toxin, were associated with adjuvant activity; however, the adjuvant effect was due in most of the cases to contaminating traces of wild-type toxin (Tamura *et al.*, 1994; Blanchard *et al.*, 1998). When recombinant LTB and CTB became available, it was clear that B subunits were very poor mucosal adjuvants. Mutation in position 33 (Gly to Asp) blocked the ability of LTB to bind the receptor as well as its immunogenicity, suggesting that an intact receptor-binding site is necessary both for binding and immunogenicity (Nashar *et al.*, 1996). These LTB mutants lose also other immune-modulating activities including the ability to induce apoptosis of CD4+ and CD8+ cells (Nashar *et al.*, 1996; Truitt *et al.*, 1998). Whether LT mutants defective in receptor binding, with and without enzymatic activity, are still active as adjuvants is controversial (De Haan *et al.*, 1998; Guidri *et al.*, 1997).

Recombinant A Subunit

An alternative approach to separate the adjuvant activity of LT and CT from toxicity has been the use of the A subunit only. The gene coding for the A1 subunit of CT has been fused to the gene coding for the immunoglobulin binding domain of protein A of *Staphylococcus aureus* (CTA1-DD fusion protein). This molecule retains the adjuvant activity of CT following mucosal and systemic administration due to its ability to direct the enzymatic activity of the A subunit to B cells (Agren *et al.*, 1997, 1999 and 2000). This fusion protein represents a new strategy for the targeted delivery of adjuvant activity to a selected group of cells. However, a possible limitation of this approach is that it may not induce a broad immune response by targeting the antigen only to B cells. Enzymatically inactive CTA1-DD molecules failed to induce an adjuvant response following systemic immunization showing that the adjuvant effect of CTA1-DD depends on the enzymatic activity (Agren *et al.*, 1999).

The His-tagged form of LTA, and the His-tagged form of a genetically detoxified derivative, LTA-K112, have been reported to retain the mucosal adjuvant properties of the wild-type toxin, suggesting that the adjuvant effect is independent from ADP-ribosylation (De Haan *et al.*, 1996). The mechanism by which a His-tagged A subunit can be internalized in the absence of a receptor-binding domain is unclear. It is possible that the polycationic histidine peptide tail may provide a non-specific cell binding activity (Blanke *et al.*, 1996).

Genetically Detoxified Mutants of LT: LTK63 and LTR72 as Strong Mucosal Adjuvants

Computer modelling and site-directed mutagenesis of the A subunit have allowed the identification of residues located in or around the catalytic site, and which have a key role on the enzymatic activity or on the structure of the active site (Pizza *et al.*, 1994a). Amino acid substitutions of these residues generated LT and CT mutants, which have no toxicity *in vitro* and *in vivo*, and mutants that retain a residual toxicity *in vitro* and *in vivo*. Among them, the LTK63 and LTR72 have been characterized in detail for their biochemical and immunological properties. LTK63 contains a serine 63 to lysine substitution in the A subunit and is devoid of any enzymatic and toxic activity. The mutant is assembled in the AB5 structure efficiently, retains the ability to bind the receptor and to interact with ARF (Pizza *et al.*, 1994a; 1994b; Magagnoli *et al.*, 1996; Stevens *et al.*, 1999). Its X-ray structure has shown a complete identity to wild-type LT, with the exception of the catalytic site where the introduced lysine fills the cavity making it unsuitable for the enzymatic activity (Van den Akker *et al.*, 1997).

LTR72 contains an alanine 72 to arginine substitution in the A subunit. This mutant is partially detoxified, retaining 1% of the wild-type ADP ribosylating activity, a toxicity *in vitro* on Y1 cells reduced by a factor of 10^4-10^5 and a toxicity *in vivo* in the rabbit ileal loop model reduced by 25- to 100-fold (Giuliani *et al.*, 1998).

LTK63 and LTR72 are highly immunogenic following systemic and mucosal immunization, and able to induce antibodies neutralizing the toxic activity of wild-type LT both, *in vitro* and *in vivo* supporting their potential as components of vaccines against enterotoxigenic *E.coli* (Giuliani *et al*, 1998). LTK63 and LTR72 have been extensively characterized for their ability to act as mucosal adjuvants. As shown in Table 1, the adjuvant activity has been tested with a wide range of co-administered antigens (bacterial and viral antigens and synthetic peptides), using different routes of immunizations and different animal models. The two mutants are not only able to behave as strong mucosal adjuvants, but are also able to favor protective immunity in appropriate animal models of challenge. The potency of LTK63 and LTR72 is not affected by the presence of pre-existing immunity to the adjuvant (Ugozzoli *et al.*, 2001).

LTR72, the mutant retaining a residual enzymatic activity, is a stronger adjuvant as compared to the fully non toxic LTK63 mutant, inducing antigen-specific antibodies titers comparable to those induced by wild-type LT (Giuliani *et al.*, 1998). On the other hand, the LTK63 is a stronger adjuvant as compared to the B subunit (Douce *et al.*, 1998; Giuliani *et al.*, 1998), suggesting that ADP-ribosylation activity is important but not necessary for adjuvanticity. The presence of an enzymatically inactive A subunit, which can interact with regulatory proteins inside the cells, confers to the AB complex an adjuvanticity higher than that present in the B subunit. (Giuliani *et al.*, 1998).

These mutant molecules represent not only promising adjuvants for human use, but also an interesting tool to dissect the mechanism of mucosal adjuvanticity and to evaluate the role and the relative contribution of the B subunit, the AB complex, and the enzymatic activity to adjuvanticity. Clinical trials have been planned to evaluate the safety, immunogenicity and adjuvanticity profiles of LTK63 and LTR72.

Using a similar approach, non-toxic or partially detoxified mutants of CT have been also obtained (Fontana *et al.*, 1995). Of these, the best characterized are the CTK63 (containing a Ser to Lys substitution in position 63, the same mutation present in the LTK63), which is fully non-toxic, and the CTS106 (containing a Pro to Ser substitution in position 106), which retains a residual enzymatic activity. Surprisingly, the CTK63 exhibited a very weak adjuvant activity following intranasal immunization in mice, as compared to the strong adjuvanticity of the homologous LTK63 mutant (Douce *et al.*, 1997). The best adjuvant activity was observed with the CTS106 molecule, retaining a residual enzymatic activity comparable to that observed with the LTR72 mutant (Douce *et al.* 1997). These data suggest

Table 1. Adjuvant activity of LTK63 and LTR72 with a variety of antigens by different routes of immunization and in different animal models

Adjuvant: LTK63 LTR72	Antigen	Route of Immunization	Animal Model	Reference
+ +	Ovalbumin	Intranasal		Douce *et al.*, 1997; Giuliani *et al.*, 1998
+	Fragment C of tetanus toxin	Intranasal	Mice	Douce *et al.*, 1997
+	CTL epitope of measles virus.	Intranasal	Mice	Partidos, 1996; Partidos *et al.*, 1999
+	Diphtheria, Tetanus, acellular Pertussis	Intranasal	Mice	Ryan *et al.*, 1999
+	Acellular pertussis	Intranasal	Mice	Ryan *et al.*, 1999
+ +	FHA, 69K and PT9K/129G of *Bordetella pertussis*	Intranasal	Mice	Ryan *et al.*, 1999; 2000
+	Subunit influenza vaccine	Intranasal	Mice	Barackman *et al.*, 1999 Barchfeld *et al.*, 1999
+ +	Subunit influenza vaccine	Intranasal	Mice	Pizza and Del Giudice (unpublished)
+	gD2 of Herpes Simplex Virus	Intranasal	Mice and guinea pigs	Ugozzoli *et al.*, 1998; O'Hagan *et al.*, 1999
+	p24 and gp120 of HIV	Intranasal	Mice	O'Hagan (unpublished)
+	Meningococcus C conjugate	Intranasal	Mice and pigs	Ugozzoli *et al.*, 2001

+ +	Pneumococcus polysaccharide	Intranasal	Mice	Jakobsen *et al*, 1999
+	Ovalbumin	Intravaginal	Mice	Di Tommaso *et al.*, 1996
+	Subunit influenza vaccine	Intranasal	Rabbits and minipigs	O'Hagan (unpublished)
+	CagA, VacA and urease of *H. pylori*	Oral	Mice and beagle dogs	Ghiara *et al.*, 1997; Marchetti *et al.*, 1998; Rappuoli and Del Giudice (unpublished)
+	KLH	Oral	Mice	Douce *et al.*, 1999
+ +	Gag p55 of HIV	Intranasal, oral	Mice	Neidleman *et al.*, 2000
+	CTL peptide of respiratory Syncytial virus	Intranasal	Mice	Simmons *et al.*, 2001
+	HPV-6b virus-like particles	Intranasal	Mice	Greer *et al.*, 2000
+ +	Influenza hemagglutinin	Oral	Mice	Barackman *et al.*, 2001

that enzymatic activity is necessary for the adjuvanticity of cholera toxin. The qualitatively different immunological properties exhibited by the two molecules could be due to different receptor-binding activities of LT and CT. However, in a different study, non-toxic mutants of CT were reported to maintain the adjuvant properties of the wild-type toxin (Yamamoto *et al*, 1997; Hagiwara *et al.*, 1999). These contrasting results may reflect the different doses of adjuvant and antigen used and the route of delivery.

An alternative approach to detoxify LT has been based on the idea to make the protease sensitive loop located between the A1 and A2 resistant to proteases, rendering the toxin not susceptible to the activation necessary for enzymatic activity and toxicity. LTG192, in which arginine 192 is replaced by a glycine, is the best characterized (Grant *et al.*, 1994; Dickinson and Clements, 1995; Giannelli *et al.*, 1997). *In vitro,* the mutant toxin is resistant to trypsin cleavage. *In vivo*, proteases other than trypsin can cleave the loop and activate the toxin, since toxicity is detectable. This molecule is indistinguishable from wild-type toxin both in terms of immunogenicity and adjuvanticity. In humans, the mutant was safe at very low doses, but induced diarrhoea at 100 µg/dose (De Noon, 1997). LTR72, which is much less toxic than LTG192, and LTK63, which is totally devoid of toxicity, are expected to have a better safety profile.

MECHANISM OF ADJUVANTICITY

The immunomodulatory effects of LT and CT are still unclear and their mechanism remains to be defined. Despite their high degree of homology, CT and LT seem to exert their adjuvanticity through different mechanisms. CT-mediated adjuvanticity appears to be accompanied by a preferential activation of Th2 type CD4+ cell populations. This comes from the observation that mucosal immunization with antigens plus CT induces increased production of IL-4, IL-5, and IL-10, predominant production of IgG1 isotype, and induction of antigen-specific IgE (Marinaro *et al.*, 1995). This polarization of the immune response towards a Th2 functional phenotype is due to the ability of CT to inhibit the production of IL-12 p70 and the expression of the $\beta 1$ and $\beta 2$ chains of the IL-12 receptor, leading to the functional suppression of Th1 cell differentiation (Braun *et al.*, 1999). The ability of CT to polarize the immune response towards Th2 is maintained also by enzymatically inactive mutants such as CTK112 and this has been attributed to the up-regulation of B7-2 expression on antigen presenting cells (Cong *et al.*, 1997). When LT is used as a mucosal adjuvant, both Th1 and Th2 cells are activated (Takahashi *et al.*, 1996).

The LT mutants described, LTR72 and LTK63, have been used as tools to investigate the role of the enzymatic activity and the non toxic holotoxin on the adjuvant and immunomodulatory activities of LT. Low doses of the fully nontoxic LTK63 mutant enhanced the Th1/Th2 profile, whereas the LTR72 mutant, which retains a residual enzymatic activity, enhanced the Th2 response but suppressed the Th1 response. LTK63 enhanced IL-12 and TNF-α production and NFkB translocation, whereas LT R72, as well as wild-type LT failed to active NF-kB, but stimulate cAMP production. Therefore, the ability of LT to induce a Th2 response and suppress the Th1 response is linked to the effect of the enzymatic activity on NFkB activation and cAMP production (Ryan *et al.*, 2000).

CONCLUSIONS

A better understanding of the mechanism of action of the adjuvants described as well as the identification of factors that promote specific activation of the immune response is of primary importance in the design of new vaccines. Such knowledge could allow to define the best adjuvant-antigen combination that is able to induce the type of immune response required for protection against a specific infection.

The current availability of new molecules with adjuvant activity opens up an opportunity for their evaluation in humans. To date there are no evidences that most of them can act as effective and safe adjuvants in humans and clinical trials are expected to answer this question.

REFERENCES

Aderem, A., and Ulevitch, C.A. 2000. Toll-like receptors in the induction of the innate immune response. Nature 406: 782-787.

Agren, L.C., Ekman, L., Lowenadler, B., and Lycke, N.Y. 1997. Genetically engineered nontoxic vaccine adjuvant that combines B cell targeting with immunomodulation by cholera toxin A1 subunit. J. Immunol. 158: 3936-3946.

Agren, L.C., Ekman, L., Lowenadler, B., Nedrud, J.G., and Lycke, N.Y. 1999. Adjuvanticity of the cholera toxin A1-based gene fusion protein, CTA1-DD, is critically dependent on the ADP-ribosyltransferase and Ig-binding activity. J. Immunol. 162: 2432-2440.

Agren, L., Sverremark, E., Ekman, L., Schon, K., Lowenadler, B., Fernandez, C., and Lycke, N. 2000. The ADP-ribosylating CTA1-DD adjuvant enhances T cell-dependent and independent responses by direct action on B cells involving anti-apoptotic Bcl-2- and germinal center-promoting effects. J. Immunol. 164: 6276-6286.

Allison, A.C., and Byars, N.E. 1986. An adjuvant formulation that selectively elicits the formation of antibodies of protective isotypes and of cell-mediated immunity. J. Immunol. Methods. 95: 157-168.

Alving, C.R. 1992. Immunologic aspects of liposomes: presentation and processing of liposomal protein and phospholipid antigens. Biochim. Biophys. Acta. 1113: 307-322.

Ambrosch, F., Wiedermann, G., Jonas, S., Althaus, B., Finkel, B., Gluck, R., Herzog, C. 1997. Immunogenicity and protectivity of a new liposomal hepatitis A vaccine. Vaccine 15: 1209-1213.

Barackman, J.D., Ott, G., and O'Hagan, D.T. 1999. Intranasal immunization of mice with influenza vaccine in combination with the adjuvant LT-R72 induces potent mucosal and serum immunity which is stronger than that with traditional intramuscular immunization. Infect. Immun. 67: 4276-4279.

Barackman, J.D., Ott, G. Pine, S. and O'Hagan, D. 2001. Oral administration of influenza vaccine in combination with the adjuvants LT-K63 and LTR72 induces potent immune responses comparable to or stronger than traditional intramuscular immunization. Clin. Diagn. Lab. Immunol. 8: 652-657.

Barchfeld, G.L., Hessler, A.L., Chen, M., Pizza, M., Rappuoli, R. and Van Nest, G.A. 1999. The adjuvants MF59 and LT-K63 enhance the mucosal and systemic immunogenicity of subunit influenza vaccine administered intranasally in mice. Vaccine 17: 695-704.

Bastiaens, P.I.H., Majoul, I.V., Verveer, P.J., Soeling, H.D., and Jovin, T.M. 1996. Imaging the intracellular trafficking and state of the AB5 quaternary structure of cholera toxin. EMBO J. 15: 4246-4253.

Bates, J., Ackland, J., Coulter, A., Cox, J., Drane, D., Macfarlan, R., Varigos, J., Wong, T-Y., and Woods, W. 1996. IscomT adjuvant - a promising adjuvant for influenza virus vaccines. In: Options for the Control of Influenza III. L.E, Brown, A.W. Hampson, and R.G. Webster, eds. Elsevier Science B.V. p.661-667.

Bird, A.P. 1986. CpG-rich islands and the function of DNA methylation. Nature 321: 209-213.

Blanchard, T.G., Lycke, N., Czinn, S.J. and Nedrud, J.G. 1998. Recombinant cholera toxin B subunit is not an effective mucosal adjuvant for oral immunization of mice against *Helicobacter felis*. Immunology 94: 22-27.

Blanke, S.R., Milne, J.C., Benson, E.L. and Collier, R.J. 1996. Fused polycationic peptide mediates delivery of diphtheria toxin A chain to the cytosol in the presence of anthrax protective antigen. Proc. Natl. Acad. Sci. USA. 93: 8437-8442.

Booth, B.A., Boesman-Finkelstein, M., and Finkelstein, R.A. 1984. Comparative study of *Vibrio cholerae* non-O1 protease and soluble hemagglutinin with those of *Vibrio cholerae* O1. Infect. Immun. 45: 558-560.

Braun, M.C., He, J., Wu, C.Y., and Kelsall, B.L. 1999. Cholera toxin suppresses interleukin (IL)-12 production and IL-12 receptor beta1 and beta2 chain expression. J. Exp. Med. 189: 541-552..

Cherwinski, H.M., Schumacher, J.H., Brown, K.D., and Mosmann, T.R. 1987. Two types of mouse helper T cell clone. III. Further differences in lymphokine synthesis between Th1 and Th2 clones revealed by RNA hybridization, functionally monospecific bioassays, and monoclonal antibodies.J. Exp. Med. 166: 1229-1244.

Childers, N.K., Miller, K.L., Tong, G., Llarena, J.C., Greenway, T., Ulrich, J.T., Michalek, S.M., and Moingeon, P. 2000. Adjuvant activity of monophosphoryl lipid A for nasal and oral immunization with soluble or liposome-associated antigen. Infect. Immun. 68: 5509-5516.

Cong, Y., Weaver, C.T. and Elson, C.O. 1997. The mucosal adjuvanticity of cholera toxin involves enhancement of costimulatory activity by selective up-regulation of B7.2 expression. J. Immunol. 159: 5301-5308.

Cox, J.C., and Coulter, A.R. 1997. Adjuvants - a classification and review of their mode of action. Vaccine. 15: 248-256.

Cox, J.C., Sjolander A., Barr, I.G. 1998. ISCOMs and other saponin based adjuvants. Adv. Drug Del. Rev. 32: 247-271.

Dallas, W. S., and Falkow, S. 1980. Amino acid homology between cholera toxin and *Escherichia coli* heat labile toxin. Nature 288: 499-501.

Davis, H.L., Weeranta, R., Waldschmidt, T.J., Tygrett, L., Schorr, J., and Krieg, A.M. 1998. CpG DNA is a potent enhancer of specific immunity in mice immunized with recombinant hepatitis B surface antigen. J. Immunol.160: 870-876.

De Becker, G., Moulin, V., Pajak, B., Bruck, C., Francotte, M., Thiriart, C., Urbain, J., Moser, M., and Moingeon, P. 2000. Monophosphoryl lipid A as an adjuvant. Past experiences and new directions. Int.Immunol.12: 807-815.

De Donato, S., Granoff, D., Minutello, M., Lecchi, G., Faccini, M., Agnello, M., Senatore, F., Verweij, P., Fritzell, B., and Podda, A. 1999. Safety and immunogenicity of MF59-adjuvanted influenza vaccine in the elderly. Vaccine 17: 3094-3101.

de Haan, L., Feil, I.K., Verweij, W.R., Holtrop, M., Hol, W.G., Agsteribbe, E., and Wilschut, J. 1998. Mutational analysis of the role of ADP-ribosylation activity and GM1-binding activity in the adjuvant properties of the *Escherichia coli* heat-labile enterotoxin towards intranasally administered keyhole limpet hemocyanin. Eur. J. Immunol. 28: 1243-1250.

de Haan, L., Verweij, W.R., Feil, I.K., Holtrop, M., Hol, W.G., Agsteribbe, E., and Wilschut, J. 1996. Role of GM1 binding in the mucosal immunogenicity and adjuvant activity of the *Escherichia coli* heat-labile enterotoxin and its B subunit. Infect. Immun. 64: 5413-5416.

De Noon, D.D. 1997. Conference Coverage (ICAAC) in Vaccine Weekly (Nov3). p. 4.

Di Tommaso, A., Saletti, G., Pizza, M., Rappuoli, R., Dougan, G., Abrignani, S., Douce, G. and De Magistris, M.T. 1996. Induction of antigen-specific antibodies in vaginal secretions by using a nontoxic mutant of heat-labile enterotoxin as a mucosal adjuvant. Infect. Immun. 64: 974-979.

Dickinson, B.L. and Clements, J.D. 1995. Dissociation of *Escherichia coli* heat-labile enterotoxin adjuvanticity from ADP-ribosyltransferase activity. Infect. Immun. 63: 1617-1623.

Douce, G., Turcotte, C., Cropley, I., Roberts, M., Pizza, M., Domenghini, M., Rappuoli, R. and Dougan, G. 1995. Mutants of *Escherichia coli* heat-labile toxin lacking ADP-ribosyltransferase activity act as nontoxic, mucosal adjuvants. Proc. Natl. Acad. Sci. USA. 92: 1644-1648.

Douce, G., Fontana, M.R., Pizza, M., Rappuoli, R., and Dougan, G. 1997. Intranasal immunogenicity and adjuvanticity of site-directed mutant derivatives of cholera toxin. Infect. Immun. 65: 2821-2828.

Douce, G., Giuliani, M.M., Giannelli, V., Pizza, M., Rappuoli, R., and Dougan, G.. 1998. Mucosal immunogenicity of genetically detoxified derivatives of heat labile toxin from *Escherichia coli*. Vaccine 16: 1065-1073.

Douce, G., Giannelli, V., Pizza, M., Lewis, D., Everest, P., Rappuoli, R., and Dougan, G. 1999. Genetically detoxified mutants of heat-labile toxin from *Escherichia coli* are able to act as oral adjuvants. Infect. Immun. 67: 4400-4406.

Dupuis, M., Murphy, T.J., Higgins, D., Ugozzoli, M., Van Nest, G., Ott, G., and McDonald, D.M. 1998. Dendritic cells internalize vaccine adjuvant after intramuscular injection. Cell. Immunol. 186: 18-27.

Eldridge, J.H., Staas, J.K., Meulbroek, J.A., Tice, T.R., and Gilley, R.M. 1991. Biodegradable and biocompatible poly(DL-lactide-co-glycolide) microspheres as an adjuvant for staphylococcal enterotoxin B toxoid which enhances the level of toxin-neutralizing antibodies. Infect. Immun. 59: 2978-2986.

Ennis, F.A., Cruz, J., Jameson, J., Klein, M., Burt, D., and Thipphawong, J. 1999. Augmentation of human influenza A virus-specific cytotoxic T lymphocyte memory by influenza vaccine and adjuvanted carriers (ISCOMS). Virology 259: 256-261.

Fearon, D.T., and Locksley, R.M. 1996. The instructive role of innate immunity in the acquired immune response. Science 272: 50-53.

Field, M., Rao, M.C., and Chang, E. B. 1989. Intestinal electrolyte transport and diarrheal disease (1). N. Engl. J. Med. 321: 800-806.

Fontana, M.R., Manetti, R., Giannelli, V., Magagnoli, C., Marchini, A., Domenighini, M., Rappuoli, R., and Pizza, M. 1995. Construction of nontoxic derivatives of cholera toxin and characterization of the immunological response against the A subunit. Infect. Immun. 63: 2356-2360.

Germain, R.N. 1994. MHC-dependent antigen processing and peptide presentation, providing ligands for lymphocyte activation. Cell 76: 287-299.

Ghiara, P., Rossi, M., Marchetti, M., Di Tommaso, A., Vindigni, C., Ciampolini, F., Covacci, A., Telford, J.L., De Magistris, M.T., Pizza, M., Rappuoli, R., and Del Giudice, G. 1997. Therapeutic intragastric vaccination against *Helicobacter pylori* in mice eradicates an otherwise chronic infection and confers protection against reinfection. Infect. Immun. 65: 4996-5002.

Giannelli, V., Fontana, M.R., Giuliani., M.M., Guancai, D., Rappuoli, R., and Pizza, M. 1997. Protease susceptibility and toxicity of heat-labile enterotoxins with a mutation in the active site or in the protease-sensitive loop. Infect. Immun. 65: 331-334.

Gill, D.M., and Rappaport, R.S. 1979. Origin of the enzymatically active A1 fragment of cholera toxin. J. Infect. Dis. 139: 674-680.

Gill, D.M., and Woolkalis, M. J. 1991. Cholera toxin-catalyzed [32P]ADP-ribosylation of proteins. Methods. Enzymol. 195: 267-280.

Giuliani, M.M., Del Giudice, G., Giannelli, V., Douce, G., Dougan, G., Rappuoli, R., and Pizza, M. 1998. Mucosal Adjuvanticity and immunogenicity of LTR72, a mutant of *Escherichia coli* heat-labile enterotoxin with partial knockout of ADP-ribosyltranseferase activity. J. Exp. Med. 187: 1123-1132.

Granoff, D.M., McHugh, Y.E., Raff, H.V., Mokatrin, A.S., and Van Nest, G.A. 1997. MF59 adjuvant enhances antibody responses of infant baboons immunized with *Haemophilus influenzae* type b and *Neisseria meningitidis* group C oligosaccharide-CRM197 conjugate vaccine. Infect Immun . 65: 1710-1715.

Grant, C.C., Messer, R.J., and Cieplak, W.J. 1994. Role of trypsin-like cleavage at arginine 192 in the enzymatic and cytotonic activities of *Escherichia coli* heat-labile enterotoxin. Infect. Immun. 62: 4270-4278.

Greer, C.E., Petracca, R., Buonamassa, D.T., Di Tommaso, A., Gervase, B., Reeve, R.L., Ugozzoli, M., Van Nest, G., De Magistris, M.,T. and Bensi, G. 2000. The comparison of the effect of LTR72 and MF59 adjuvants on mouse humoral response to intranasal immunisation with human papillomavirus type 5b (HPV-6b) virus-like particles. Vaccine 19: 1008-1012.

Gregoriadis, G. 1990. Immunological adjuvants: a role for liposomes. Immunol. Today. 11: 89-97.

Griffiths, S.L., Finkelstein, R.A., and Critchley, D.R. 1986. Characterization of the receptor for cholera toxin and *Escherichia coli* heat-labile toxin in rabbit intestinal brush borders. Biochem. J. 238: 313-322.

Guidry, J.J., Cardenas, L., Cheng, E., and Clements, J.D. 1997 Role of receptor binding in toxicity, immunogenicity, and adjuvanticity of *Escherichia coli* heat-labile enterotoxin. Infect. Immun. 65: 4943-4950.

Gupta, R.K., Chang, A.C., Griffin, P., Rivera, R., and Siber, G.R. 1996. *In vivo* distribution of radioactivity in mice after injection of biodegradable polymer microspheres containing 14C-labeled tetanus toxoid.Vaccine14: 1412-1416.

Gupta, R.K. 1998 Aluminum compounds as vaccine adjuvants. Adv. Drug. Deliv. Rev . 32: 155-172.

Gupta, R.K., Singh, M., and O'Hagan, D.T. 1998. Poly(lactide-co-glycolide) microparticles for the development of single-dose controlled-release vaccines. Adv. Drug. Deliv. Rev. 32: 225-246.

Gustafson, G.L., and Rhodes, M.J. 1992. Bacterial cell wall products as adjuvants: early interferon gamma as a marker for adjuvants that enhance protective immunity. Res. Immunol. 143: 483-488.

Hagiwara, Y., Komase, K., Chen, Z., Matsuo, K., Suzuki, Y., Aizawa, C., Kurata, T., and Tamura, S. 1999. Mutants of cholera toxin as an effective and safe adjuvant for nasal influenza vaccine. Vaccine 17: 2918-2926.

Hartmann, G., Weeratna, R.D., Ballas, Z.K., Payette, P., Blackwell, S., Suparto, I., Rasmussen, W.L., Waldschmidt, M., Sajuthi, D., Purcell, R.H., Davis, H.L., and Krieg, A.M. 2000. Delineation of a CpG phosphorothioate oligodeoxynucleotide for activating primate immune responses *in vitro* and *in vivo*. J. Immunol. 164: 1617-1624.

Heath, A.W. 1995. Cytokines as immunological adjuvants. In: Vaccine Design: The Subunit and Adjuvant Approach. M.F. Powell and M.J. Newman, eds. Plenum Press, New York. p. 645-658.

Hedley, M.L., Curley, J., and Urban, R. 1998. Microspheres containing plasmid-encoded antigens elicit cytotoxic T-cell responses. Nat. Med. 4: 365-368.

Holmgren, J., Lonnroth, I., and Svennerholm, L. 1973. Tissue receptor for cholera exotoxin: postulated structure from studies with GM1 ganglioside and related glycolipids. Infect. Immun. 8: 208-214.

Holmgren, J. 1981. Actions of cholera toxin and the prevention and treatment of cholera. Nature 292: 413-417.

Holmgren, J., Fredman, P., Lindblad, M., Svennerholm, A.M., and Svennerholm, L. 1982. Rabbit intestinal glycoprotein receptor for *Escherichia coli* heat-labile enterotoxin lacking affinity for cholera toxin. Infect. Immun. 38: 424-433.

Holmgren, J., Lindblad, M., Fredman, P., Svennerholm, L., and Myrvold, H. 1985. Comparison of receptors for cholera and *Escherichia coli* enterotoxins in human intestine. Gastroenterology 89: 27-35.

Hsieh, C.S., Macatonia, S.E., Tripp, C.S., Wolf, S.F., O' Garra, A., and Murphy, K.M. 1993. Development of Th1 CD4+ T cells through IL-12 produced by *Listeria*-induced macrophages. Science 260: 547-549.

Jakobsen, H., Schulz, D., Pizza, M., Rappuoli, R. and Jonsdottir, I. 1999. Intranasal immunization with pneumococcal polysaccharide conjugate vaccines with nontoxic mutants of *Escherichia coli* heat-labile enterotoxins as adjuvants protects mice against invasive pneumococcal infections. Infect. Immun. 67: 5892-5897.

Johnson, D.A., Keegan, D.S., Sowell, C.G., Livesay, M.T., Johnson, C.L., Taubner, L.M., Harris, A., Myers, K.R., Thompson, J.D., Gustafson, G.L., Rhodes, M.J., Ulrich, J.T., Ward, J.R., Yorgensen, Y.M., Cantrell, J.L., Brookshire, V.G., and Moingeon P. 1999. 3-O-Desacyl monophosphoryl lipid A derivatives: synthesis and immunostimulant activities. J. Med. Chem. 42: 4640-4649.

Kagi, D., Ledermann, B., Burki, K., Zinkernagel, R.M., and Hengartner, H. 1996. Molecular mechanisms of lymphocyte-mediated cytotoxicity and their role in immunological protection and pathogenesis *in vivo*. Ann. Rev. Immunol. 14: 207-232.

Kahn, J.O., Sinangil, F., Baenziger, J., Murcar, N., Wynne, D., Coleman, R.L., Steimer, K.S., Dekker, C.L., and Chernoff, D. 1994. Clinical and immunologic responses to human immunodeficiency virus (HIV) type 1SF2 gp120 subunit vaccine combined with MF59 adjuvant with or without muramyl tripeptide dipalmitoyl phosphatidylethanolamine in non-HIV-infected human volunteers. J. Infect. Dis. 170: 1288-1291.

Karlsson, K.-A., Tenenberg, S., Angstrom, J., Kjellberg, A., Hirst, T.R., Bergstrom, J., and Miller-Prodaza, H. 1996. Unexpected carbohydrate cross-binding by *Escherichia coli* heat-labile enterotoxin. Recognition of human and rabbit target cell glycoconjugates in comparison with cholera toxin. Bioorg. Med. Chem. 4: 1919-1928.

Kazzaz, J., Neidleman, J., Singh, M., Ott, G., and O'Hagan, D.T. 2000. Novel anionic microparticles are a potent adjuvant for the induction of cytotoxic T lymphocytes against recombinant p55 gag from HIV-1. J. Control. Release 67: 347-356.

Keefer, M.C., Wolff, M., Gorse, G.J., Graham, B.S., Corey, L., Clements-Mann, M.L., Verani-Ketter, N., Erb, S., Smith, C.M., Belshe, R.B., Wagner, L.J., McElrath, M.J., Schwartz, D.H., Fast, P., and Moingeon, P. 1997. Safety profile of phase I and II preventive HIV type 1 envelope vaccination: experience of the NIAID AIDS Vaccine Evaluation Group. AIDS Res. Hum. Retroviruses 13: 1163-1177.

Kensil, C.R., Soltysik, S., Wheeler, D.A., and Wu, J. 1996. Structure/function studies on QS-21, a unique immunological adjuvant from *Quillaja saponaria*. Y. Adv. Exp. Med. Biol. 404: 165-172.

Kensil, CR. 1996. Saponins as vaccine adjuvants. Crit. Rev. Ther. Drug Carrier Syst. 13: 1-55.

Klinman, D.M., Barnhart, K.M., and Conover, J. 1999. CpG motifs as immune adjuvants. Vaccine 17: 19-25.

Krieg, A.M., Yi, A.K., Matson, S., Waldschmidt, T.J., Bishop, G.A., Teasdale, R., Koretzky, G.A., and Klinman, D.M. 1995. CpG motifs in bacterial DNA trigger direct B-cell activation. Nature 374: 546-549.

Langenberg, A.G., Burke, R.L., Adair, S.F., Sekulovich, R., Tigges, M., Dekker, C.L., and Corey, L. 1995. A recombinant glycoprotein vaccine for herpes simplex virus type 2: safety and immunogenicity. Ann. Intern. Med. 122: 889-898.

Levine, M.M., Kaper, J.B., Black, R.E. and Clements, M.L. 1983. New knowledge on pathogenesis of bacterial enteric infections as applied to vaccine development. Microbiol. Rev. 56: 622-647.

Lovgren-Bengtsson, K., and Morein B. 2000. The ISCOM^{TM} Technology. In: Vaccine Adjuvants: Preparation methods and research protocols, D. O'Hagan, ed. Humana Press, Totowa, NJ. p. 239-258.

Lycke, N., Tsuji, T. and Holmgren, J. 1992. The adjuvant effect of *Vibrio cholerae* and *Escherichia coli* heat-labile enterotoxins is linked to their ADP-ribosyltransferase activity. Eur. J. Immunol. 22: 2277-2281.

Magagnoli, C., Manetti, R., Fontana, M.R., Giannelli, V., Giuliani, M.M., Rappuoli, R., and Pizza, M. 1996. Mutations in the A subunit affect yield, stability, and protease sensitivity of nontoxic derivatives of heat-labile enterotoxin. Infect. Immun. 64: 5434-5438.

Majoul, I.V., Bastiaens, P.I.H., and Soeling, H.D. 1996. Transport of an external Lys-Asp-Glu-Leu (KDEL) protein from the plasma membrane to the endoplasmic reticulum: studies with cholera toxin in Vero cells.

J. Cell Biol. 133: 777-789.

Marchetti, M., Rossi, M., Giannelli, V., Giuliani, M.M., Pizza, M., Censini, S., Covacci, A., Massari, P., Pagliaccia, C., Manetti, R., Telford, J.L., Douce, G., Dougan, G., Rappuoli, R., and Ghiara, P. 1998. Protection against *Helicobacter pylori* infection in mice by intragastric vaccination with *H. pylori* antigens is achieved using a non-toxic mutant of *E. coli* heat-labile enterotoxin (LT) as adjuvant. Vaccine 16: 33-37.

Marinaro, M., Staats, H.F., Hiroi, T., Jackson, R.J., Coste, M., Boyaka, N.P., Okahashi, N., Yamamoto, M., Kiyono, H., Bluethmann, H., Fujihashi, K., and McGhee, J.R. 1995. Mucosal adjuvant effect of cholera toxin in mice results from induction of T helper 2 (Th2) cells and IL-4. J. Immunol. 155: 4621-4629.

Medzhitov, R., and Janeway, C.A. 1998. Innate immune recognition and control of adaptive immune responses. Semin. Immunol. 10: 351-333.

Mekalanos, J.J., Swartz, D.J., Pearson, G.D., Harford, N., Groyne, F., and de Wilde, M. 1983. Cholera toxin genes: nucleotide sequence, deletion analysis and vaccine development. Nature 306: 551-557.

Menegon, T., Baldo, V., Bonello, C., Dalla, C.D., Di Tommaso, A., and Trivello, R. 1999. Influenza vaccines: antibody responses to split virus and MF59-adjuvanted subunit virus in an adult population. Eur. J. Epidemiol. 15: 573-576.

Messina, J.P., Gilkeson, G.S., and Pisetsky, D.S. 1991. Stimulation of *in vitro* murine lymphocyte proliferation by bacterial DNA. J. Immunol. 147: 1759-1764.

Mills, K.G.H., Barnard, A., Watkins, J., and Redhead, K. 1993. Cell-mediated immunity to *Bordetella pertussis*: role of Th1 cells in bacterial clearance in a murine respiratory infection model. Infect.Immun. 61: 399-410.

Milon, G., Del Giudice, G., and Louis, J.A. 1995. Immunobiology of experimental coutaneous leishmaniasis. Parasitol. Today 11: 244-247.

Minutello, A., Senatore, F., Cecchinelli, G., Bianchi, M., Andreani, T., Podda, A., and Crovari, P. 1999. Safety and immunogenicity of an inactivated subunit influenza virus vaccine combined with MF59 adjuvant emulsion in elderly subjects, immunized for three consecutive influenza seasons. Vaccine 17: 99-104.

Mosmann, T.R., and Sad, S. 1996. The expanding universe of T cell subset: Th1, Th2 and more. Immunol. Today 17: 138-146.

Moss, J. and Vaughan, M. 1984. Toxin ADP-ribosyltransferases that act on adenylate cyclase systems. Methods Enzymol. 106: 411-418.

Nashar, T.O., Webb, H.M., Eaglestone, S., Williams, N.A. and Hirst, T.R. 1996. Potent immunogenicity of the B subunits of *Escherichia coli* heat-labile enterotoxin: receptor binding is essential and induces differential modulation of lymphocyte subsets. Proc. Natl. Acad. Sci. USA. 93: 226-230.

Neidleman, J.A., Vajdy, M., Ugozzoli, M., Ott, G. and O'Hagan, D. 2000. Genetically detoxified mutants of heat-labile enterotoxin from *Escherichia coli* are effective adjuvants for induction of cytotoxic T-cell responses against HIV-1 gag-p55. Immunology 101: 154-160.

Nitayaphan, S., Khamboonruang, C., Sirisophana, N., Morgan, P., Chiu, J., Duliege, A.M., Chuenchitra, C., Supapongse, T., Rungruengthanakit, K., deSouza, M., Mascola, J.R., Boggio, K., Ratto-Kim, S., Markowitz, L.E., Birx, D., Suriyanon, V., McNeil, J.G., Brown, A.E., and Michael, R.A. 2000. A phase I/II trial of HIV SF2 gp120/MF59 vaccine in seronegative thais. AFRIMS-RIHES Vaccine Evaluation Group. Armed Forces Research Institute of Medical Sciences and the Research Institute for Health Sciences. Vaccine 18: 1448-1455.

O'Hagan, D.T., Rahman, D., McGee, J.P., Jeffery, H., Davies, M.C., Williams, P., Davis, S.S., and Challacombe, S.J. 1991a. Biodegradable microparticles as controlled release antigen delivery systems. Immunology 73: 239-242.

O'Hagan, D.T., Jeffery, H., Roberts, M.J., McGee, J.P., and Davis, S.S. 1991b. Controlled release microparticles for vaccine development. Vaccine 9: 768-771.

O'Hagan, D.T., Jeffery, H., and Davis, S.S. 1993. Long-term antibody responses in mice following subcutaneous immunization with ovalbumin entrapped in biodegradable microparticles. Vaccine 11: 965-969.

O'Hagan, D.T. 1996. The intestinal uptake of particles and the implications for drug and antigen delivery. J. Anat. 189: 477-482.

O'Hagan, D.T. 1998. Microparticles and polymers for the mucosal delivery of vaccines. Adv. Drug Deliv. Rev. 34: 305-320.

O'Hagan, D.T., Goldbeck, C., Ugozzoli, M., Ott, G., and Burke, R.L. 1999. Intranasal immunization with recombinant gD2 reduces disease severity and mortality following genital challenge with herpes simplex virus type 2 in guinea pigs. Vaccine 17: 2229-2236.

O'Hagan, D.T., Ugozzoli, M., Barackman, J., Singh, M., Kazzaz, J., Higgins, K., VanCott, T.C., and Ott, G. 2000. Microparticles in MF59, a potent adjuvant combination for a recombinant protein vaccine against HIV-1.Vaccine.18: 1793-1801.

O'Hagan, D.T. 2001. Induction of potent immune responses by cationic microparticles with adsorbed human immunodeficiency virus DNA vaccines. J. Virol. 75: 9037-9043.

Okada H, and Toguchi H. 1995. Biodegradable microspheres in drug delivery. Crit. Rev. Ther. Drug Carrier Syst. 12: 1-99.

Ott, G., Barchfeld, G.L., Chernoff, D., Radhakrishnan, R., van Hoogevest, P., and Van Nest G. 1995. MF59: Design and evaluation of a safe and potent adjuvant for human vaccines. In: Vaccine Design: The Subunit and Adjuvant Approach, M.F. Powell and M.J. Newman, eds. Plenum Press, New York. p. 277-296.

Partidos, C.D., Salani, B.F., Pizza, M., and Rappuoli, R. 1999. Heat-labile enterotoxin of *Escherichia coli* and its site-directed mutant LTK63 enhance the proliferative and cytotoxic T-cell responses to intranasally co-immunized synthetic peptides. Immunol. Lett. 67: 209-216.

Partidos, C.D., Pizza, M., Rappuoli, R., and Steward, M.W. 1996. The adjuvant effect of a non-toxic mutant of heat-labile enterotoxin of *Escherichia coli* for the induction of measles virus-specific CTL responses after intranasal co-immunization with a synthetic peptide. Immunology 89: 483-487.

Pass, R.F., Duliege, A.M., Boppana, S., Sekulovich, R., Percell, S., Britt, W., and Burke, R.L. 1999. A subunit cytomegalovirus vaccine based on recombinant envelope glycoprotein B and a new adjuvant. A subunit cytomegalovirus vaccine based on recombinant envelope glycoprotein B and a new adjuvant. J. Infect. Dis. 180: 970-975.

Pizza, M., Domenighini, M., Hol, W., Giannelli, V., Fontana, M.R., Giuliani, M.M., Magagnoli, C., Peppoloni, S., Manetti, R., and Rappuoli, R. 1994a. Probing the structure-activity relationship of *Escherichia coli* LT-A by site-directed mutagenesis. Mol. Microbiol. 14: 51-60.

Pizza, M., Fontana, M.R., Giuliani, M.M., Domenighini, M., Magagnoli, C., Giannelli, V., Nucci, D., Hol, W., Manetti, R., and Rappuoli, R. 1994b. A genetically detoxified derivative of heat-labile *Escherichia coli* enterotoxin induces neutralizing antibodies against the A subunit. J. Exp. Med. 6: 2147-2153.

Pizza, M., Masignani, V., and Rappuoli, R. 1999. Molecular, functional and evolutionary aspects of ADP-ribosylating toxins. In: The Comprehensive Sourcebook of Bacterial Protein Toxins. J. Alouf and J. Freer, eds. Academic Press, New York. p.45-72.

Polakos, N.K., Drane, D., Cox, J., Ng, P., Selby, M.J., Chien, D., O'Hagan, D.T., Houghton, M., and Paliard, X. 2001. Characterization of hepatitis C virus core-specific immune responses primed in rhesus macaques by a nonclassical ISCOM vaccine. J. Immunol. 166: 3589-3598.

Putney, S.D., and Burke, P.A. 1998. Improving protein therapeutics with sustained-release formulations. Nat. Biotechnol. 16: 153-157.

Quan, W.D.Jr, Dean, G.E., Spears, L., Spears, C.P., Groshen, S., Merritt, J.A., Mitchell, M.S. 1997. Active specific immunotherapy of metastatic melanoma with an antiidiotype vaccine: a phase I/II trial of I-Mel-2 plus SAF-m. J. Clin. Oncol. 15: 2103-2110.

Ramon, G. 1924. Sur la toxine et sur l'anatoxine diphtheriques. Ann. Inst. Pasteur. 38: 1-18.

Rank, R.G., Ramsey, K.H., Pack, E.A., and Williams, D.M. 1992. Effect of gamma interferon on resolution of murine *Chlamydia* genital infection. Infect. Immun. 60: 4427-4429.

Reiner, S.L., and Locksley, R.M. 1995. The regulation of immunity to *Leishmania major*. Ann. Rev. Immunol. 13: 151-177.

Relyveld, E.H., Bizzini, B., and Gupta, R.K. 1998. Vaccine rational approaches to reduce adverse reactions in man to vaccines containing tetanus and diphtheria toxoids.16: 1016-1023.

Rimmelzwaan, G.F., Baars, M., van Beek, R., van Amerongen, G., Lovgren-Bengtsson, K., Claas, E.C., and Osterhaus, A.D. 1997. Induction of protective immunity against influenza virus in a macaque model: comparison of conventional and iscom vaccines. J. Gen. Virol. 78: 757-765.

Romagnani, S. 1994. Lymphokine production by human T cells in disease states. Ann. Rev Immunol. 12: 227-257.

Ryan, E.J., McNeela, E., Murphy, G.A., Stewart, H., O'Hagan, D., Pizza, M., Rappuoli, R., and Mills, K.H.G. 1999. Mutants of *Escherichia coli* heat-labile toxin act as effective mucosal adjuvants for nasal delivery of an acellular pertussis vaccine: differential effects of the nontoxic AB complex and enzyme activity on Th1and Th2 cells. Infect. Immun. 67: 6270-6280.

Ryan, E.J., McNeela, E., Pizza, M., Rappuoli, R., O'Neil, L., and Mills, K.H.G. 2000. Modulation of innate and acquired immune responses by *Escherichia coli* heat-labile toxin: distinct pro and anti-infalmmatory effects of the nontoxic AB complex and the enzyme activity. J. Immunol. 165: 5750-5759.

Sasaki, S., Tsuji, T., Hamajima, K., Fukushima, J., Ishii, N., Kaneko, T., Xin, K.Q., Mohri, H., Aoki, I., Okubo, T., Nishioka, K., and Okuda, K. 1997. Monophosphoryl lipid A enhances both humoral and cell-mediated immune responses to DNA vaccination against human immunodeficiency virus type 1. Infect. Immun. 65: 3520-3528.

Sasaki, S., Sumino, K., Hamajima, K., Fukushima, J., Ishii, N., Kawamoto, S., Mohri, H., Kensil, C.R., and Okuda, K. 1998. Induction of systemic and mucosal immune responses to human immunodeficiency virus type 1 by a DNA vaccine formulated with QS-21 saponin adjuvant via intramuscular and intranasal routes. J. Virol. 72: 4931-4939.

Simmons, C.P., Hussel, T., Sparer, T., Walzl, G., Openshaw, P., and Dougan, G. 2001. Mucosal delivery of a respiratory syncytial virus CTL peptid with enterotoxin-based adjuvants elicits protective, immunopathogenic, and immunoregulatory antiviral CD8+ Tcell responses. J. Immunol. 166: 1106-1113.

Singh, M., McGee, J.P., Li, X.M., Koff, W., Zamb, T., Wang, C.Y., and O'Hagan, D.T. 1997. Biodegradable microparticles with an entrapped branched octameric peptide as a controlled-release HIV-1 vaccine. J. Pharm. Sci. 86:1229-1233.

Singh, M., Briones, M., Ott, G., and O'Hagan, D. 2000. Cationic microparticles: A potent delivery system for DNA vaccines. Proc. Natl. Acad. Sci. USA. 97: 811-816.

Sixma, T.K., Pronk, S.E., Kalk, K.H., Wartna, E.S., van Zanten, B.A., Witholt, B., and Hol, W.G. 1991. Crystal structure of a cholera toxin related heat-labile enterotoxin from *E. coli*. Nature 351: 371-377.

Sixma, T.K., Kalk, K.H., Vanzanten, B.A.M., Dauter, Z., Kingma, J., Witholt, B., and Hol, W.G.J. 1993a. Refined structure of *Escherichia-coli* heat-labile enterotoxin, a close relative of cholera toxin. J. Mol. Biol. 230: 890-918.

Sixma, T.K., Stein, P.E., Hol, W.G., and Read, R.J. 1993b. Comparison of the B-pentamers of heat-labile enterotoxin and verotoxin-1: two structures with remarkable similarity and dissimilarity. Biochemistry 32: 191-198.

Sjolander, A., Drane, D., Maraskovsky, E., Scheerlinck, J., Suhrbier, A., Tennent, J., Pearse, M. 2001. Intranasal immunisation with influenza-ISCOM induces strong mucosal as well as systemic antibody and cytotoxic T-lymphocyte responses. Vaccine 19: 2661-2665.

Smith, R.E., Donachie, A.M., Grdic, D., Lycke, N., and Mowat, A.M. 1999. Immune-stimulating complexes induce an IL-12-dependent cascade of innate immune responses. J. Immunol. 162: 5536-5546.

Soltysik, S., Wu, J.Y., Recchia, J., Wheeler, D.A., Newman, M.J., Coughlin, R.T., and Kensil, C.R. 1995. Structure/function studies of QS-21 adjuvant: assessment of triterpene aldehyde and glucuronic acid roles in adjuvant function. Vaccine 13: 1403-1410.

Spangler, B.D. 1992. Structure and function of cholera toxin and the related *Escherichia coli* heat-labile enterotoxin. Microbiol. Rev. 56: 622-647.

Spicer, E.K., Kavanaugh, W.M., Dallas, W.S., Falkow, S., Konigsberg, W.H., and Shafer, D. 1981. sequence homologies between A subunits of *E. coli* and *V. cholerae* enterotoxin. Proc. Natl. Acad. Sci. USA. 78: 50-54.

Stevens, L., Moss J., Vaughan, M., Pizza, M., and Rappuoli R. 1999. Effects of site-directed mutagenesis of *Escherichia coli* heat-labile enterotoxin on ADP-ribosyltransferase activity and interaction with ADP-ribosylation factors. Inect. Immun. 67: 259-265.

Strober, W., Kelsall, B., and Marth, T. 1998. Oral tolerance. J. Clin. Immunol. 18: 1-30.

Sugii, S. T. 1989. Binding specificities of heat-labile enterotoxins isolated from porcine and human enterotoxigenic *Escherichia coli* for different gangliosides. Can. J. Microbiol. 35: 670-673.

Sun, S., Kishimoto, H., and Sprent, J. 1998. DNA as an adjuvant: capacity of insect DNA and synthetic oligodeoxynucleotides to augment T cell responses to specific antigen. J. Exp. Med. 187: 1145-1150.

Takahashi, I., Marinaro, M., Kiyono, H., Jackson, R.J., Nakagawa, I., Fujihashi, K., Hamada, S., Clements, J.D., Bost, K.L., and McGhee, J. 1996. Mechanisms for mucosal immunogenicity and adjuvancy of *Escherichia coli* labile enterotoxin J. Infect. Dis. 173: 627-635.

Tamura, S., Yamanaka, A., Shimohara, M., Tomita, T., Komase, K., Tsuda, Y., Suzuki, Y., Nagamine, T., Kawahara, K., Danbara, H., Aizawa, C. Oya, A. and Kurata, T. 1994. Synergistic action of cholera toxin B subunit (and *Escherichia coli* heat-labile toxin B subunit) and a trace amount of cholera whole toxin as an adjuvant for nasal influenza vaccine. Vaccine 12: 419-426.

Tenenberg, S., Hirst, T.R., Angstrom, J., and Karlsson, K. 1994. Comparison of the glycolipid-binding specificities of cholera toxin and porcine *Escherichia coli* heat-labile enterotoxin: identification of a receptor-active non-ganglioside glycolipid for the heat-labile toxin in infant rabbit small intestine. Glycoconj. 11: 533-540.

Thoelen, S., Van Damme, P., Mathei, C., Leroux-Roels, G., Desombere, I., Safary, A., Vandepapeliere, P., Slaoui, M., and Meheus, A. 1998. Safety and immunogenicity of a hepatitis B vaccine formulated with a novel adjuvant system. Vaccine 16: 708-714.

Tokunaga T, Yamamoto H, Shimada S, Abe H, Fukuda T, Fujisawa Y, Furutani Y, Yano O, Kataoka T, and Sudo T. 1984. Antitumor activity of deoxyribonucleic acid fraction from *Mycobacterium bovis* BCG. I. Isolation, physicochemical characterization, and antitumor activity. J. Natl. Cancer Inst. 72: 955-962.

Truitt, R.L., Hanke, C., Radke, J., Mueller, R., and Barbieri, J.T. 1998. Glycosphingolipids as novel targets for T-cell suppression by the B subunit of recombinant heat-labile enterotoxin. Infect. Immun. 66: 1299-1308.

Tsai, S.C., Noda, M., Adamik, R., Moss, J., and Vaughan, M. 1988. Stimulation of choleragen enzymatic activities by GTP and two soluble proteins purified from bovine brain. J. Biol. Chem. 263: 1768-1772.

Ugozzoli, M., O'Hagan, D.T., and Ott, G.S. 1998. Intranasal immunization of mice with herpes simplex virus type 2 recombinant gD2: the effect of adjuvants on mucosal and serum antibody responses. Immunol. 93: 563-

571.

Ugozzoli, M., Santos, G. and O'Hagan, D.T. 2001. Potency of a genetically detoxified mucosal adjuvant derived from heat-labile enterotoxin of *Escherichia coli* (LTK63) not adversely affected by the presence of preexisting immunity to the adjuvant. J. Infect. Dis. 18: 351-354.

Ulanova, M., Tarkowski, A., Hahn-Zoric, M., Hanson, L.A., and Moingeon, P. 2001. The Common vaccine adjuvant aluminum hydroxide up-regulates accessory properties of human monocytes via an interleukin-4-dependent mechanism. Infect. Immun. 69: 1151-1159.

Ulrich, J.T., and Myers, K.R. 1995. Monophosphoryl lipid A as an adjuvant. Past experiences and new directions. Pharm. Biotechnol. 6: 495-524.

Van den Akker, F., Pizza, M., Rappuoli, R., and Hol, W.G.J. 1997. Crystal structure of a non-toxic mutant of heat-labile enterotoxin which is a potent mucosal adjuvant. Protein Sci. 6: 2650-2654.

Van Nest, G.A., Steimer, K.S., Haigwood, N.L., Burke, R.L., and Ott, G. 1992. Advanced adjuvant formulation for use with recombinant subunit vaccines. In: Vaccines 92. F. Brown, R. Chanock, H.S. Ginsberg, and R. Lerner R., eds. Cold Spring Harbor Laboratoy Press, Cold Spring Harbor, New York. p. 57-62.

Waite, D.C., Jacobson, E.W., Ennis, F.A., Edelmann, R., White, B., Kammer, R., Anderson, C., and Kensil, C.R. 2001. Three-double blind randomized trial evaluating the safety and tolerance of different formulations of the saponin adjuvant QS-21. Vaccine 19: 3957-3967.

Yamamoto, S., Kiyono, H., Yamamoto, M., Imaoka, K., Yamamoto, M., Fujihashi, K., Van Ginkel, F.W., Noda, M., Takeda, Y., and McGhee, J.R. 1997. A nontoxic mutant of cholera toxin elicits Th2-type responses for enhanced mucosal immunity. Proc. Natl. Acad. Sci. USA. 94: 5267-5272.

From: *Vaccine Delivery Strategies*
Edited by: Guido Dietrich and Werner Goebel

Chapter 3

Transcutaneous Immunization

Gregory M. Glenn

ABSTRACT

Transcutaneous immunization (TCI) is a novel immunization strategy by which antigen and adjuvant are applied topically to induce potent antibody and cell-mediated immune responses specific for both the antigen and the adjuvant. TCI therefore combines the advantages of needle-free delivery with targeting of the immunologically rich milieu of the skin. In animal studies, this simple technique induces robust systemic and mucosal immune responses against vaccine antigens. The first clinical studies confirmed that large antigens can be delivered to the skin to induce systemic immune responses, and that the adjuvant plays a critical role in the induction of robust responses in conjunction with delivery of antigens in a patch. These results provide an excellent basis for further development of TCI for use in humans.

INTRODUCTION

Adjuvant scientists and vaccinologists have long recognized that the method of vaccine delivery and the tissue targeted for delivery can have a profound impact on the subsequent immune response, phenomena well illustrated by vaccine delivery to the mucosa. Recently, it has been shown that the skin contains an accessible and competent immune system that is highly desirable for vaccine delivery and that targeting the skin may prove to have a uniquely useful set of immune response outcomes with distinctive advantages such as safety and tolerability of adjuvant use.

We have coined the term transcutaneous immunization (TCI) to denote the passive delivery of vaccines to the skin via a patch or other topical formulation, which differentiates the technique from transdermal drug delivery or device-based vaccine delivery techniques. Recent studies suggest that transcutaneous immunization and related vaccine delivery methods are likely to have a major impact on future approaches to immunization. Previously, the skin was bypassed using needles to deliver vaccines to deeper tissues. In terms of passive delivery of vaccines, the skin was seen as an impervious barrier to large protein molecules such as antigens and thus primarily as an obstacle for vaccine delivery. Active targeting of the skin using intradermal immunization required considerable skill and was fraught with inconsistencies, and has been followed more recently by as yet unproven device-based concepts for delivery to the skin immune system. TCI as a passive skin delivery technique using a patch or similar means of delivery is both a practical and powerful method of immunization, with a growing body of preclinical and clinical data supporting its feasibility.

The skin contains a highly accessible and extensive population of dendritic cells that are an appealing target for vaccine delivery. As a theoretical concept, the combination of immunostimulating compounds (adjuvants) and dendritic cells may only be exceeded by live viral vaccines for the magnitude and duration of the immune responses elicited. Thus, many new vaccine delivery strategies utilize adjuvants for enhancing immune responses to vaccines. As might be expected, immune stimulation by adjuvants is often accompanied by side effects, mostly from bystander events. As a result, there are various strategies to detoxify adjuvants, for example, for use intranasally or orally (Dickinson and Clements, 1995; Rappuoli *et al.*, 1999). The outer layers of the skin represent a focused adjuvant target in terms of the dense population of antigen-presenting cells; the compartmentalization of the immune stimulatory events associated with the use of adjuvants on the skin has been clearly shown to allow the safe use of the most potent adjuvants (Glenn *et al.*, 2000; Güereña-Burgueño *et al.*, 2002). Thus, TCI allows vaccinologists to employ the advantages of immunostimulation without the acute safety risks associated with systemic adverse reactions to the immunostimulating compounds. The primary reason for considering the skin as a target for vaccine delivery, therefore, is its potential for safe and potent immunostimulation.

There are also many practical aspects to patch-based skin delivery strategies that make vaccine delivery using a patch or passive delivery system attractive. The CDC, WHO, and others have rated needle-free delivery as a priority for new technology developments in vaccine delivery due to the risk of needle-born transmission of disease and hopes for increased compliance (Aylward *et al.*, 1995; W.H.O., 1996; Fletcher and Saliou, 2000). The simplicity of skin patch delivery strategies may alleviate needle-born disease and the potential risks of disease transmission associated with device-based skin delivery (Whittle *et al.*, 1987; Mason *et al.*, 1993). If accompanied by cold chain-free formulations, transcutaneous immunization may lead to improved vaccine access, especially in the developing world.

In this chapter, we briefly describe the scientific paradigm for TCI, including aspects of skin anatomy and Langerhans cell studies relevant to TCI. We then discuss immune responses seen after TCI, including a summary of preclinical efficacy studies and mucosal responses. Finally, we present the clinical observations made to date using TCI and outline some of the important opportunities that lie ahead.

THE SKIN AS A BARRIER AND TARGET FOR TRANSCUTANEOUS IMMUNIZATION

Mammalian skin is covered by the stratum corneum (SC), an outer protective layer of quiescent, keratin-filled epidermal cells encased in a mortar of surrounding lipids and keratin filaments that have been secreted by the maturing keratinocytes. The living epidermis that underlies the SC is composed primarily (95%) of epidermal keratinocytes, but also includes a significant population (1-3%) of immune surveillance cells (Jakob and Udey, 1999) called Langerhans cells (LCs), which are a special subset of dendritic cells. Their immune surveillance role is consistent with the remarkable fact that 25% of the total skin surface area in humans is uniformly undergirded by LCs that are distributed among the epidermal cells (keratinocytes) (Yu *et al.*, 1994). LCs thus form an extensive, highly superficial network barrier of immune cells at the very surface of the skin. The extensive dedication of biological resources committed to immune surveillance in the superficial layers of the skin suggests that the SC is often penetrated by microbes, and makes the skin an attractive target for vaccine delivery.

In the context of transdermal drug delivery, the stratum corneum (SC) is widely accepted as the principal barrier to penetration of the skin (Barry, 1985) and continues to be judged as impervious to large molecules over 500 Daltons (Barry, 1985; Wester and Maibach, 1992; Rietschel and Fowler, 1995; Bos and Meinardi, 2000). The maxims on molecular size limits for skin penetration that apply to drugs (Bos and Meinardi, 2000) are clearly different for antigen delivery. Whole viruses (Hammond *et al.*, 2000), large proteins (Glenn *et al.*, 2000), and even larger recombinants (Güereña-Burgueño *et al.*, 2002; Yu *et al.*, 2002) readily pass through the SC into the epidermis, where they evoke immune responses. These seemingly disparate observations between transdermal and transcutaneous barriers are likely a figment of the site of the target tissue (distant vs local), target cell reaction (limited effects vs highly amplified immune responses), and the biological readout (ELISA detecting minute amounts of antibody vs drug effects).

Langerhans cells are a special class of bone marrow-derived dendritic cells that migrate to the skin, where they carry out immune surveillance. There is constant traffic at low levels by LCs into the lymphatics that is markedly increased in the face of stimulatory signals (Macatonia *et al.*, 1987; Kripke *et al.*, 1990). Several studies have described the depletion of the epidermal LCs, increased activation state, and increased numbers of LCs found after transcutaneous or device-based skin delivery of vaccines. Thus vaccines, vaccine adjuvants (Jakob *et al.*, 1999; Vassell *et al.*, 1999; Ban *et al.*, 2000; El-Ghorr *et al.*, 2000), microbial infections (Johnston *et al.*, 2000), and trauma using controlled skin manipulation (Watabe *et al.*, 2001) (e.g. tape stripping), or tissue disruption (Chen *et al.*, 2001b) ('gene guns'), provide a danger signal for amplification of immune responses against invasion at the level of the skin, resulting in increased numbers of activated LCs going to the draining lymph node. Mature (activated) LCs are extremely effective antigen-presenting cells (APCs) with high levels of costimulatory molecules and cytokine production (Jakob and Udey, 1999), and this confluence of increased numbers of activated APCs in response to a stimulatory signal results in intense, specific immune responses.

The stratum corneum is an effective but fragile barrier to skin penetration. Several well established strategies have emerged for penetration of the SC.

Occlusion, wetting of the skin, and other techniques lead to hydration of the SC. Hydration of the SC results in swelling of the keratinocytes, pooling of fluid in the inter-cellular spaces, and marked microscopic changes in the SC structure (Roberts and Walker, 1993). Hydrated SC clearly allows antigens to pass through the skin, although the transit pathways utilized by antigens to traverse the stratum corneum are difficult to characterize and are unknown at this time. Transdermal drug delivery of polar drugs is thought to occur through aqueous intercellular channels formed between the keratinocytes, and it is reasonable to presume similar pathways for antigen delivery (Roberts and Walker, 1993). As mentioned above, it has been important to conceptually differentiate transcutaneous immunization, the passive delivery of antigens (which are relatively large molecules) through the SC to the epidermal immune cells, from transdermal drug delivery, which generally delivers relatively small molecules through the epidermis, the basement membrane, into the dermis and into blood vessels where the drug is adsorbed and carried to distant sites. However, because the SC is the limiting barrier for penetration by both transcutaneous and transdermal methods, the techniques and materials utilized (patches, formulations, and packaging) have provided a wealth of practical strategies for vaccine delivery to the skin.

Other barrier disruption strategies have been employed to enhance the efficiency of antigen transit into the skin. The use of physical disruption techniques can assist the delivery of antigen formulations. For example stripping, a procedure that may entirely disrupt the stratum corneum, has been used to deliver peptides or naked DNA into the epidermis to induce CTLs (Seo *et al.*, 2000; Watabe *et al.*, 2001). Other techniques such as the use of delipidating agents (Gockel *et al.*, 2000) or other penetration enhancers may be employed. It seems to be clinically acceptable to pretreat the skin prior to TCI in a clinical setting (Güereña-Burgueño *et al.*, 2002), as is standard practice for needle-based injections, and it seems likely that skin pretreatment methods will be incorporated into future TCI protocols.

ADJUVANTS, IMMUNE RESPONSES IN THE SKIN

As a strategy, the use of adjuvants for augmentation of the immune response to vaccines stretches back to the 1920s (Ramon, 1925) or before and is of considerable interest today, especially where adjuvants may address particular problems in vaccine coverage. For example, there is a clear need for improvement in the vaccine responses in the elderly population where the morbidity and mortality from diseases such as influenza and pneumococcal disease is related to the general immune suppression seen in this population (Goronzy *et al.*, 2001). The elderly are known to have depressed humoral and T cell responses to influenza antigens, including cytotoxic T cell responses to influenza, and have fewer T cell subsets that can respond to influenza antigens (Fagiolo *et al.*, 1993; Swenson *et al.*, 1996). With estimates of influenza vaccine efficacy ranging from 15-34% for decreasing hospitalizations and 27-75% for mortality (Patriarca *et al.*, 1985; Strassburg *et al.*, 1986; Fedson *et al.*, 1993; Van Hoecke *et al.*, 1996), there has been considerable interest in overcoming the poor response rates to the vaccine using adjuvants. There have been a number of evaluations of adjuvant strategies in the context of flu in younger adults (Hashigucci *et al.*, 1996; Gluck *et al.*, 2000) and some studies using adjuvants with influenza vaccines in the elderly (Keitel *et al.*, 1993; Baldo *et al.*, 2001). The earliest adjuvanted flu vaccine study using incomplete Freund's provided good evidence that adjuvants can clearly and safely augment the immune response and improve efficacy (Salk *et al.*, 1953). Other more recent studies have confirmed this effect in the elderly to a lesser degree (Gasparini *et al.*, 2001). We have employed several strategies to evaluate the potential for the use of adjuvants to enhance the immune response in the context of influenza. Some groups have explored the use of synthetic peptide epitopes derived from the HA and NP surface proteins of influenza and shown protection against influenza challenge (Shapira *et al.*, 1984). Using an MHC class I restricted CTL epitope derived from the NP protein of influenza, we immunized mice with a simple topical formulation containing the peptide, and a helper epitope with and without adjuvant (Hammond, unpublished observations). As shown in Figure 1, specific killing of peptide-loaded targets by CTLs was achieved, but only in animals receiving adjuvant. Using more conventional split-virus subunit formulations, neutralizing titers for influenza can readily be obtained. As shown in Table 1, mice immunized on the skin using cholera toxin (CT) as adjuvant and an influenza A/Sydney split virus preparation readily produce measurable antibodies that are neutralizing at levels equivalent to antibodies produced using needle-based delivery. Similar data have been shown using gun based immunization using flu antigens and plasmid DNA with adjuvants, and also confirm the role of adjuvants in enhancing the immune response by this method (Chen *et al.*, 2001a; Watabe *et al.*, 2001).

In most studies, adjuvants are a universal requirement of effective immunization via topical application (Glenn *et al.*, 1999; Baca-Estrada *et al.*, 2000; El-Ghorr *et al.*, 2000; Gockel *et al.*, 2000; Scharton-Kersten *et al.*, 2000; Güereña-Burgueño *et al.*, 2002). Although antigens such as tetanus toxoid (TTx) can induce antigen-specific antibodies that are detectable, the

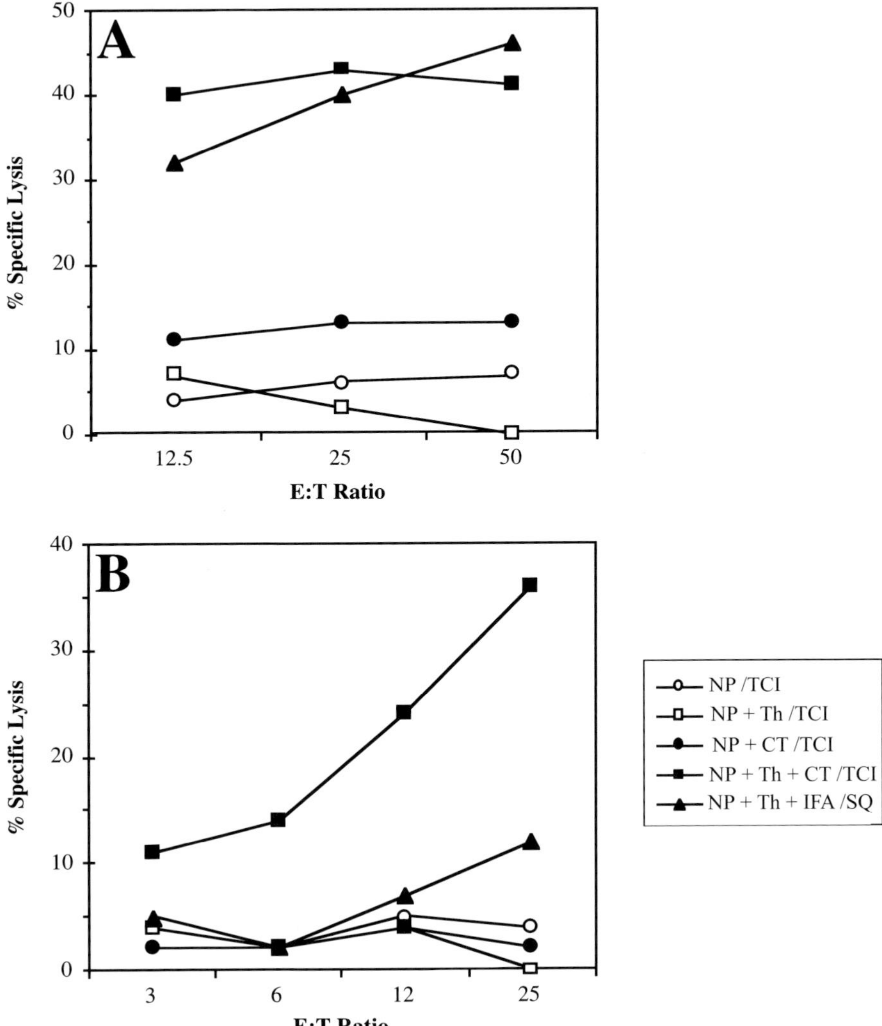

Figure 1. Influenza nucleoprotein (NP) peptide specific CTL responses induced by skin immunization (TCI). 100 µg of peptide derived from Influenza A/PR/8/34 NP (aa 147-155; TYQRTRALV) and/or 100 µg of a T helper (Th) peptide (SFERFEIFPKE) with or without adjuvant (50µg of cholera toxin) were applied to saline hydrated skin of BALB/c mice (n=5) three times at two week intervals. A separate control group of mice were subcutaneously immunized (SQ) with 100 µg of NP peptide, 100 µg of Th peptide, and adjuvanted with incomplete Freund's adjuvant (IFA). Spleens (A) and inguinal lymph nodes (B) were removed, pooled, cultured for 6 days in the presence of NP peptide, and assayed for NP-specific cytolytic activity. The net percent specific lysis is graphed (experimental lysis minus naïve lysis) for each group.

Table 1. Transcutaneous immunization of mice with influenza split virus and CT

Immunization[a]	HAI[b] Titers (Individual Mice)					Flu A[c] IgG (EU[d])(Individual Mice)					Geometric Mean
Flu A (25)/CT(1) – TCI[e]	5120	1280	80	1280	10	72351	39735	11821	138201	23	10155
Flu A (25) – TCI	10	10	10	10	10	28	29	29	49	40	34
CT (25) – TCI	10	10	10	10	10	32	21	45	46	19	31
Flu A (1.5) – SQ[f]	160	1280	1280	1280	160	16404	55638	53530	42728	8365	28081

[a] The dose of antigen and adjuvant in micrograms is listed in parenthesis for each group.
[b] Hemagglutinin inhibition
[c] Influenza A/Sydney/5/97 split virus
[d] ELISA unit is the inverse dilution at which the sera yields an optical density of 1.0
[e] Transcutaneous immunization
[f] Subcutaneous immunization

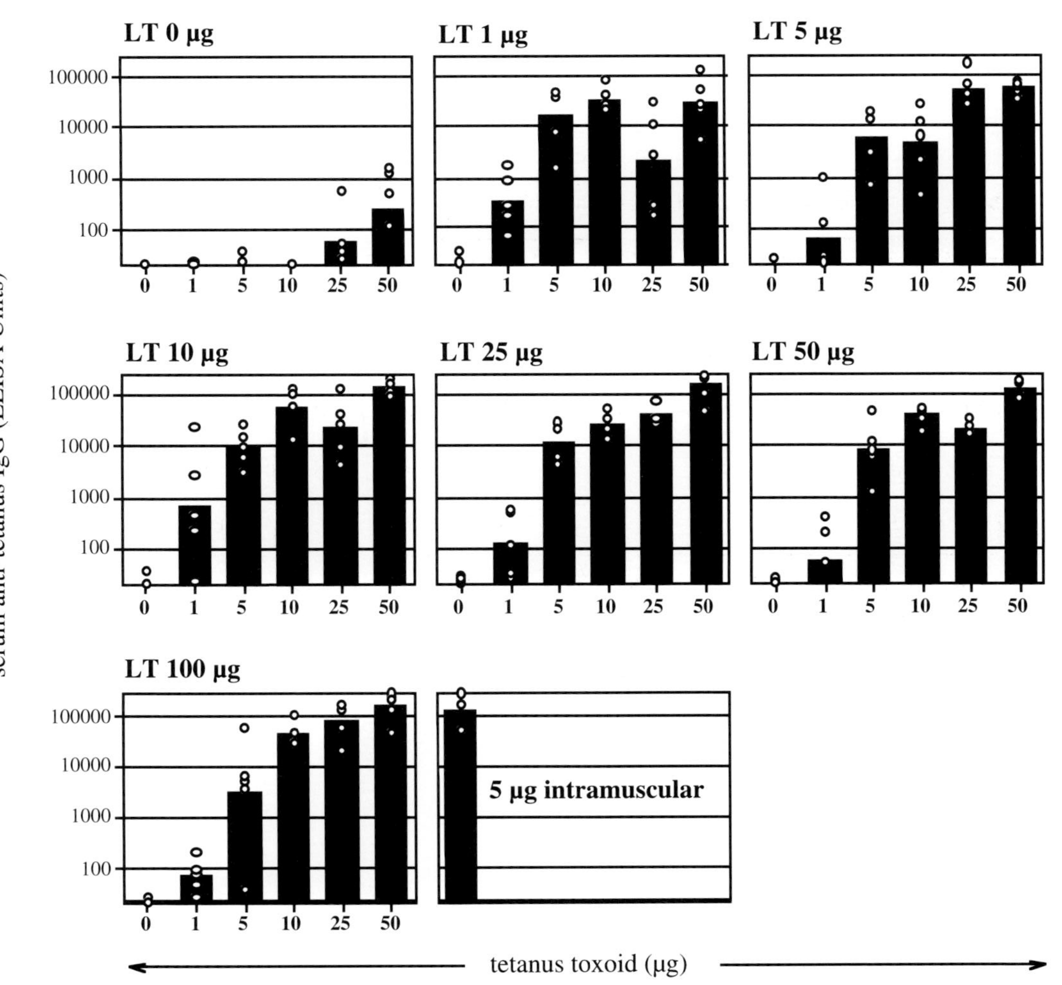

Figure 2. Anti-tetanus toxoid (TTx) response in mice immunized with varying doses of antigen and adjuvant. C57BL/6 mice (n=5) were immunized on the skin with LT (doses indicated above each panel) and TTx (doses indicated on the x-axis) at 0, 4 and 7 weeks. The IM group was immunized with alum and TTx (5 µg) doses at 0, 4, and 8 weeks. Serum collected two weeks after the final immunization was assayed for TTx specific IgG by ELISA. The geometric mean (bar) and individual values (open circles) are shown for each group. Reprinted with permission from Scharton-Kersten et al., 2000, Infect. Immun. 68: 5306-5313.

addition of even small amounts of adjuvant results in a several log increase in antibody titers (Scharton-Kersten *et al.*, 2000) (Figure 2). The addition of adjuvant results in complete protection in tetanus toxin challenge studies, whereas even large doses of antigen alone delivered topically result in immune responses that provide scant to no protection (Scharton-Kersten *et al.*, 2000). Significant enhancement of the immune response using adjuvants has also been shown using gun delivery of antigens (Chen *et al.*, 2001a) and DNA (Watabe *et al.*, 2001). The lack of a robust immune response in the absence of an adjuvant appears to be an important limitation of other approaches to topical immunization (Paul *et al.*, 1995; Shi *et al.*, 1999). Although most published data on TCI have focused on the bacterial ADP-ribosylating exotoxins such as *E. coli* heat-labile toxin (LT) and CT, we and others have found that a wide variety of adjuvants have the same effect topically, i.e. they enhance the immune response to a coadministered antigen (Baca-Estrada *et al.*, 2000; Scharton-Kersten *et al.*, 2000; Watabe *et al.*, 2001). The mechanisms by which the bacterial ADP-ribosylating exotoxins function are not entirely known, although the binding activity of the B-subunit (de Haan *et al.*, 1998; Glenn *et al.*, 1999; Beignon *et al.*, 2001) and some residual ribosyl-transferase activity (Scharton-Kersten *et al.*, 2000) appear to be important for the induction of robust responses when used in the skin as is required in the mucosa (O'Hagan, 2000). These data support our working hypothesis that TCI requires an adjuvant for a robust immune response and that this is a general observation in the context of the skin immune system not restricted to CT or LT.

The immunostimulation that results from parenteral, intranasal or oral adjuvant use may be accompanied by adverse side effects, most frequently local inflammation at the site of injection (Jacobs *et al.*, 1982), rhinorrhea (Cryz and Glück, 1998), or diarrhea in the case of oral use of LT (Michetti *et al.*, 1999) and its mutants (Kotloff *et al.*, 2001). The immunostimulation created by adjuvants delivered systemically has raised potential safety concerns for long-term effects regarding induction of cancer and autoimmunity. However, 35-year follow-up of emulsion-based (i.e. adjuvanted) influenza vaccines failed to demonstrate such an effect (Beebe *et al.*, 1972; Page *et al.*, 1993). These data are reassuring, as emulsion-based adjuvants are extremely potent. However, the acute toxicities of adjuvants delivered systemically or mucosally illustrate a potential advantage of topical administration to the skin, where systemic toxicities related to immunization have not been seen (Glenn *et al.*, 2000; Güereña-Burgueño *et al.*, 2002; Yu *et al.*, 2002) and would not be expected. In fact, large doses of one of the most potent adjuvants (LT), well beyond that which can be used by other routes, have been safely used on the skin without systemic side effects (Glenn *et al.*, 2000; Güereña-Burgueño *et al.*, 2002) Concerns regarding the parenteral use of LPS or LPS derivatives are not likely to be as relevant for topical preparations because the adjuvants are apparently not absorbed into the systemic circulation. In fact, the presence of LPS in antigen preparations may even be beneficial, adding adjuvant properties to the antigen. Similarly, while oral use of native LT is known to be diarrheagenic in human trials (Michetti *et al.*, 1999), in clinical trials using TCI, no vaccine related diarrhea has been seen (Glenn *et al.*, 2000). Although there are a variety of mutant toxins designed to alleviate this side effect of oral use, it appears that native toxins, unmatched for their adjuvanticity, may be safely used by the topical route. The safe use of highly potent and inexpensive adjuvants opens new and previously restricted possibilities for vaccine development.

Immune Responses To TCI

The use of the skin as a target tissue has raised questions as to whether immune responses typical of standard vaccines might be expected. At this time, it is clear that TCI can induce systemic antibodies and T cell responses. Antibodies to tetanus and diphtheria toxoids (Glenn *et al.*, 1998a, 1999; Gockel *et al.*, 2000), inactivated viruses (El-Ghorr *et al.*, 2000), gene products of carrier viruses (Hammond *et al.*, 2000; Shi *et al.*, 2001), influenza matrix (M) protein encoded by plasmids (Watabe *et al.*, 2001), large recombinant proteins (Yu *et al.*, 2002) and toxins (Glenn *et al.*, 1998a, 1998b, 1999, and 2000) have been observed. Typical boosting kinetics are seen (Glenn *et al.*, 1999) and adjuvants exert their effects with repeated use with different antigens as has been shown in the context of nasal immunization (Tamura *et al.*, 1989; Glenn *et al.*, 1999). As discussed below, TCI also readily induces antigen specific mucosal IgG and IgA. As might be expected, vaccine formulations delivered to the skin induce T cell responses (El-Ghorr *et al.*, 2000; Gockel *et al.*, 2000; Beignon *et al.*, 2001; Hammond *et al.*, 2001) as well as CTLs (Seo *et al.*, 2000; Watabe *et al.*, 2001) (Figure 1). Although DTH responses may occur locally at the site of immunization (Güereña-Burgueño *et al.*, 2002), this appears to be the exception (Glenn *et al.*, 2000; Gockel *et al.*, 2000; Yu *et al.*, 2002) and generally, TCI results in robust immune responses systemically in the absence of local immune sequelae in the skin (Beignon *et al.*, 2001).

PRECLINICAL EFFICACY STUDIES

The skin immune system has traditionally been seen as a site for immunodermatopathology and not a site for the induction of 'useful' immune responses. We first demonstrated that skin immunization could protect mice against a pulmonary toxin challenge model (Glenn *et al.*, 1998b). We then confirmed the relevance of the original study using an enteric toxin challenge that simulates the disease process found in traveler's diarrhea and cholera and replicates previous protection studies using immunization by other routes (Pierce *et al.*, 1972; Pierce and Reynolds, 1974; Yu *et al.*, 2002). As shown in Figure 3, mice were given intragastric holotoxin, which results in a measurable fluid accumulation in the small intestine. When previously immunized transcutaneously with LT, the mice were solidly protected against this rigorous challenge. Others have similarly shown that mice can be protected against intraperitoneal toxin challenge after topical immunization with LT (Beignon *et al.*, 2001). Protection against tetanus toxin challenge, a systemic disease caused by toxin effects at the neuromuscular junction, was seen after immunization with CT and TTx via the skin (Scharton-Kersten *et al.*, 2000). Incomplete protection against live clostridial challenge was also seen using an adenovirus carrier system after topical immunization (Shi *et al.*, 2001).

In previous studies, our group (Hammond *et al.*, 2000) had shown that immunization with a whole virus vector (mengovirus) could induce antibodies to the F1 protein of *Yersinia pestis*. El-Ghorr *et al.* (2000) found that immunization with inactivated herpes virus (HSVi) or HSV-1 antigens extracted from infected Vero cells (HSVag) using CT as adjuvant resulted in serum and mucosal (fecal) antibodies to HSV, with the CT+HSVi vaccine being a more potent stimulator of humoral immunity. The CT inactivated virus vaccine, however, was the more potent stimulator of cell-mediated immunity, giving rise to a strong delayed type hypersensitivity response and lymphocyte proliferation *in vitro*. When the mice were challenged by epidermal inoculation of HSV, the CT+HSVag vaccine induced a higher level of protection than the CT+HSVi vaccine, confirming that HSV vaccines are most likely to be protective via stimulation of cell-mediated rather than humoral responses. In a similar study, Johnston *et al.* (1996 and 2000) studied the effect of intradermal live viral infection. LCs respond to cutaneous viral infections, which are effectively cleared by the immune system. Using the arthropod-borne viruses, West Nile virus or Semliki Forest virus, the investigators found that major histocompatibility complex class II+/NLDC145+/E-cadherin+ LCs are increased in the draining lymph nodes of intradermally challenged mice, and this increase is accompanied by a

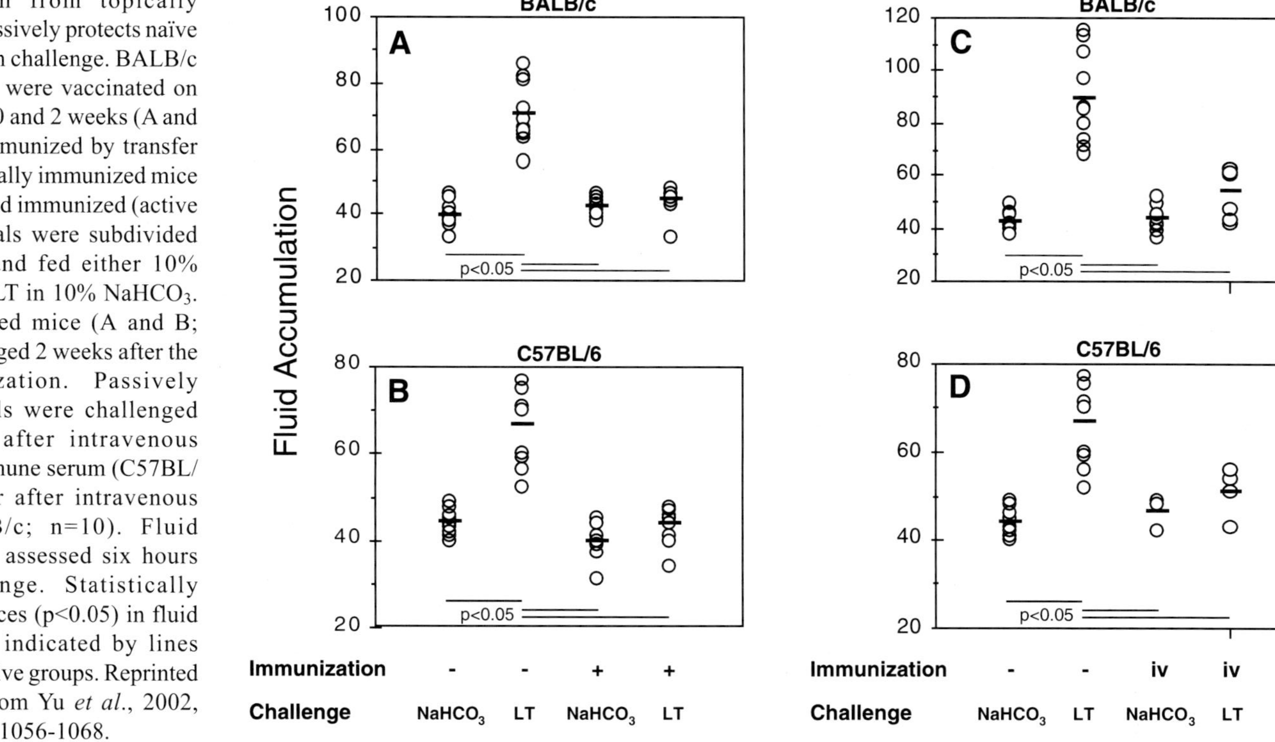

Figure 3. Serum from topically immunized mice passively protects naïve mice from oral toxin challenge. BALB/c and C57BL/6 mice were vaccinated on the skin with LT at 0 and 2 weeks (A and B), or passively immunized by transfer of serum from topically immunized mice (C and D). Naïve and immunized (active and passive) animals were subdivided into two groups and fed either 10% $NaHCO_3$ alone or LT in 10% $NaHCO_3$. Actively immunized mice (A and B; n=10) were challenged 2 weeks after the second immunization. Passively vaccinated animals were challenged either 12 hours after intravenous injection of the immune serum (C57BL/6; n=4) or 1 hour after intravenous injection (BALB/c; n=10). Fluid accumulation was assessed six hours after the challenge. Statistically significant differences (p<0.05) in fluid accumulation are indicated by lines between the respective groups. Reprinted with permission from Yu et al., 2002, Infect. Immun. 70: 1056-1068.

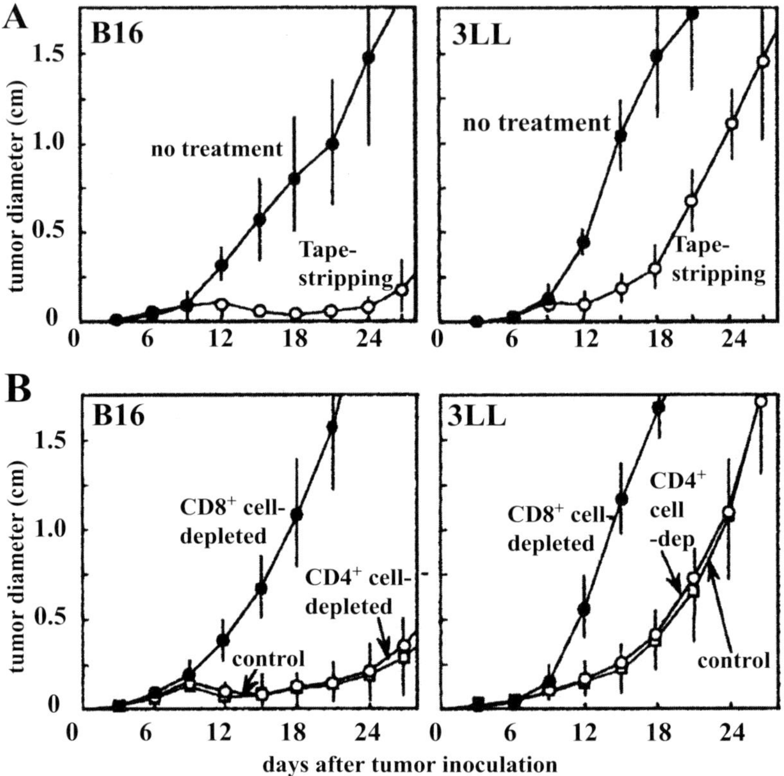

Figure 4. Protection against tumor cell challenge after peptide immunization via barrier-disrupted skin. (A) Mice (n=10) were treated with TRP-2 or MUT1 on untreated or tape-stripped skin. B16 or 3LL tumor cells (1 x 10^5 cells per mouse) were inoculated s.c. into TRP-2 or MUT1-treated mice, respectively, and tumor sizes were measured every 3 days. (B) CD4+ or CD8+ cell-depleted, or control rat IgG-treated mice (n=10) were painted with TRP-2 or MUT1 on tape-stripped skin. B16 or 3LL tumor cells (1 x 10^5 cells per mouse) were inoculated s.c. into TRP-2 or MUT1-treated mice, respectively, and tumor sizes were measured every 3 days. Reprinted with permission from Seo *et al.*, 2000, PNAS 97: 371-376.

concomitant decrease in the LC density in the epidermis. LC migration was associated with an accumulation of leukocytes in the lymph node, which is one of the earliest events in the initiation of an immune response. Both, the LC migratory response and the draining lymph node leukocyte accumulation, were abrogated if ultraviolet-inactivated instead of live viruses were used, suggesting the activation and subsequent migration of LCs requires a live, replicating antigen. These findings suggested that the use of a live replicating virus may provide high level danger signals to enhance the immune response, similar to adjuvants. However, live replicating viral vectors are accompanied by safety risks and are generally modified to avoid replication (Moingeon, 2001), and the repeated use of viral vectors seems to diminish the response to antigens of interest in boosting regimens, including their transcutaneous use (Shi *et al.*, 2001). Consistent with the protection and immune responses seen after immunization with protein-based formulations, others have shown that topical immunization with plasmid DNA encoding for the influenza M protein can induce protective immunity against respiratory challenge (see below) (Watabe *et al.*, 2001).

Using well established tumor challenge models, Seo *et al.* used topically applied peptide immunization on tape-stripped skin and clearly demonstrated the induction of tumor peptide specific CD8+ CTLs, protection against tumor challenge (Figure 4), and more impressively, survival in mice with established tumors subsequently immunized with peptide topically (Figure 5) (Seo *et al.*, 2000). Although adjuvants were not used, our data would suggest that the immune responses would be enhanced by the use of adjuvants (see Figure 1). The same group also presented evidence that the immunization is mediated by LCs, and that the LCs are activated by tape stripping (Takigawa *et al.*, 2001), as has been previously described (Katoh *et al.*, 1997).

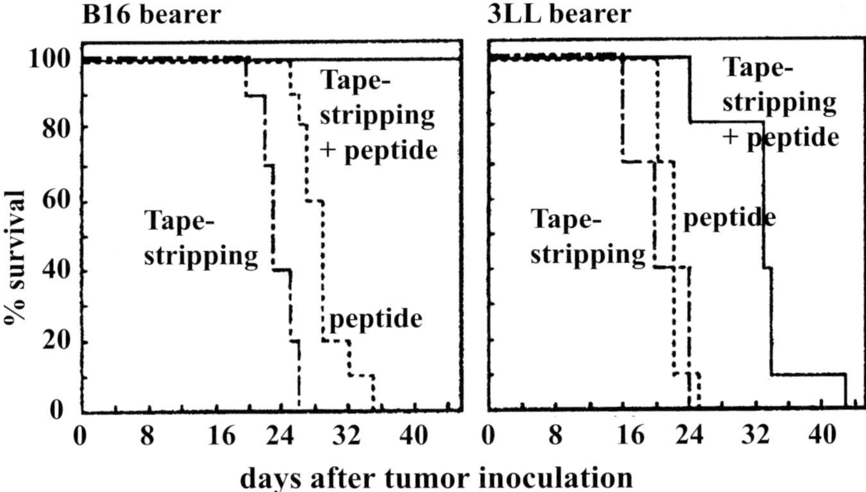

Figure 5. Tumor immunotherapy by peptide application to barrier-disrupted skin. Mice inoculated with B16 (n=20) or 3LL (n=20) were treated with TRP-2 or MUT1, respectively, on tape-stripped earlobes and then abdomen 2 days later. Percentage survival of the mice treated with peptide at tape-stripped skin (solid line), treated with tape-stripping only (dash-dot line), or treated with peptide at intact skin (dotted line) was monitored.Reprinted with permission from Seo *et al.*, 2000, PNAS 97: 371-376.

MUCOSAL RESPONSES TO TCI

In multiple studies it has been shown that topical immunization with LT and CT as adjuvants clearly induces both IgG and IgA antibodies in mucosal secretions (Glenn *et al.*, 1998b; El-Ghorr *et al.*, 2000; Enioutina *et al.*, 2000; Glenn *et al.*, 2000; Gockel *et al.*, 2000; Watabe *et al.*, 2001). We have suggested that the skin immune system may be an extension of the mucosal immune system. The mucosa and skin share similar elements, including LCs and secretory organs, and IgA can be found in the sweat glands (Gebhart *et al.*, 1987; Okada *et al.*, 1988), most likely the origin of the secretory IgA that coats microorganisms found on the skin (Hard, 1969; Metze *et al.*, 1991). Thus, the skin immune system has immunological responses to microbes that are mucosal-like, suggesting that the skin shares elements of the mucosal immune system.

The topical application of bacterial ADP-ribosylating exotoxins (bAREs), such as LT, CT, and co-administered antigens, induces antibodies that can be detected at the mucosa (Glenn *et al.*, 1998b; El-Ghorr *et al.*, 2000; Scharton-Kersten *et al.*, 2000) as well as mucosal cellular responses (Gockel *et al.*, 2000). Mice immunized transcutaneously with CT produce anti-CT IgG and IgA antibodies in the stool and pulmonary secretions (Figure 6) that are toxin-neutralizing (Glenn *et al.*, 1998b; Yu *et al.*, 2002). IgG antibodies to the co-administered antigen have been detected in the mucosa in several settings (Glenn *et al.*, 1999; El-Ghorr *et al.*, 2000; Scharton-Kersten *et al.*, 2000), and IgA to tetanus and herpes antigens have been detected in mice immunized topically with CT and TTx or inactivated herpes virus (El-Ghorr *et al.*, 2000; Gockel *et al.*, 2000). The detection of antibodies in the stool and lung wash of immunized mice suggests that antibody secreting cells have homed to the mucosa; it has been shown that anti-TTx antibody secreting cells (ASCs) can be detected in the vaginal mucosa of mice immunized topically using CT and TTx (Gockel *et al.*, 2000), but migration of LCs to the gut may also explain these findings (Enioutina *et al.*, 2000). Alternatively, antibodies may represent transudates into the mucosal secretions, although recent data has shown that anti-LT antibodies detected in the stool and lung wash contain the secretory component of IgA, indicating that local antibody production occurs as well (Yu *et al.*, 2002). Berneman *et al.* (1998) have shown that mucosal IgG may be locally produced; the relevance of this observation in the context of TCI needs to be confirmed. Plasmid DNA immunization delivered by TCI similarly induces both serum IgG and fecal IgA against the influenza M protein encoded in the plasmid, and elicited a protective immune response on

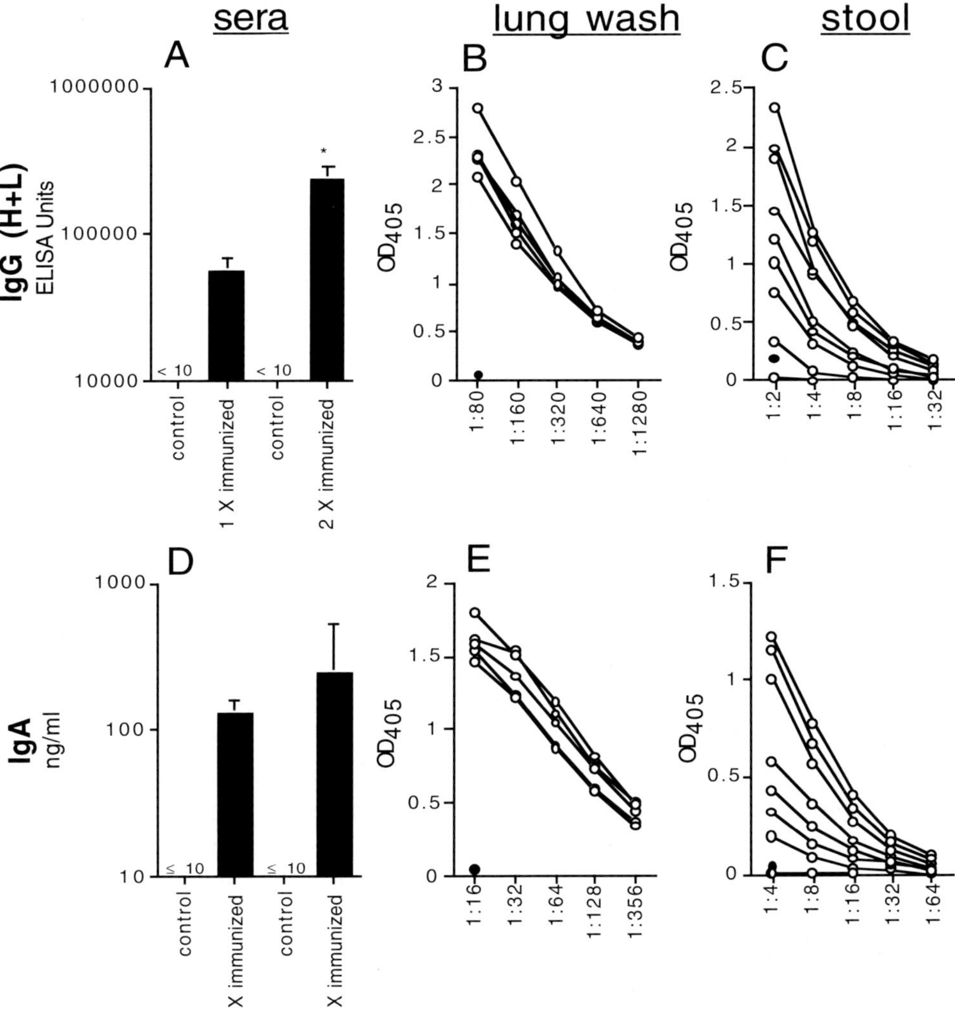

Figure 6. Sera (A and D), mucosal lung (B and E), and stool (C and F) Ab responses to CT after TCI. A and D, C57BL/6 mice (17-22 animals per group) were immunized transcutaneously at 0 or at 0 and 3 wk with 100 μg of CT. Sera were collected at 3 and 6 wk. Data shown are the geometric mean + SEM for ELISA measurements from five individual animals. *, a statistically significant (p<0.05) difference between the titers measured in the 1X and 2X immunization groups. B and E, C57BL/6 mice were immunized transcutaneously at 0 wk; lung washes were collected from vaccinated, unchallenged mice (n=5) on the day of challenge (3 wk). •, indicates the OD detected from control lung washes from mice immunized with an irrelevant protein. IgG and IgA levels were assessed by ELISA; the titers (OD = 405 nm) from individual animals are shown. C and F, C57BL/6 mice were immunized transcutaneously at 0 wk. Single stool pellets were collected immediately after defecation on the day before toxin challenge (6 wk). IgG and IgA levels were assessed in fecal homogenates by ELISA; the dilution curves from eight (f) or nine (c) individual animals are shown. •, the maximal level of anti-CT IgG or anti-CT IgA detected in 1/2 dilutions of stool from unimmunized mice (background). Reprinted with permission from Hammond *et al.*, 2001, Therapeutic Drug Delivery Systems 18: 503-526.

influenza virus challenges (Watabe *et al.*, 2001). Anti-LT IgG and IgA antibodies were found in humans immunized topically with LT, which is consistent with the repeated observations in mice (Glenn *et al.*, 2000). The presence of antibodies in the secretions of animals immunized by TCI raises many mechanistic questions, but the data suggest that induction of mucosal and systemic responses by TCI may be used to enhance vaccine efficacy.

DELIVERY OF ANTIGENS IN HUMANS

The delivery of a large molecule (86kD) such as LT is counter to existing paradigms of human skin delivery (Bos *et al.*, 2000). In order to test the hypothesis that a large antigen could pass through the SC into the epidermis to elicit an immune response, we elected to deliver LT in a simple 'wet' patch. As LT acts both as antigen and adjuvant, we could evaluate the outcome by measuring serum antibodies to LT. A dose escalation study was done in 18 healthy volunteers to assess the safety and immune response to simple liquid application of LT to skin without any skin preparation steps (Glenn *et al.*, 2000). Volunteers received 25, 50, 250 or 500 µg of an LT solution that was added to a gauze pad under an adhesive patch and applied to the upper arm for six hours. They were monitored for systemic or local reactions after vaccination and were boosted at 12 weeks. The six that received 500 µg LT returned for a third immunization 35 weeks after the first immunization. No serious vaccine-related adverse reactions were observed, either systemically or at the site of immunization. One volunteer developed a mild dermatitis at the adhesive site. Histologic sections of biopsies taken at the dosing sites and matched control sites were normal, consistent with the absence of DTH clinically. Consistent with a host of preclinical observations (Aiba and Katz, 1990; Johnston *et al.*, 1996; Vassell *et al.*, 1999), LCs visualized in the same biopsy using anti-CD1a staining consistently demonstrated enlarged or rounded LC cell bodies at the site of immunization at 24 and 48 hours compared to the control biopsies from the opposite arm.

Systemic and mucosal immune responses to LT were detected in all subjects in the high-dose group. This group had a 14.6 and 7.2 mean fold rise in serum anti-LT IgG and IgA, respectively, at 44 weeks. The antibodies against LT were durable and clearly persisted after the second immunization. There were minimal responses in other dosing groups. All individuals in the 500 µg group also had detectable IgG or IgA antibodies against LT in either the

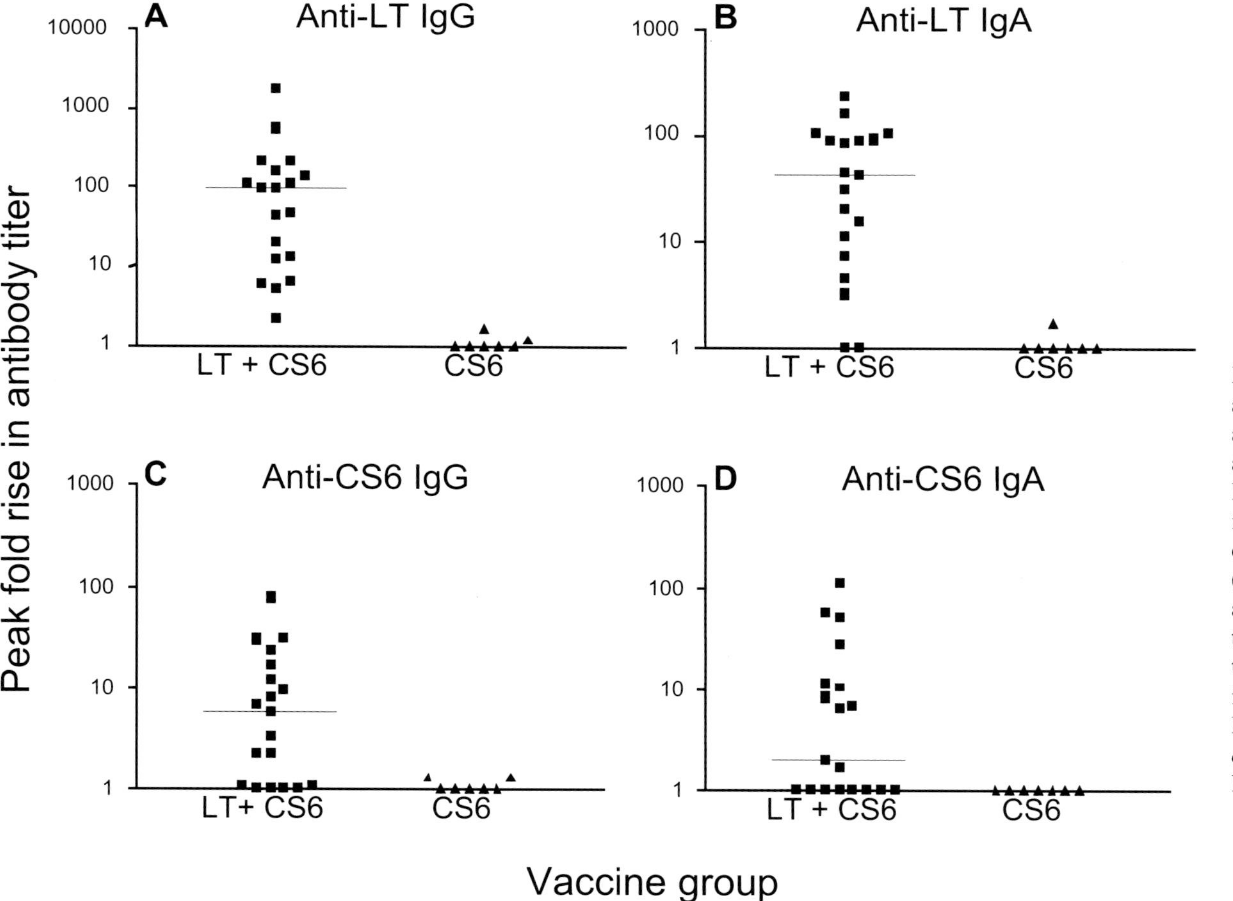

Figure 7. Individual IgG and IgA peak fold rise in antibody titer to LT (A and B) and CS6 (C and D) among volunteers immunized with adjuvant combined with antigen (LT+CS6), or with antigen alone (CS6). The transverse bar represents the median peak fold rise in antibody titer. Reprinted from Guereña *et al.*, 2002, Infect. Immun. 70: 1874-1880.

urine or stool, although there was no clear correlation between the magnitude of the individual serum responses and antibodies detected in the urine or stool.

Preclinical studies of candidate ETEC-related traveler's diarrhea vaccine antigens have shown good immunogenicity when delivered with adjuvants by TCI. We have initiated a development program for an ETEC vaccine beginning with the colonization factor CS6, a multi-subunit intestinal epithelial cell-binding protein (Wolf *et al.*, 1997) augmented by anti-toxin immunity (Clemens *et al.*, 1988). This trial also afforded the opportunity to test the hypothesis that the adjuvant plays an important role in the induction of an immune response to coadministered antigens, as has been observed extensively in preclinical studies (Glenn *et al.*, 1998a and 1999; Baca-Estrada *et al.*, 2000; El-Ghorr *et al.*, 2000; Gockel *et al.*, 2000; Scharton-Kersten *et al.*, 2000; Yu *et al.*, 2002). Healthy adult volunteers were enrolled in a dose-escalating study of 250, 500, 1000 or 2000 µg CS6 alone or with 500 µg LT dosed at 0, 1, and 3 months (Güereña-Burgueño *et al.*, 2002). Fourteen of 19 volunteers (74%) in the combined groups had mild delayed-type hypersensitivity skin reactions with the second or third dose, suggesting sensitization to the CS6. No other adverse events correlated with vaccine administration. Volunteers receiving LT as adjuvant produced serum anti-CS6 IgG and IgA (Figure 7). The anti- LT response was approximately 10 times greater in comparison to the previous trial (above) and may be explained by the use of simple skin preparation steps in application of the patch. Overall, when CS6 was given with LT, 68% and 53% had anti-CS6 IgG and IgA, respectively, and 100% and 90% had anti-LT IgG and IgA responses, respectively. This anti-CS6 response compares favorably to a protective challenge infection using the B7A ETEC strain, where 35% and 31% developed anti-CS6 IgG and IgA, respectively (Levine *et al.*, 1979; Wolf *et al.*, 1999). The anti-LT response to TCI, not measured in the challenge study, will likely contribute to protection against LT toxin-induced diarrheal disease as well (Trach *et al.*, 1997). Antibody secreting cells (ASCs) were also measured in the peripheral blood. In the combined dose TCI groups, 37% and 42% developed anti-CS6 IgG and IgA ASCs, respectively, compared to 50% that developed anti-CS6 IgA ASCs following challenge, historically (Wolf *et al.*, 1999). There were no immune responses seen in the CS6 alone groups. The lack of response to CS6 without LT and clear responses in the presence of LT confirmed the universal finding in animal studies that the adjuvant plays a critical role in TCI. Favorable induction of an immune response in comparison with the one seen after a live challenge suggests the vaccination may provide a similar degree of protection.

These studies have confirmed the extensive preclinical observations that large antigens can be delivered to the skin to induce systemic immune responses, and that the adjuvant plays a critical role in the induction of robust responses in conjunction with delivery of antigens in a patch. Remarkably, these studies were conducted with simple formulation, patches and skin preparation strategies. Future studies, using more sophisticated techniques will be expected to build on this initial data set. Clearly, the efficiency of antigen utilization in the clinical setting will need to follow the trend in preclinical studies, where the robust immune responses have been seen with antigen/adjuvant doses as low as 5/0.5 µg respectively, down from 100-200 µg in initial studies (Glenn *et al.*, 1998a). Product specifications will dictate the many aspects of patch and formulation materials, as well as antigen and adjuvant doses.

CONCLUSIONS

Transcutaneous immunization is an established method of immunization with emerging data suggesting the feasibility of this approach. In the past few years there has been an explosion of the interest in targeting the skin immune system. Although variolation for smallpox may in truth be considered the first innovation regarding skin targeted immunization, the first modern description of the concept of a device-free passive delivery system for immunization was by Paul and Cevc (1995). Our group may claim the first invention of a passive vaccine delivery system (Alving *et al.*, 1996), use of the skin immune system with vaccine antigens, as well as the first human vaccine study showing the feasibility of passive vaccine delivery to the skin (Glenn *et al.*, 2000). There is much recent data that has validated these observations, and while many mechanistic questions remain, it appears quite certain that Langerhans cells are the primary targets for transcutaneous immunization techniques, and the activation of Langerhans cells by the immunization process appears to be a critical feature for eliciting useful, strong immune responses. The observation that adjuvants can act safely and effectively on the skin immune system and the advantages of needle-free delivery suggest that this technique has the ample robustness and practicality required for formulation as a product.

ACKNOWLEDGEMENTS

I thank Ms. Wanda Hardy for assistance in preparation of the manuscript and Dr. Scott Hammond for a critical review of the manuscript.

REFERENCES

Aiba, S., and Katz, S.I. 1990. Phenotypic and functional characteristics of *in vivo*-activated Langerhans cells. J. Immunol. 145: 2791-2796.

Alving, C.R., and Glenn, G.M. 1996. Transdermal delivery system for antigen. U.S. Patent #5,910,306.

Aylward, B., Lloyd, J., Zaffran, M., McNair-Scott, R., and Evans, P. 1995. Reducing the risk of unsafe injections in immunization programmes: financial and operational implications of various injection technologies. Bull. World Health Org. 73: 531-540.

Baca-Estrada, M.E., Foldvari, M., Ewen, C., Badea, I., and Babiuk, L.A. 2000. Effects of IL-12 on immune responses induced by transcutaneous immunization with antigens formulated in a novel lipid-based biphasic delivery system. Vaccine 18: 1847-1854.

Baldo, V., Menegon, T., Bonello, C., Floreani, A., Trivello, R., and Collaborative, G. 2001. Comparison of three different influenza vaccines in institutionalised elderly. Vaccine 19: 3472-3475.

Ban, E., Dupre, L., Hermann, E., Rohn, W., Vendeville, C., Quatannens, B., Ricciardi-Castagnoli, P., Capron, A., and Riveau, G. 2000. CpG motifs induce Langerhans cell migration *in vivo*. Int. Immunol. 12: 737-745.

Barry, B.W. 1985. Dermatologic formulations. In: Percutaneous Absorption: Methods, Methodology, Drug Delivery. R. L. Bronaugh and H. I. Maibach, eds., Marcel Dekker, New York. p. 33.

Beebe, G.W., Simon, A.H., and Vivona, S. 1972. Long-term mortality follow-up of Army recruits who received adjuvant influenza virus vaccine in 1951-1953. Am. J. Epidemiol. 95: 337-346.

Beignon, A.S., Briand, J.P., Muller, S., and Partidos, C.D. 2001. Immunization onto bare skin with heat-labile enterotoxin of *Escherichia coli* enhances immune responses to coadministered protein and peptide antigens and protects mice against lethal toxin challenge. Immunology 102: 344-351.

Berneman, A., Belec, L., Fischetti, V.A., and Bouvet, J.P. 1998. The specificity patterns of human immunoglobulin G antibodies in serum differ from those in autologous secretions. Infect. Immun. 66: 4163-4168.

Bos, J.D., and Meinardi, M.M. 2000. The 500 Dalton rule for the skin penetration of chemical compounds and drugs. Exp. Dermatol. 9: 165-169.

Chen, D., Erickson, C.A., Endres, R.L., Periwal, S.B., Chu, Q., Shu, C., Maa, Y.F., and Payne, L.G. 2001a. Adjuvantation of epidermal powder immunization. Vaccine 19: 2908-2917.

Chen, D., Weis, K.F., Chu, Q., Erickson, C., Endres, R., Lively, C.R., Osorio, J., and Payne, L.G. 2001b. Epidermal powder immunization induces both cytotoxic T-lymphocyte and antibody responses to protein antigens of influenza and hepatitis B viruses. J. Virol. 75: 11630-11640.

Clemens, J.D., Sack, D.A., Harris, J.R., Chakraborty, J., Neogy, P.K., Stanton, B., Huda, N., Khan, M.U., Kay, B.A., Khan, M.R., *et al.* 1988. Cross-protection by B subunit-whole cell cholera vaccine against diarrhea associated with heat-labile toxin-producing enterotoxigenic *Escherichia coli*: results of a large-scale field trial. J. Infect. Dis. 158: 372-377.

Cryz, S.J., Jr., and Gluck, R. 1998. Immunopotentiating reconstituted influenza virosomes as a novel antigen delivery system. Dev. Biol. Stand. 92: 219-223.

de Haan, L., Verweij, W.R., Feil, I.K., Holtrop, M., Hol, W.G., Agsteribbe, E., and Wilschut, J. 1998. Role of GM1 binding in the mucosal immunogenicity and adjuvant activity of the *Escherichia coli* heat-labile enterotoxin and its B subunit. Immunology 94: 424-430.

Dickinson, B.L., and Clements, J.D. 1995. Dissociation of *Escherichia coli* heat-labile enterotoxin adjuvanticity from ADP-ribosyltransferase activity. Infect. Immun. 63: 1617-1623.

El-Ghorr, A.A., Williams, R.M., Heap, C., and Norval, M. 2000. Transcutaneous immunisation with herpes simplex virus stimulates immunity in mice. FEMS Immunol. Med. Microbiol. 29: 255-261.

Enioutina, E.Y., Visic, D., and Daynes, R.A. 2000. The induction of systemic and mucosal immune responses to antigen- adjuvant compositions administered into the skin: alterations in the migratory properties of dendritic cells appears to be important for stimulating mucosal immunity. Vaccine 18: 2753-2767.

Fagiolo, U., Amadori, A., Cozzi, E., Bendo, R., Lama, M., Douglas, A., and Palu, G. 1993. Humoral and cellular immune response to influenza virus vaccination in aged humans. Aging (Milano). 5: 451-458.

Fedson, D.S., Wajda, A., Nicol, J.P., Hammond, G.W., Kaiser, D.L., and Roos, L.L. 1993. Clinical effectiveness of influenza vaccination in Manitoba. J.A.M.A. 270: 1956-1961.

Fletcher, M.A., and Saliou, P. 2000. Vaccines and infectious disease. EXS 89: 69-88.

Gasparini, R., Pozzi, T., Montomoli, E., Fragapane, E., Senatore, F., Minutello, M., and Podda, A. 2001. Increased immunogenicity of the MF59-adjuvanted influenza vaccine compared to a conventional subunit vaccine in elderly subjects. Eur. J. Epidemiol. 17: 135-140.

Gebhart, W., Metze, D., and Jurecka, W. 1987. IgA in human skin appendages. In: Immunodermatology. R. Caputo, ed., CIC Edizioni Internationali. p. 185.

Glenn, G.M., Rao, M., Matyas, G.R., and Alving, C.R. 1998a. Skin immunization made possible by cholera toxin. Nature 391: 851.

Glenn, G.M., Scharton-Kersten, T., Vassell, R., Mallett, C.P., Hale, T.L., and Alving, C.R. 1998b. Transcutaneous immunization with cholera toxin protects mice against lethal mucosal toxin challenge. J. Immunol. 161: 3211-3214.

Glenn, G.M., Scharton-Kersten, T., Vassell, R., Matyas, G.R., and Alving, C.R. 1999. Transcutaneous immunization with bacterial ADP-ribosylating exotoxins as antigens and adjuvants. Infect. Immun. 67: 1100-1106.

Glenn, G.M., Taylor, D.N., Li, X., Frankel, S., Montemarano, A., and Alving, C.R. 2000. Transcutaneous immunization: A human vaccine delivery strategy using a patch. Nat. Med. 6: 1403-1406.

Gluck, R., Mischler, R., Durrer, P., Furer, E., Lang, A.B., Herzog, C., and Cryz, S.J., Jr. 2000. Safety and immunogenicity of intranasally administered inactivated trivalent virosome-formulated influenza vaccine containing *Escherichia coli* heat-labile toxin as a mucosal adjuvant. J. Infect. Dis. 181: 1129-1132.

Gockel, C.M., Bao, S., and Beagley, K.W. 2000. Transcutaneous immunization inducesmucosal and systemic immunity: A potent method for targeting immunity to the female reproductive tract. Mol. Immunol. 37: 537-544.

Goronzy, J.J., Fulbright, J.W., Crowson, C.S., Poland, G.A., O'Fallon, W.M., and Weyand, C.M. 2001. Value of immunological markers in predicting responsiveness to influenza vaccination in elderly individuals. J. Virol. 75: 12182-12187.

Güereña-Burgueño, F., Hall, E.R., Taylor, D.N., Cassels, F.J., Scott, D.A., Wolf, M.K., Roberts, Z.J., Nesterova, G.V., Alving, C.R., and Glenn, G.M. 2002. Safety and immunogenicity of a prototype enterotoxigenic *Escherichia coli* vaccine administered transcutaneously. Infect. Immun. 70: 1874-1880.

Hammond, S.A., Tsonis, C., Sellins, K., Rushlow, K., Scharton-Kersten, T., Colditz, I., and Glenn, G.M. 2000. Transcutaneous immunization of domestic animals: opportunities and challenges. Adv. Drug Delivery Rev. 43: 45-55.

Hammond, S.A., Walwender, D., Alving, C.R., and Glenn, G.M. 2001. Transcutaneous immunization: T-cell responses and boosting of existing immunity. Vaccine 19: 2701-2707.

Hard, G.C. 1969. Electron microscopic examination of *Corynebacterium ovis*. J. Bacteriol. 97: 1480-1485.

Hashigucci, K., Ogawa, H., Ishidate, T., Yamashita, R., Kamiya, H., Watanabe, K., Hattori, N., Sato, T., Suzuki, Y., Nagamine, T., Aizawa, C., Tamura, S., Kurata, T., and Oya, A. 1996. Antibody responses in volunteers induced by nasal influenza vaccine combined with *Escherichia coli* heat-labile enterotoxin B subunit containing a trace amount of the holotoxin. Vaccine 14: 113-119.

Jacobs, R.L., Lowe, R.S., and Lanier, B.Q. 1982. Adverse reactions to tetanus toxoid. J.A.M.A. 247: 40-42.

Jakob, T., and Udey, M.C. 1999. Epidermal Langerhans cells: from neurons to nature's adjuvants. Adv. Dermatol. 14: 209-258.

Jakob, T., Walker, P.S., Krieg, A.M., von Stebut, E., Udey, M.C., and Vogel, J.C. 1999. Bacterial DNA and CpG-containing oligodeoxynucleotides activate cutaneous dendritic cells and induce IL-12 production: implications for the augmentation of Th1 responses. Int. Arch. Allergy Immunol. 118: 457-461.

Johnston, L.J., Halliday, G.M., and King, N.J. 1996. Phenotypic changes in Langerhans' cells after infection with arboviruses: a role in the immune response to epidermally acquired viral infection. J. Virol. 70: 4761-4766.

Johnston, L.J., Halliday, G.M., and King, N.J. 2000. Langerhans cells migrate to local lymph nodes following cutaneous infection with an arbovirus. J. Invest. Dermatol. 114: 560-568.

Katoh, N., Hirano, S., Kishimoto, S., and Yasuno, H. 1997. Acute cutaneous barrier perturbation induces maturation of Langerhans' cells in hairless mice. Acta. Derm. Venereol. 77: 365-369.

Keitel, W., Couch, R., Bond, N., Adair, S., Van Nest, G., and Dekker, C. 1993. Pilot evaluation of influenza virus vaccine (IVV) combined with adjuvant. Vaccine 11: 909-913.

Kotloff, K.L., Sztein, M.B., Wasserman, S.S., Losonsky, G.A., DiLorenzo, S.C., and Walker, R.I. 2001. Safety and immunogenicity of oral inactivated whole-cell *Helicobacter pylori* vaccine with adjuvant among volunteers with or without subclinical infection. Infect. Immun. 69: 3581-3590.

Kripke, M.L., Munn, C.G., Jeevan, A., Tang, J.M., and Bucana, C. 1990. Evidence that cutaneous antigen-presenting cells migrate to regional lymph nodes during contact sensitization. J. Immunol. 145: 2833-2838.

Levine, M.M., Nalin, D.R., Hoover, D.L., Bergquist, E.J., Hornick, R.B., and Young, C.R. 1979. Immunity to enterotoxigenic *Escherichia coli*. Infect. Immun. 23: 729-736.

Macatonia, S.E., Knight, S.C., Edwards, A.J., Griffiths, S., and Fryer, P. 1987. Localization of antigen on lymph node dendritic cells after exposure to the contact sensitizer fluorescein isothiocyanate. Functional and morphological studies. J. Exp. Med. 166: 1654-1667.

Mason, A., Wick, M., White, H., and Perrillo, R. 1993. Hepatitis B virus replication in diverse cell types during chronic hepatitis B virus infection. Hepatology 18: 781-789.

Metze, D., Kersten, A., Jurecka, W., and Gebhart, W. 1991. Immunoglobulins coat microorganisms of skin surface: a comparative immunohistochemical and ultrastructural study of cutaneous and oral microbial symbionts. J. Invest. Dermatol. 96: 439-445.

Michetti, P., Kreiss, C., Kotloff, K.L., Porta, N., Blanco, J.L., Bachmann, D., Herranz, M., Saldinger, P.F., Corthesy-Theulaz, I., Losonsky, G., Nichols, R., Simon, J., Stolte, M., Ackerman, S., Monath, T.P., and Blum, A.L. 1999. Oral immunization with urease and *Escherichia coli* heat-labile enterotoxin is safe and immunogenic in *Helicobacter pylori*-infected adults. Gastroenterology 116: 804-812.

Moingeon, P. 2001. Cancer vaccines. Vaccine 19: 1305-1326.

O'Hagan, D.T., ed. 2000. Methods in Molecular Medicine. Humana Press, Inc., Totowa, NJ.

Okada, T., Konishi, H., Ito, M., Nagura, H., and Asai, J. 1988. Identification of secretory immunoglobulin A in human sweat and sweat glands. J. Invest. Dermatol. 90: 648-651.

Page, W.F., Norman, J.E., and, Benenson, A.S. 1993. Long-term follow-up of army recruits immunized with Freund's incomplete adjuvanted vaccine. Vaccine Res. 2: 141-149.

Patriarca, P.A., Weber, J.A., Parker, R.A., Hall, W.N., Kendal, A.P., Bregman, D.J., and Schonberger, L.B. 1985. Efficacy of influenza vaccine in nursing homes. Reduction in illness and complications during an influenza A (H3N2) epidemic. J.A.M.A. 253: 1136-1139.

Paul, A., and Cevc, G. 1995. Noninvasive administration of protein antigens: Transdermal immunization with bovine serum albumin in transfersomes. Vaccine Res. 4: 145-164.

Paul, A., Cevc, G., and Bachhawat, B.K. 1995. Transdermal immunization with large proteins by means of ultradeformable drug carriers. Eur. J. Immunol. 25: 3521-3524.

Pierce, N.F., Kaniecki, E.A., and Northrup, R.S. 1972. Protection against experimental cholera by antitoxin. J. Infect. Dis. 126: 606-616.

Pierce, N.F., and Reynolds, H.Y. 1974. Immunity to experimental cholera. I. Protective effect of humoral IgG antitoxin demonstrated by passive immunization. J. Immunol. 113: 1017-1023.

Ramon, G. 1925. Sur l'aumentation anormale de l'antitoxine chez les chevaux producteurs de serum antidipherique. Bull. Soc. Cent. Med. Vet. 101: 227-234.

Rappuoli, R., Pizza, M., Douce, G., and Dougan, G. 1999. Structure and mucosal adjuvanticity of cholera and *Escherichia coli* heat-labile enterotoxins. Immunol. Today 20: 493-500.

Rietschel, R.I., and Fowler, J.F. 1995. Fisher's Contact Dermatitis, 4th Edition. Williams & Wilkins, Baltimore, MD.

Roberts, M.S., and Walker, M. 1993. Water, the most natural penetration enhancer. Marcel Dekker, New York.

Salk, J.E., Contakos, M., Laurent, A.M., Sorensen, M., Rapalski, A.J., Simmons, H., and Sandberg, H. 1953. Use of adjuvants in studies on influenza immunization. Degree of persistence of antibody in human subjects two years after vaccination. J.A.M.A. 151: 1169-1175.

Scharton-Kersten, T., Yu, J., Vassell, R., O'Hagan, D., Alving, C.R., and Glenn, G.M. 2000. Transcutaneous immunization with bacterial ADP-ribosylating exotoxins, subunits, and unrelated adjuvants. Infect. Immun. 68: 5306-5313.

Seo, N., Tokura, Y., Nishijima, T., Hashizume, H., Furukawa, F., and Takigawa, M. 2000. Percutaneous peptide immunization via corneum barrier-disrupted murine skin for experimental tumor immunoprophylaxis. Proc. Natl. Acad. Sci. USA. 97: 371-376.

Shapira, M., Jibson, M., Muller, G., and Arnon, R. 1984. Immunity and protection against influenza virus by synthetic peptide corresponding to antigenic sites of hemagglutinin. Proc. Natl. Acad. Sci. USA. 81: 2461-2465.

Shi, Z., Curiel, D.T., and Tang, D.C. 1999. DNA-based non-invasive vaccination onto the skin. Vaccine 17: 2136-2141.

Shi, Z., Zeng, M., Yang, G., Siegel, F., Cain, L.J., van Kampen, K.R., Elmets, C.A., and Tang, D.C. 2001. Protection against tetanus by needle-free inoculation of adenovirus-vectored nasal and epicutaneous vaccines. J. Virol. 75: 11474-11482.

Strassburg, M.A., Greenland, S., Sorvillo, F.J., Lieb, L.E., and Habel, L.A. 1986. Influenza in the elderly: report of an outbreak and a review of vaccine effectiveness reports. Vaccine 4: 38-44.

Swenson, C.D., Cherniack, E.P., Russo, C., and Thorbecke, G.J. 1996. IgD-receptor up-regulation on human peripheral blood T cells in response to IgD *in vitro* or antigen *in vivo* correlates with the antibody response to influenza vaccination. Eur. J. Immunol. 26: 340-344.

Takigawa, M., Tokura, Y., Hashizume, H., Yagi, H., and Seo, N. 2001. Percutaneous peptide immunization via corneum barrier-disrupted murine skin for experimental tumor immunoprophylaxis. Ann. N. Y. Acad. Sci. 941: 139-146.

Tamura, S., Funato, H., Nagamine, T., Aizawa, C., and Kurata, T. 1989. Effectiveness of cholera toxin B subunit as an adjuvant for nasal influenza vaccination despite pre-existing immunity to CTB. Vaccine 7: 503-505.

Trach, D.D., Clemens, J.D., Ke, N.T., Thuy, H.T., Son, N.D., Canh, D.G., Hang, P.V., and Rao, M.R. 1997. Field trial of a locally produced, killed, oral cholera vaccine in Vietnam. Lancet 349: 231-235.

Van Hoecke, C., Prikazsky, V., Uto, I., and Menschikowski, C. 1996. Immunogenicity of an inactivated split influenza vaccine in institutionalized elderly patients. Gerontology 42: 190-198.

Vassell, R., Glenn, G.M., Udey, M.C., Scharton-Kersten, T., Alving, C.R., and Jakob, T. 1999. Activation of Langerhans Cells Following Transcutaneous Immunization. In 5th National Symposium, Basic Aspects of Vaccines, Bethesda, MD.

W.H.O. 1996. Reducing the risk of unsafe injections in immunization programmes: The role of injection equipment. In. World Health Organization, Geneva, Switzerland.

Watabe, S., Xin, K., Ihata, A., Liu, L., Honsho, A., Aoki, I., Hamajima, K., Wahren, B., and Okuda, K. 2001. Protection against influenza virus challenge by topical application of influenza DNA vaccine. Vaccine 19: 4434-4444.

Wester, R.C., and Maibach, H.I. 1992. Percutaneous absorption of drugs. Clin. Pharmacokinet. 23: 253-266.

Whittle, H.C., Lamb, W.H., and Ryder, R.W. 1987. Trials of intradermal hepatitis B vaccines in Gambian children. Ann. Trop. Paediatr. 7: 6-9.

Wolf, M., Hall, E., Taylor, D., Coster, T., Trespalacios, F., Cassels, F., deLorimier, A., and McQueen, C. 1999. Use of the human challenge model to characterize the immune response to the colonization factors of enterotoxigenic *Escherichia coli* (ETEC). In The 35th Joint Conference of the U.S.-Japan Cooperative Medical Science Program, Baltimore, MD.

Wolf, M.K., de Haan, L.A., Cassels, F.J., Willshaw, G.A., Warren, R., Boedeker, E.C., and Gaastra, W. 1997. The CS6 colonization factor of human enterotoxigenic *Escherichia coli* contains two heterologous major subunits. FEMS Microbiol. Lett. 148: 35-42.

Yu, J., Scharton-Kersten, T., Vassell, R., Cassels, F., Lyon, J., and Glenn, G.M. 2002. Mucosal protection from toxin challenge and production of *E. coli* colonization factor CS6 antibodies in mice vaccinated in a multivalent vaccine using transcutaneous immunization. Infect. Immun. 70: 1056-1068.

Yu, R.C., Abrams, D.C., Alaibac, M., and Chu, A.C. 1994. Morphological and quantitative analyses of normal epidermal Langerhans cells using confocal scanning laser microscopy. Br. J. Dermatol. 131: 843-848.

From: *Vaccine Delivery Strategies*
Edited by: Guido Dietrich and Werner Goebel

Chapter 4

Virosomes and Liposomes in Vaccinology

Rinaldo Zurbriggen

ABSTRACT

Liposomes and virosomes have been used for the delivery of a wide range of vaccines. Liposomes are vesicular structures limited by a bilayer membrane composed of phospholipids and cholesterol and were successfully employed the delivery of subunit vaccines. Recently, a novel vaccine antigen delivery system, so-called virosomes, has been developed by incorporating the hemagglutinin from influenza virus into liposomes. This influenza virus surface glycoprotein guides the virosomes to antigen-presenting cells and leads to fusion with their endosomal membrane. This process provides optimal processing and presentation of the antigens to immunocompetent cells and results in the elicitation of humoral and cellular immune responses.

INTRODUCTION

Immunization represents the most effective defense tool against microbial infections today. Although highly effective vaccines are currently available for a number of infectious diseases, vaccine formulations can still be improved. The induction of antigen-specific humoral and especially cell mediated immunity is crucial to the development of effective prophylactic and therapeutic vaccines. To achieve this immunity, a good combination of biochemical, immunological and virological concepts is needed.

Subunit immunogens, or peptides containing subsets of proteins from pathogens, represent powerful tools for manipulating the immune response in reaction to complex pathogens as an alternative to traditional vaccine formulations. Unfortunately, these antigens are often weakly immunogenic, or non-immunogenic. In addition, they are costly or are often only available in small quantities. Consequently, there is a definite need for new, effective, and safe adjuvants, as well as antigen carrier systems.

Possible vehicles for the presentation of antigens to the immune system include many substances (see Table 1), from the traditional aluminum-containing adjuvants which originated in 1926 (Glenny *et al.*, 1926) with their drawbacks and limitations (Collier *et al.*, 1979; Frost *et al.*, 1985; Clemmenson and Knudsen, 1980; Durand *et al.*,1992), to new promising preparations, like polymeric microspheres (Johansen *et al.*, 2000), ISCOMS (Horzinek, 1973; Morein *et al.*, 1984; Kersten, 1990) and liposomes (Ostro, 1987; Klausner *et al.*, 1984; Varkleij, 1984; Litzinger and Huang, 1992; Sato and Sunamoto, 1992; Storm *et al.*, 1991; Parker *et al.*, 1996; Rott *et al.*,1995).

Many studies have been carried out since the demonstration that liposomes could be used to enhance antibody responses (Allison and Gregoriadis, 1974). Today, the role of liposomes as adjuvants in vaccinology has gained much attention, especially with their characteristic of immune potentiation for a large number of different antigens (Morein and Simons, 1985; Boudreault and Thobodeau, 1985).

In this chapter I describe the development and present status of the use of liposomes as adjuvants and delivery systems in modern vaccinology.

Table 1. Vehicles for the presentation of antigens

Vehicle	Composition
Complete Freund's adjuvant	Drakeol 6VR (mineral oil), Arlacel (emulsifier), killed mycobacteria
Incomplete Freund's adjuvant	Drakeol 6VR (mineral oil) Arcacel (emulsifier)
Adjuvant 65	Peanut oil, Arcacel (emulsifier) Aluminium monostearate (stabilizer)
Titermax	Nonionic block polymer, squalene, stabilizer (unknown)
Ribi adjvant	Monophosphoryl lipid A, trehalose dicorynomycolate, squalene, Tween-80
Syntex adjuvant formulation	Pluronic L121 (Nonionic block polymer), squalene, Tween-80, muramyl dipeptide derivative
MF59	Microfluidized detergent-stabilized oil-in-water emulsion
QS-21	Purified saponin
Aluminium salts	Aluminium hydroxide or phosphate
Polymeric microspheres	Poly lactide-glycolide polymers (a.o.)
Liposomes	Phospholipids, cholesterol
ISCOMS	Quil A (saponin), cholesterol, phospholipid
AS02 (SBAS2)	Oil-in-water emulsion + MPL[®1] + QS-21
Montanide ISA-51	Stabilized oil-in-water emulsion
Montanide ISA-720	Stabilized water-in-oil emulsion

[2] MPL[®] - Monophosphoryl Lipid A

CLASSICAL ADJUVANTS

Adjuvants include a large group of compounds, which administered together with an antigen, stimulate the immune response against that antigen. Many substances are known to have such characteristics, such as some bacterial species (*Bordetella pertussis, Mycobacterium tuberculosis*); bacterial components (lipopolysaccharides, lipid A); natural adjuvants like saponins, or synthetic ones like non-ionic block polymers.

Most of the currently available vaccines are adjuvanted using aluminium salts. The adjuvant activity of aluminium salts was discovered around 1920, rather casually, during purification attempts of diphtheria toxoid, when it was seen that aluminium contamination of the antigen precipitated after the procedure induced a stronger antibody reaction than the untreated antigen. It is common to mix aluminum precipitates with weak antigens like in vaccines against diphtheria, tetanus, pertussis, meningococcal meningitis, hepatitis A and B, and more.

Although the mode of action of alum is still not fully understood, its adjuvant activity is mainly based on both serving as an antigen depot and inducing a localized inflammatory response (Gupta *et al.*, 1993). However, this is often accompanied by undesirable local adverse reactions, like erythema, subcutaneous nodules, contact hypersensitivity and granulomatous inflammation , as well as several systemic complications (Good *et al.*, 1992; Hendrick *et al.*, 1994).

Effective vaccines for certain infectious diseases need the induction of a cellular immune response and for the development of therapeutic vaccines, a stimulation of cytotoxic and helper T-lymphocytes is very important. Since alum-adjuvanted vaccines are not able to induce such a cell mediated immune response, there is a need for new adjuvants.

Several studies have shown that liposomes, artificial lipid vesicles formed by allowing phospholipids to swell in aqueous media which were first described in 1965 (Bangham *et al.*, 1965), are effective adjuvants for the induction of humoral and cellular immunity against a large number of antigens (Thérien *et al.*, 1990; Garçon and Six, 1991; Glück *et al.*, 1992; Alving, 1992).

Table 2. Nomenclature and description of various liposomes (from Szoka and Papahadjopoulos, 1980)

Liposome type	Abbreviation	Size (nm)	Mode of Preparation
Small unilamellar vesicles	SUV	25-50 30-100 100-200	Sonication Ethanol injection Detergent dialysis
Large unilamellar vesicles	LUV	150-250 200-1000	Ether infusion Calcium-induced fusion
LUV/reverse phase evaporation	REV	100-1000	Reverse phase evaporation
Large unilamellar vesicles by extrusion	LUVET	100-1000	Membrane extrusion
Multilamellar vesicles	MLV	25-100 400-5000	French Press extrusion Rotoevaporation
Freeze and thaw multilamellar vesicles	FT-MLV	100-500	Freeze and thaw MLV
Stable plurilamellar vesicles	SPLV	100-1000	Ether infusion/osmotic buffers

LIPOSOMES

Liposomes are artificial lipid vesicles, usually made up of biodegradable, non-toxic, non-immunogenic materials such as phospholipids, whose composition, size and specific targeting devices can be modified depending on their specific use. The formation of such artificial vesicles by allowing phospholipids to swell in aqueous media was first described by Bangham *et al.* (1965). Based on particle size and type of preparation, they can be classified into various types, as shown in Table 2.

The most common component is phosphatidylcholine (PC), a zwitterionic phospholipid, used as the basic phospholipid for the preparation of liposomes. The net surface charge can be changed depending on the incorporation of negatively charged lipids as dicetylphosphate, phosphatidylglycerol or phosphatidylserine or positively charged stearylamine.

Table 3. Examples of liposomal adjuvants (from R. Glueck, 2000)

Antigen	Reference
Diphtheria toxoid	Allison and Gregoriadis, 1974
Streptococcus mutans	Wachsmann *et al.*, 1986
Streptococcus sobrinus	Gregory *et al.*, 1986
Bacillus subtilis	Antimisiaris *et al.*, 1993
Plasmodium falciparum	Alving and Richards, 1990
Hepatitis A	Glueck, 1992
Hepatitis B	Manesis *et al.*, 1979
Influenza A and B	Glueck *et al.*, 1994
Herpes simplex virus	Lawman *et al.*, 1981
Adenovirus	Kramp *et al.*, 1982
Rabies virus	Perrin *et al.*, 1984
Rubella virus	Trudel *et al.*, 1982
Measles virus	Garnier *et al.*, 1991
Semliki Forest virus	Morein *et al.*, 1978
Sendai virus	Goodman-Snitkoff *et al.*, 1991
Synthetic peptides	Lifshitz *et al.*,1981; Friede *et al.*,1993

Liposomes have been initially used as model of lipid bilayers to investigate ion transport across cell membranes and furthermore for studying the reconstitution of membrane transport proteins and enzymes, the mode of action of ionophoric peptides and a variety of anesthetics and other drugs (Bangham, 1968; Bangham *et al.*, 1974). They have also played an important role in research areas such as membrane fusion, antigen-antibody interactions, the complement system, blood coagulation and arteriosclerosis (Brotherus *et al.*, 1981; Duzzqunes and Papahadjopoulos, 1983; Lüscher-Mattli *et al.*, 1993; Honegger *et al.*, 1980; Müller-Eberhard, 1988; Small and Shipley, 1974).

Since the first studies were published about their adjuvant properties (Allison and Gregoriadis, 1974), liposomes have been evaluated in various vaccine formulations based on many bacterial, viral or toxin antigens (Gregoriadis, 1990; Buiting *et al.*, 1992) and Table 3 shows a representative selection of such combinations.

Liposomes are able to elicit humoral and cellular immune responses (Pietrobon, 1995). In order to understand the adjuvantal activity of liposomes, many studies have been carried out on the interaction between liposomes and cells of the immune system. Macrophages play a key role in the immune-stimulatory action of the liposomes, being able, after phagocytosis of the carrier vesicles, to present antigenic material in the context of the MHC class II molecules to T helper cells, thus producing a humoral immune response (Gregoriadis, 1992; Szoka, 1992; Su and van Rooijen, 1989).

Another mechanism of action of liposomes is based on a prolonged retention of the antigen at the inoculation site and a depot mechanism responsible for slow release and presentation to macrophages and eventually also to other professional antigen presenting cells (APCs) such as dendritic cells.

Many studies were carried out as to the influence of several parameters in order to optimize the immune enhancement of liposomes. The influence of liposome type, size, epitope density (Kinsky *et al.*, 1983; Tadakuma *et al.*, 1980), phase transition temperature of the phospholipids (Dancey *et al.*, 1978), membrane fluidity (Grover and Sundharadas, 1986), cholesterol content (Bakouche and Gerlier, 1986), effect of encapsulation and covalent association with the bilayer and type of adjuvants have been tested. Unfortunately, the results of the different groups give no conclusive answer about the parameters affecting liposomal immunogenicity.

Liposomes may present antigens to immunocompetent cells by different ways. The antigen can be delivered at the surface of the liposomes, it can be entrapped into the liposomes or hydrophobic antigens can be intercalated in the liposomal membrane. The different delivery mechanisms affect the type of immune response that will be induced. If the antigen is cross-linked to the surface of the liposome, a humoral immune response will predominantly be induced. However, the insertion of a certain antigen into the liposome or into the liposomal bilayer may enhance its ability to stimulate the cellular immune response.

VIROSOMES

Virosomes represent a unique system for presentation of antigens to the immune system. First, virosomes closely resemble the envelope of the virus they are derived from and therefore constitute an antigen-presentation form superior to isolated surface antigens. In addition, properly assembled virosomes retain the membrane fusion activity of the naive virus and therefore, may be used to deliver encapsulated, unrelated, antigens to the cytosol of antigen-presenting cells. In this respect, virosomes differ from conventional liposomes which will target enclosed antigens primarily to the phagolysosomal system of macrophages. Both aspects of influenza derived

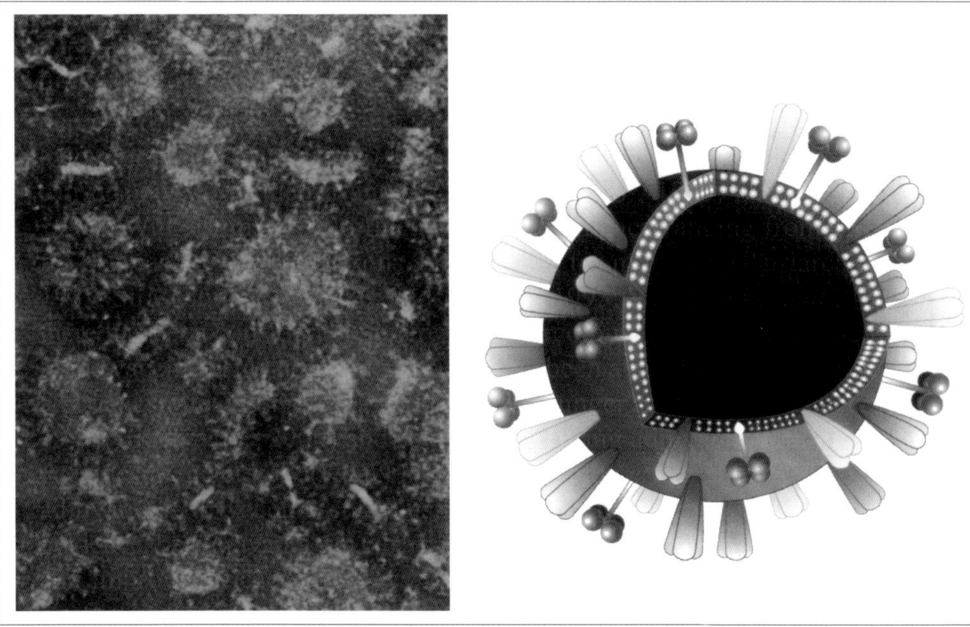

Figure 1. Electron microscopic image (magnification: x 500'000) and a schematic illustration of IRIVs. Source: Th. Wyler, Institute of Zoology, University of Berne, Switzerland.

virosomes have been exploited, to induce - firstly - enhanced influenza-specific antibody responses, and - secondly - CTL activity against virosome-encapsulated antigens.

Virosomes As An Antigen-Carrier System

Virosomes are vesicular particles reconstituted from viral envelopes (Glück *et al.,* 1992; Glück, 1995a, and 1995b; Glück and Wälti, 1996). They can be prepared in various ways, generally involving detergent-mediated disassembly of viral membranes, followed by separation of the viral capsid containing the genetic material from the dissolved membrane components, and, after optional addition of excess lipids, final removal of the detergent from the membrane components to induce reassembly of membranous vesicles carrying the viral surface proteins. By virtue of the fact that reconstituted viral envelopes closely mimic the outer surface of the virus they are derived from, virosomes represent a very useful system for presentation of antigens to induce antibody responses against the native virus (Almeida *et al.,* 1975; Glück *et al.,* 1994; Ando *et al.,* 1997; Boudreault and Thibodeau, 1985; El Guink *et al.,* 1989).

Immunopotentiating Reconstituted Influenza Virosomes (IRIV)

Immunostimulating reconstituted influenza virosomes (IRIVs) are spherical, unilamellar vesicles with a mean diameter of approx. 150 nm. IRIVs are prepared by detergent removal from influenza surface glycoproteins and a mixture of natural and synthetic phospholipids containing 70% egg yolk phosphatidylcholine (EYPC), 20% phosphatidylethanolamine (PE) and 10% envelope phospholipids originating from H1N1 influenza virus [A/Singapore/6/86] (Figure 1).

The approach adapted for virosomal vaccines is of particular interest, as it combines several components that are known to contribute to immunostimulation and that are at the same time harmless:

EYPC is known to be well tolerated in man and is an important constituent in commercial solutions for i.v. applications in undernourished persons. EYPC has been used in nearly all liposomal preparations which were produced for the enhancement of immune responses. PE was chosen for two reasons: First it is known that the hepatitis A virus (HAV) attachment to host cells occurs via binding to PE regions of the cell membrane (Seganti *et al.*, 1989). Furthermore, it has been shown that liposomes containing PE are able to directly stimulate B cells to produce antibodies without any T cell determinant being present (Garçon and Six, 1991). There were several reasons for including influenza virus envelope glycoproteins: The hemagglutinin (HA) plays a key role in the mode of action of the IRIVs. HA is the major antigen of influenza virus, containing epitopes on both HA1 and HA2 polypeptides, and is responsible for the fusion of the virus with the endosomal membrane (Durrer *et al.,* 1996; Tsurudome *et al.*, 1992). The HA1 globular head groups contain the sialic acid site for HA and it is therefore assumed that the IRIVs bind to such receptors of antigen presenting cells (e.g. macrophages, lymphocytes) initiating a successful immune response. The entry of influenza viruses into cells occurs through HA-receptor mediated endocytosis (Matlin *et al.,* 1981). It is likely that this mechanism also functions with the IRIV particles. The HA2 subunit of HA mediates the fusion of viral and endosomal membranes, which is required to initiate infection of cells. At the low pH of the host cell endosome (approx. pH 5), a conformational change occurs in the HA that is a prerequisite for fusion to occur. Fusion activity tests have shown that there was no difference of activity between natural influenza virus and virosomes. It is expected that this mediates the rapid release of the transported antigen into the membranes of

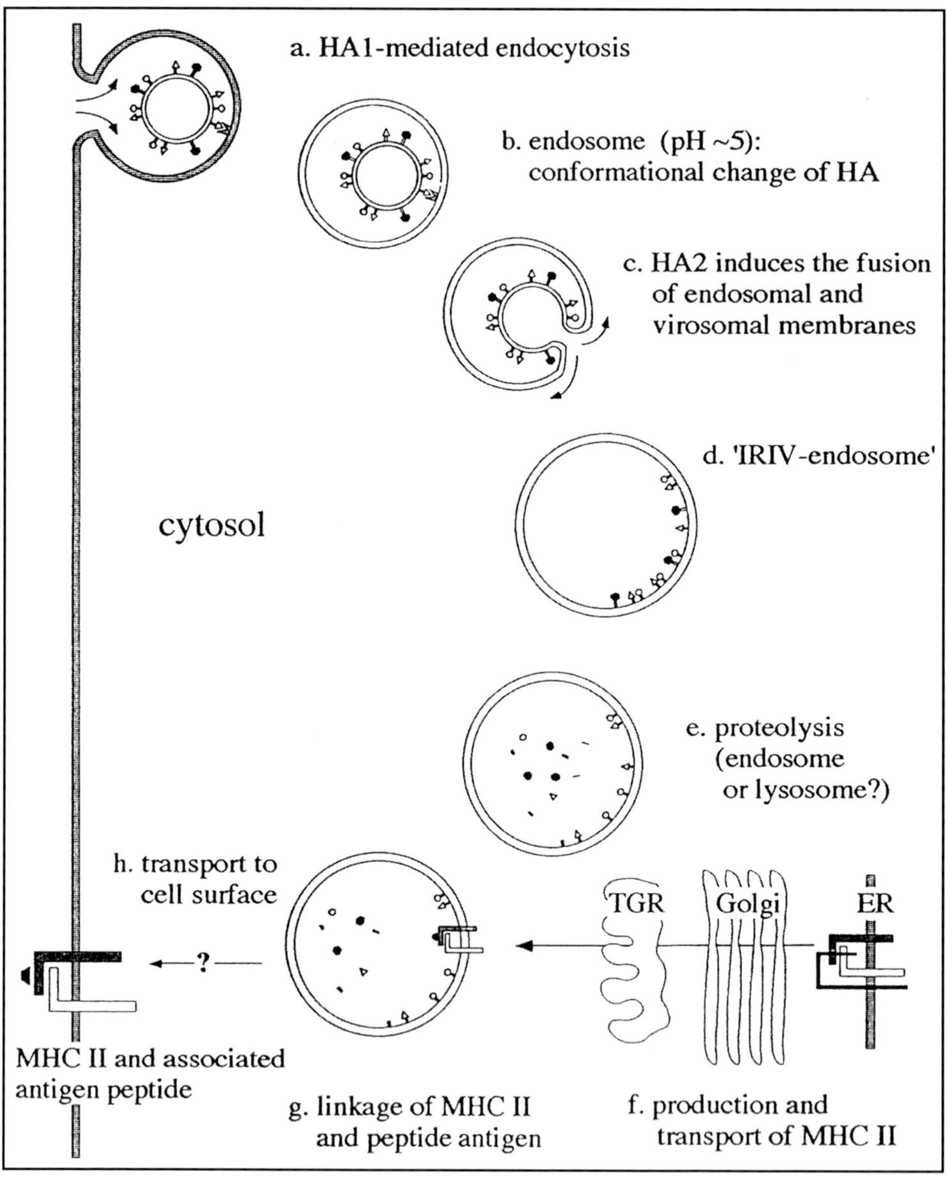

Figure 2. Immunological basis of immunostimmulation of IRIV-based Vaccines. A detailed description is provided in the text.

Table 4. Antibody response to different vaccine formulations

	Streptavidin	Streptavidin mixed with IRIV's	Strepavidin bound to IRIV's
Number of mice	5	5	5
Day 52 (GMT) [a]	15	61	71316

[a] Results are expressed as the geometric mean of reciprocal serum dilutions.

the target cells (Glück, 1995a). Figure 2 shows schematically the fusion mechanism of virosomes.

Using streptavidin as a model antigen, the adjuvant activity of the virosomal carrier system was shown (Zurbriggen *et al.,* 2000). In the mouse model, a mixture of the antigen with virosomes induced a 4-fold higher antibody immune response than strepavidin given alone. Delivery of the antigen via biotinilated virosomes led to an approximately 4500-fold higher antibody titer (in comparison to the antigen given alone and demonstrated the powerful capability of virosomes (Table 4).

Vaccines using conformationally defined, proteolytically stable, and highly immunogenic, artificial B-cell epitopes in small synthetic peptides or proteins could have a dramatic impact in medicinal chemistry. Synthetic peptide vaccines are currently under investigation to combat malaria, HIV, schistosomiasis, foot-and-mouth disease, and influenza, amongst others. Synthetic, conformational B-cell epitopes would offer a number of advantages over conventional protein-based vaccines including, a) ease of handling and storage of small inherently stable molecules rather than proteins, b) ease of synthesis, c) avoidance of problems associated with materials produced in cells, d) avoidance of other immune reactions associated with intact foreign proteins. The development of such synthetic peptide vaccines needs a delivery system that presents these epitopes to the immune system in a natural-like way and does not destroy the conformation of the epitopes. It has been shown that IRIVs are suitable for this purpose (Moreno *et al.,* 2001). Using the virosomal delivery system in the mouse model, synthetic, conformational malaria B-cell epitopes induced highly specific antibodies that cross-react with the parasite. In contrast, antibodies induced by the alum-formulated vaccine did not cross-react with the parasite.

Co-administered with the mucosal adjuvant *Escherichia coli* heat labile toxin (HLT), the virosomal vaccines induce a strong mucosal and systemic immune response. In clinical trials a nasal influenza vaccine was shown to be safe and highly immunogenic (Glück *et al.,* 1999).

Virosomes are also suitable as a DNA / RNA carrier system, since these fusogenic particles mimic a virus. The genetic material is enclosed in the virosome and is therefore protected from DNAase and RNAase. After the above described fusion event, the DNA / RNA is delivered into the cytosol of the „infected" cell and the expression of the coding antigen will start. In combination with the mucosal adjuvant HLT, even a mucosal application of this DNA / RNA-carrier is possible (Cusi *et al.,* 2000).

IRIV BASED LICENSED VACCINES

Although Paul Ehrlich mentioned the "magic bullet" about 75 years ago, the first liposomal vaccine for human use was licensed in 1996, a virosomal hepatitis A vaccine. This vaccine contains formalin-inactivated and highly purified hepatitis A viruses (HAV) of strain RG-SB, cultured on human diploid cells, which are coupled to the IRIV vesicle. Compared with a conventional aluminum adsorbed hepatitis A vaccine, the IRIV-based vaccine provided higher antibody titers and less local adverse events than an alum-adjuvanted formulation (Glück *et al.,* 1992). This vaccine is now registered in nearly all countries of the EU, the Americas and Asia.

The trivalent IRIV-formulated commercially available influenza vaccine has shown a very good immunogenicity in all age groups and also excellent tolerability (Conne *et al.,* 1997). The purified influenza membrane glycoproteins are incorporated into the lipid bilayer and are presented to the immune system in a natural way. The influenza hemagglutinin acts to physically stabilize the virosomes so they will maintain an appropriate particle size allowing for efficient uptake by macrophages and other antigens presenting cells.

These IRIV based vaccines are safe and do not engender any anti-phospholipid antibodies against the liposome components of the IRIV (Cryz *et al.,* 1996). The IRIV adjuvant represents the first alternative to the problematic old chemical aluminum salts.

IRIVs have shown their potential to induce a good and long lasting humoral immune response. In preclinical studies, the IRIV-based antigen delivery system is able to induce a cytotoxic T-cell response, an immune response necessary for therapeutic vaccines. The use of monoclonal antibodies, crosslinked to the IRIV's surface, could even target this cellular immune response to infected cells or to tumor cells.

ACKNOWLEDGEMENTS

I thank M. Zanoni and S. Rosenfellner for their help to prepare this manuscript

REFERENCES

Allison, A.C., and Gregoriadis, G. 1974. Liposomes as immunological adjuvants. Nature 252: 252-255.

Almeida, J.D., Edwards, D.C., Brands, C.M., and Heath, T.D. 1975. Formation of virosomes from influenza subunits and liposomes. The Lancet 2: 899-901.

Alving, C.R. 1992. Immunologic aspects of liposomes. Presentation and processing of liposomal protein and phospholipid antigens. Biochim. Biophys. Acta 1113: 307-322.

Alving, C.R., and Richards, R.L. 1990. Liposomes containing lipid A: A potent nontoxic adjuvant for a human malaria sporozoite vaccine. Immunol. Lett. 25: 275-280.

Ando, S., Tsuge, H., and Mayumi, T. 1997. Preparation of influenza virosome vaccine with muramyldipeptide derivative B30-MDP. J. Microencaps 14: 79-90.

Antimisiaris, S.G., Javasekera, P., and Gregoriadeis, G. 1993. Liposomes as vaccine carriers-incorporation of soluble and particulate antigens in giant vesicles. J. Immunol. Meth. 166: 271-280.

Bakouche, O., and Gerlier, D. 1986. Enhancement of immunogenicity of tumour virus antigen by liposomes: the effect of lipid composition. Immunology 58: 507-513.

Bangham, A.D. 1968. Membrane models with phospholipids. Prog. Biophys Mol. Biol. 18: 29-37.

Bangham. A.D., Hill, M.W., and Miller, N.G.A. 1974. Preparation and use of liposomes as models of biological membranes. In: Methods in Membrane Biology, E.D. Korn, ed. Plenum Press, New York. P. 1-23.

Bangham, A.D., Standish, M.M., and Watkins, J.C.D. 1965. Diffusion of univalent ions across the lamellae of swollen phospholipids. J. Mol. Biol. 13: 238-252.

Boudreault, A., and Thibodeau, L. 1985. Mouse response to influenza immunosomes. Vaccine 3: 231-234.

Brotherus, J.R., Griffith, O.H., and Brotherus, M.O. 1981. Lipid-protein multiple binding equilibria. Biochemistry 20: 5261-5267.

Buiting, A.M.J., van Rooijen, N., and Claassen, E. 1992. Liposomes as antigen carriers and adjuvants *in vivo*. Res. Immunol. 143: 541-548.

Clemmenson, O., and Knudsen, H.E. 1980. Contact sensitivity to aluminium in a patient hyposensitized with aluminum precipitated grass pollen. Contact Dermatitis 6: 305-308.

Collier, L.H., Polakoff, S., and Mortimer, J. 1979. Reactions and antibody responses to reinforcing doses of adsorbed and plain tetanus vaccines. Lancet 1: 1364-1368.

Conne, P., Gauthey, L., Vernet, P., Althaus, B., Que, J.U., Finkel, B., Glück, R., and Cryz, S.J. Jr. 1997. Immunogenicity of trivalent subunit versus virosome-formulated influenza vaccines in geriatric patients. Vaccine 15: 1675-1679.

Cryz, S.J., Que, J.U., and Glück, R. 1996. A virosome vaccine antigen delivery system does not stimulate an antiphospholipid antibody response in humans. Vaccine 14: 1381-1383.

Cusi, M.G., Zurbriggen, R., Valassina, M., Bianchi, S., Durrer, P., Valensin, P.E., Donati, M., and Glück, R. 2000. Intranasal Immunization with Mumps Virus DNA Vaccine Delivered by Influenza Virosomes Elicits Mucosal and Systemic Immunity. Virology 277(1): 111-118.

Dancey, G.F., Yasuda, T., and Kinsky, S.C., 1978. Effect of liposomal model membrane composition on immunogenicity. J. Immunol. 120: 1109-1113

Durand, C., Pineau, A., Bureau, B., and Stalder, J.F. 1992. Complications cutanée des vaccinations diphthérie, tétanus, coqueluche, poliomyélite (tetracoq), rôle de l'hydroxide d'alumine. Nuov. Dermatol. 11: 523-526.

Durrer, P., Galli, C., Hoenke, S., Corti, C., Glück, R., Vorherr, T., and Brunner, J. 1996. H+-induced membrane insertion of influenza virus hemagglutinin involves the HA2 amino-terminal fusion peptide but not the coiled coil region. J. Biol. Chem. 271: 13417-13421.

Duzzqunes, N., and Papahadjopoulos, D. 1983. Ionotropic effects on phosholipid membranes: calcium/magnesium specificity in binding, fluidity and fusion. In: Membrane Fluidity in Biology. R.C. Aloia, ed. Academic Press, New York. p.187-197.

El Guink, N., Kris, R.M., Goodman-Snitkoff, G., Small, P.A. Jr., Mannino, R.J. 1989. Intranasal immunization with proteoliposomes protects against influenza. Vaccine 7: 147-151.

Friede, M., Mueller, S., Briand, J.P., Van Regenmortel, M.H.V., and Schuber, F. 1993. Induction of immune response against a short synthetic peptide antigen coupled to small neutral liposomes containing monophospharyl lipid A. Mol. Immunol. 30: 539-547.

Frost, L., Johansen, P., Pedersen, S., Seien, N., Ostergaard, P.A., and Nielsen, M.M. 1985. Persistent subcutaneous nodulus in children hyposensitized with aluminium-containing allergen extracts. Allergy 40: 368-373.

Garçon, N.M., and Six, H.R. 1991. Universal Vaccine Carrier. Liposomes that provide T-dependent help to weak antigen. J. Immunol. 146: 3697-3702.

Garnier, F., Forquet, F., Bertolino, P., and Gerlier, D. 1991. Enhancement of *in vivo* and *in vitro* T-cell response against measles virus hemagglutinin after its incorporation into liposomes: Effect of the phospholipid composition. Vaccine 9: 340-345.

Glenny, A.T., Pope, C.G., Waddington, H., and Wallaca, U. 1926. The antigenic value of toxoid precipitated by potassium alum. J. Pathol. Bacteriol. 29: 31-40.

Glück, R. 1992. Immunopotentiating reconstituted influenza virosomes (IRIVs) and other adjuvants for improved presentation of small antigens. Vaccine 10: 915-919.

Glück, R. 1995a. Liposomal Presentation of Antigens for Human Vaccines. In: Vaccine Design. M.R. Powell, M.J., Newman, eds. Plenum Publishing Corporation, New York and London. p. 325-345.

Glück, R. 1995b. Liposomal hepatitis A vaccine and liposomal multiantigen combination vaccines. J. Liposome Res. 5: 467-479.

Glück, R., Mischler, R., Brantschen, S., Just, M., Althaus, B., and Cryz, S. Jr. 1992. Immunopotentiating reconstituted influenza virosome (IRIV) as vaccine delivery system for immunization against hepatitis Am. J. Clin. Invest. 90: 2491-2495.

Glück, R., Mischler, R., Finkel, B., Que, J.U., Scarpa, B., and Cryz, S.J. 1994. Immunogenicity of new virosome influenza vaccine in elderly people. Lancet 344: 160-163.

Glück, R., and Wälti, E. 1996. Are anti-phospholipid antibodies to be expected after proteoliposomal hepatitis A vaccination? J. Liposome Res. 6: 415-439.

Glück, U., Gebbers, J.O., and Glück, R. 1999. Phase 1 evaluation of intranasal virosomal influenza vaccine with and without *Escherichia coli* heat-labile toxin in adult volunteers. J. Virol. 73(9): 7780-7786.

Goodman-Snitkoff, G., Good, M.F., Berzofsky, J.A., and Mannino, R.J. 1991. Role of intrastructural/intermolecular help in immunization with peptide-phospholid complexes. J. Immunol. 147: 410-415.

Good, P.F., Perl, D.P., Bierer, L.M., and Schmeidler, J. 1992. Selective accumulation of aluminium and iron in the neurofibrillary tangles of

Alzheimer's disease: a laser microprobe (LAMMA) study. Ann. Neurol. 31: 286-292.

Gregoriadis, G. 1990. Immunological adjuvants: A role for liposomes. Immunol. Today 11: 89-97.

Gregoriadis, G. 1992. Liposomes as immunological adjuvants: approaches to immunopotentiation including ligand-mediated tergeting to macrophages. Res. Immunol. 143: 178-185.

Gregory, R.L., Michalek, S.M., Richardson, G., Harmon, C., Hilton, T., and McGhee, J.R. 1986. Characterization of immune response to oral administration of *Streptococcus sobrium* ribosomal preparation in liposomes. Infect. Immun. 54: 780-786.

Grover, A., and Sundharadas, G., 1986. Effect of liposomes on lymphocytes: induction of proliferation of B lymphocytes and potentiation of the cytotoxic response of T lymphocytes to alloantigens. Eur. J. Immunol. 16: 665-670

Gupta, R.K., Relyveld, E.H., Lindblad, E.B., Bizzini, B., Ben-Efraim, S., and Gupta, C.K. 1993. Adjuvants - a balance between their toxicity and adjuvanticity. Vaccine 11: 293-305.

Hendrick, M.J., Kass, P.H., Mc Gill, L.D., and Tizard, I.R. 1994. Postvaccinal sarcomas in cats. J. Natl. Cancer Inst. 86: 314-343.

Herzog, C. Abstracts, 37 the Interscience Conference on Antimicrobial Agents and Chemotherapy (ICCAC) / September 28 – October 1; 1997, Toronto, Canada.

Honegger, J.L., Isakron, P.C., and Kinsky, S.C. 1980. Murine immunogenicity of N-substituted phosphatidylethanolamine derivatives in liposomes: response to the hapten phosphocholine. J. Immunol. 124: 669-675.

Horzinek, M.C. 1973. The structure of togaviruses. Progress in Medical Virology. 16: 109-156

Johansen, P., Estevez, F., Zurbriggen, R., Merkle, H.P., Glück, R., Corradin, G., and Gander, B. 2000. Towards clinical testing of a single-administration tetanus vaccine based on PLA/PLGA microspheres. Vaccine 19(9-10): 1047-54.

Kersten, G., and Crommelin, D.J.A. 1995. Liposomes and ISCOMS as vaccine formulations. Biochim. Biophys. Acta. 1241: 117-138.

Kersten, G. 1990. Thesis. University of Utrecht, The Netherlands.

Kinsky, S.C., Loader, J.E., and Benson, A.L. 1983. An alternative procedure for the preparation of immunogenic liposomal model membranes. J. Immunol. Methods 65: 295-306.

Klausner, R.D., van Renswoude, J., and Rivnay, B. 1984. Reconstitution of membrane proteins. Methods Enzymol. 104: 340-347.

Kramp, W.J., Six, H.R., and Kasel, J.A. 1982. Post-immunization clearance of liposomes-entrapped adenovirus type 5 hexon. Proc. Soc. Exp. Biol. Med. 16: 135-139.

Lawman, M.J.P., Naylar, P.T., Huang, L., Courtney, R.J., and Rouse, B.T. 1981. Cell-mediated immunity to herpes simplex virus: Inductio of cytotoxic T-lymphocyte response by viral antigens incorporated into liposomes. J. Immunol. 126: 304-308.

Lifshitz, R., Gitler, C., and Mozes, E. 1981. Liposomes as immunological adjuvants in eliciting antibodies specific to the synthetic polypeptide Poly (L-Tyr, L-Glu) - Poly (DL-Ala) - Poly (L-Lys) with high frequency of site-associated idiotypic determinants, Eur. J. Immunol. 11: 398-410.

Litzinger, D.C., and Huang, L. 1992. Phosphatidylethanolamine liposomes: drug delivery, gene transfer and immunodiagnostic applications. Biochim. Biophys. Acta 1113: 201-227.

Lüscher-Mattli, M., Glück, R., Kempf, C., and Zanoni-Grassi, M.A. 1993. Comparative study on the effect of dextran sulfate on the fusion and *in vitro* replication of influenza A and B, Semliki Forest, vesicular stomatitis, rabies, Sendai and mumps virus. Arch Virol. 130: 317-326.

Matlin, K.S., Reggio, H., Helenius, A. and Simmons, K. 1981. Infections entry pathway of influenza virus in a canine kidney cell line. J. Cell. Biol. 91: 601-613

Morein, B., Helenius, A., Simons, K., Petterson, R., Kääriäinen, L., and Schirrmacher, V. 1978. Effective subunit vaccines against an enveloped virus. Nature 276: 715-718.

Morein, B., and Simons, K. 1985. Subunit vaccines against enveloped viruses: virosomes, micelles and other protein complexes. Vaccine 3: 83-93.

Morein, B., Sundquist, B., Hoglund, B., Dalsgaard, K., and Osterhaus, A.D.M.E. 1984. Iscom a novel structure for antigenic presentation of membrane proteins from enveloped viruses. Nature 308: 457-460.

Moreno, R., Jiang, L., Moehle, K., Zurbriggen, R., Glück, R., Robinson, J. A., and Pluschke, G. Exploiting conformationally constrained peptidomimetics and an efficient human compatible delivery system in synthetic vaccine design. ChemBioChem 2 838-834.

Müller-Eberhard, H.J. 1988. Molecular organization and function of the complement system. Ann. Rev. Biochem. 57: 321-347.

Ostro M.J. 1987. Liposomes. Sci. Am. 256: 90-99.

Parker, E.E., and Gould, K.G. 1996. Influenza A virus - a model for viral antigen presentation to cytotoxic T lymphocytes. Virology 7: 61-73.

Perrin, P., Thibodeau, L., Dauguet, C., Fritsch, A., and Sureau, P. 1984. Amplification des propriétés immunogènes de la glycoprotéine rabique par ancrage sur des liposomes préformés. Ann. Virol. (Inst. Pasteur) 135: 183-199.

Pietrobon, P.J.F. 1995. Liposome design and vaccine development. In: Vaccine Design. M.R. Powell, M.J., Newman, eds. Plenum Publishing Corporation, New York and London. p. 347-361.

Rott, O., Charreire, J., Semichonm M,, Bismuthm G., and Cash E. 1995. B cell superstimulatory influenza virus (H2-subtype) induces B cell proliferation by a PKC-activating Ca2+-independent mechanism. J. Immunology 154: 2092-2102.

Sato, T., and Sunamoto, J. 1992. Recent aspects in the use of liposomes in biotechnology and medicine. Prog. Lipid Res. 31: 345-372.

Seganti, L., Superti, F., Orsini, N., Gabrielli, R., Divizia, M., and Panà, A. 1989. Membrane lipid components interacting with hepatitis A virus. Microbiologica 12: 225-230.

Small, D.M., and Shipley, G.G. 1974. Physical-chemical basis of the lipid deposition in arteriosclerosis. Science 185: 222-229.

Storm, G., Wilms, H.P., and Crommelin, D.J.A. 1991. Liposomes and biotherapeutics. Biotherapy 3: 25-42.

Su, D., and Van Rooijen, N. 1989. The role of macrophages in the immunoadjuvant action of liposomes: effects of elimination of splenic macrophages on the immune response against intravenously injected liposome associated albumin antigen. Immunology 66: 466-470.

Szoka, F.C. Jr. 1992. The macrophage as the principal antigen-presenting cell for liposome-encapsulated antigens. Res. Immunol. 143: 186-187.

Tadakuma, T., Yasuda, T., Kinsky, S.C., and Pierce, C.W. 1980. The effect of epitope density on the *in vitro* immunogenicity of hapten-sensitized liposomal model membranes. J. Immunol. 124: 2175-2179.

Thérien, H.M., Lair, D., and Shahum, E. 1990. Liposomal vaccine: influence af antigen association on the kinetics of the humoral response. Vaccine 8: 558-562.

Trudel, M., Nadon, F., Comtois, R., Ravacarinoro, M., and Payment, P. 1982. Antibody response to rubella virus proteins in different physical forms. Antiviral Res. 2: 347-352.

Tsurudome, M., Glück, R., Graf, R., Falchetto, R., Schaller, U., and Brunner, J. 1992. Lipid interactions of the hemagglutinin HA2NH$_2$-terminal segment during influenza virus-induced membrane fusion. J. Biol. Chemistry 267, 28: 20225-20232.

Verkleij, A.J. 1984. Lipidic intramembranous particles. Biochim. Biophys. Acta. 779: 43-63.

Wachsmann, D., Klein, J.P., Schaller, M., Ogier, J., Ackermann, F., and Frank, R.M. 1986. Serum and salivery antibody response in rats orally immunized with *Streptococcus mutans* carbohydrate protein conjugate associated with liposomes. Infect. Immun. 52: 408-413.

Zurbriggen, R., Novak-Hofer, I., Seelig, A., and Glück, R. 2000. IRIV-adjuvanted hepatitis A vaccine: *in vivo* absorption and biophysical characterization. Prog. Lipid Res. 39(1): 3-18

From: *Vaccine Delivery Strategies*
Edited by: Guido Dietrich and Werner Goebel

Chapter 5

Enhancing DNA Vaccine Efficacy by Stress Protein-Facilitated Antigen Expression

Reinhold Schirmbeck and Jörg Reimann

ABSTRACT

In nucleic acid-based vaccination plasmid DNA containing antigen-encoding sequences is delivered in a way, that supports *in vivo* expression and immunogenic presentation of the protein. DNA vaccines are attractive candidates for the specific immunotherapy of extra- and intracellular pathogens and cancer because they prime neutralizing antibody and cytotoxic T cell responses. Antigen expressed from a DNA vaccine adopts its correct three-dimensional conformation (or oligomerization), ensuring the integrity of conformational epitopes binding neutralizing antibodies. DNA vaccines stimulate T cell responses to peptides generated in (endogenous or exogenous) processing pathways (without interference by viral proteins). Currently, DNA vaccines are developed that codeliver intrinsic adjuvants to enhance and/or modulate the immune response. We have developed a technology for the expression of heat shock protein (hsp)-bound chimeric proteins and their immunogenic delivery as DNA-based vaccines that is described in this review. This system illustrates the versatility of the DNA vaccination that offers exciting prospects for preclinical (experimental) and clinical (applied) immunotherapy protocols.

POLYNUCLEOTIDE-BASED VACCINES

The DNA-based vaccine in its simplest form is a 2-10 kb closed circular, double-stranded, supercoiled plasmid DNA containing a bacterial backbone (with the origin of replication and selection markers) and a transcription unit (encoding the antigen and appropriate promoter/enhancer sequences). Many commercially available expression vectors have been used successfully as DNA vaccines. The plasmid DNA has to reach the nucleus for transcription, should not replicate in eukaryotic cells, and can be designed to minimize the chances for integration into the host cell genome. Expression of protein from the antigen-encoding transcription unit is driven by strong promoter/enhancer sequences from (cytomegalo, papova or retro) viruses, bacteria (*Borrelia*), or mammalian cells (elongation factor-1α, desmin or metallothionin promoters) (Tang *et al.*, 1992; Ulmer *et al.*, 1993; Johnston and Tang, 1994; Raz *et al.*, 1994; Michel *et al.*, 1995; Simon *et al.*, 1996). Systems that amplify the level of mRNA and hence antigen expression in the cytoplasm are available, e.g. Semliki forest virus-derived vector systems (Zhou *et al.*, 1995). Vectors can be designed to co-express different antigens, or antigen and cytokine/chemokine(s). A simple example is the construction of fusion proteins as "polyepitope vaccines"(Thomson *et al.*, 1996), "multivalent minigene vaccines" (An and Whitton, 1997), antigen/cytokine fusion vaccines (Kim *et al.*, 1997c; Maecker *et al.*, 1997), or antigen/costimulator fusion constructs (Boyle *et al.*, 1998). Alternative techniques used successfully to codeliver in a DNA vaccine either different antigens, or antigen and cytokine include:

(i)   the injection of a mixture of different expression plasmids,
(ii)   the construction of large plasmids that contain multiple, independent transcription units, or
(iii) the coating of different expression plasmids on particles that are used to deliver DNA *via* the skin with the gene gun.

In some of these approaches, the codelivered cytokine, chemokine or costimulator molecule has been shown to enhance the magnitude of the immune response and/or modified its polarization (Xiang and Ertl, 1995;

Bueler and Mulligan, 1996; He *et al.*, 1996a and 1996b; Kwak *et al.*, 1996; Mahvi *et al.*, 1996; Chow *et al.*, 1997; Corr *et al.*, 1997; Geissler *et al.*, 1997; Iwasaki *et al.*, 1997; Kim *et al.*, 1997a, 1997b, 1998a, 1998b; Okada *et al.*, 1997; Tsuji *et al.*, 1997a and 1997b; Gurunathan *et al.*, 1998; Larsen *et al.*, 1998; Sin *et al.*, 1998, 1999; Kimura *et al.*, 1999; Kipps and Mendoza, 1999; Lu *et al.*, 1999). These approaches do not support the coordinated expression of different proteins (different antigens, or antigen and cytokine/chemokine) at stochiometrically defined ratios in the same antigen-presenting cell (APC). To achieve this goal, complex vector systems have to be constructed. Antigen and/or cytokine proteins can be coexpressed either in polycistronic constructs (Dirks *et al.*, 1993; Johanning *et al.*, 1995; Huang, 1996; Clarke *et al.*, 1997; Wild *et al.*, 1998), or in expression constructs using bidirectional promoters (Kwissa *et al.*, 2000). This supports the coexpression of extensive immunogenic information of a pathogen with optimal adjuvants activity in a DNA vaccine.

Antigen-encoding nucleic acid delivered in genetic immunization is usually plasmid DNA. Few examples of successful vaccination with antigen-encoding mRNA have been reported (Martinon *et al.*, 1993; Conry *et al.*, 1995; Boczkowski *et al.*, 1996; Qiu *et al.*, 1996; Hoerr *et al.*, 2000). Although the large-scale production of mRNA is difficult to achieve, the delivery of RNA instead of DNA offers the advantages of higher transfection/expression efficiency and low safety concerns.

STRATEGIES FOR DNA DELIVERY

Different delivery techniques and delivery routes have been explored to vaccinate animals and man with plasmid DNA. All delivery techniques currently available are clearly suboptimal in species other than the mouse. It is uncertain which delivery technique will eventually find its way into widespread clinical use of DNA vaccines. Four techniques have been often used to deliver DNA vaccines:

(i) The intramuscular or subcutaneous injection of non-packaged ('naked') plasmid DNA (10 µg to 100 µg per mouse) (Jiao *et al.*, 1992; Wolff *et al.*, 1992; Davis *et al.*, 1993).

(ii) The intramuscular or subcutaneous injection of plasmid DNA packaged into liposomes, lipoplexes, polymers or virosomes (1 µg to 50 µg per mouse) (Nabel *et al.*, 1992; Martinon *et al.*, 1993; Harrison *et al.*, 1995; Yokoyama *et al.*, 1996; Ishii *et al.*, 1997; Liu *et al.*, 1997; Toda *et al.*,

1997; Dow *et al.*, 1999; Klavinskis *et al.*, 1999; Goldman *et al.*, 1997; Chen *et al.*, 1998; Kwoh *et al.*, 1999). Packaged plasmid DNA can prime an immune response when injected intramuscularly, subcutaneously, intradermally, intravenously, intraperitoneally or into tumors, or when the formulation is applied onto mucosal surfaces (Plautz *et al.*, 1994; Goldman *et al.*, 1997; Ishii *et al.*, 1997; Liu *et al.*, 1997; Chen *et al.*, 1998; Dow *et al.*, 1999; Klavinskis *et al.*, 1999; Kwoh *et al.*, 1999).

(iii) The intra-epidermal delivery of 10 ng to 1 µg plasmid DNA coated onto 0.5 - 3 µm gold particles (50-300 DNA molecules per particle) 'shot' into the skin with the gene gun (Williams *et al.*, 1991; Tang *et al.*, 1992; Eisenbraun *et al.*, 1993; Fynan *et al.*, 1993; Johnston and Tang, 1994; Vahlsing *et al.*, 1994; Fuller *et al.*, 1995, 1996; Jenkins *et al.*, 1995; Pertmer *et al.*, 1995; Sun *et al.*, 1995; Yang and Sun, 1995; Zarozinski *et al.*, 1995; Haynes *et al.*, 1996; Keller *et al.*, 1996; Mahvi *et al.*, 1996; Qiu *et al.*, 1996; Choi *et al.*, 1997; Feltquate *et al.*, 1997; Leitner *et al.*, 1997; Prayaga *et al.*, 1997; Tanelian *et al.*, 1997; Torres *et al.*, 1997; Macklin *et al.*, 1998; Porgador *et al.*, 1998). The skin is the preferred site for inoculation of particle-coated plasmid DNA with the gene gun but exposed muscle surfaces and mucosal surfaces have also been successfully used for particle bombardment (Tang *et al.*, 1992; Eisenbraun *et al.*, 1993; Fynan *et al.*, 1993; Vahlsing *et al.*, 1994; Jenkins *et al.*, 1995; Pertmer *et al.*, 1995; Zarozinski *et al.*, 1995; Keller *et al.*, 1996; Qiu *et al.*, 1996; Choi *et al.*, 1997; Feltquate *et al.*, 1997; Leitner *et al.*, 1997; Prayaga *et al.*, 1997; Torres *et al.*, 1997; Macklin *et al.*, 1998).

(iv) Genetic vaccination via the mucosal route. Preferred is the intranasal immunization with plasmid DNA-lipid complexes that primes IgA/IgG antibody and cytotoxic T lymphocyte (CTL) responses in the respiratory, intestinal and genital mucosa as well as in the spleen and peripheral lymph nodes (Fynan *et al.*, 1993; Keller *et al.*, 1996; Bagarazzi *et al.*, 1997; Ban *et al.*, 1997; Etchart *et al.*, 1997; Kuklin *et al.*, 1997; Okada *et al.*, 1997; Wang *et al.*, 1997; Livingston *et al.*, 1998; Sasaki *et al.*, 1998a and 1998b; Klavinskis *et al.*, 1999; Eo *et al.*, 2001).

PRIMING AN IMMUNE RESPONSE BY DNA VACCINES

A single inoculation of a DNA vaccine using an appropriate delivery technique and a suitable route readily primes long-lasting serum antibody and T cell responses against a wide spectrum of viral, bacterial, parasitic and tumor antigens in different animal species (e.g., mice, rats, woodchuck, pig, rabbit, sheep, cattle, dogs, monkeys, chimps, fish, chicken) and in man. Because protein antigen is expressed *in situ* in its native conformation (with posttranslational modifications such as e.g. glycosylation, proteolytic processing, lipid conjugations), antibody responses against native epitopes including protective (neutralizing) antibody responses predominate the humoral immune response elicited by DNA vaccines.

DNA vaccination is furthermore an exceptionally potent strategy to stimulate a T cell response. Different mechanisms seem to be involved in priming T cells by genetic vaccination. Intramuscular vaccination with a high dose of plasmid DNA seems to depend on 'cross-priming', i.e. antigenic material produced by transiently transfected cells gains access to professional, bone marrow-derived APC (Doe *et al.*, 1996; Ulmer *et al.*, 1996; Corr *et al.*, 1996). In contrast, intradermal delivery of low amounts of plasmid DNA with the gene gun results in the transfection of resident dendritic cells (DC) that rapidly migrate to regional lymph nodes after DNA uptake where they initiate the immune response (Porgador *et al.*, 1998).

THE POLARIZATION PROFILE OF THE IMMUNE RESPONSE PRIMED BY DNA VACCINES

Alternative polarization profiles of the immune response are induced by different DNA vaccination approaches. A single injection of either a high dose (50-100 µg/mouse) of non-packaged plasmid DNA encoding antigen delivered intramuscularly or subcutaneously, or 1 µg particle-coated plasmid DNA delivered intradermally usually primes a serum antibody response of similar magnitude and longevity but strikingly different isotype profile. Priming mice by an intramuscular injection of 100 µg plasmid DNA stimulates a long-lasting T helper cell (Th) type 1 immune response that includes specific activation of a potent major histocompatibility complex (MHC)-I-restricted CTL response. In contrast, priming mice with an intradermal injection of a low dose of plasmid DNA (0.1-1 µg/mouse) stimulates a long-lasting Th2 immune response but no CTL response. This polarization pattern is confirmed by analyses on the cytokine expression profile of the primed T cells: while interferon-γ (IFN-γ)-producing T cells are preferentially primed by the injection of high doses of non-packaged plasmid DNA, IL-4-, IL-5- and IL-10-producing T cells predominate after intradermal delivery of low doses of particle-bound plasmid DNA with the gene gun (Feltquate *et al.*, 1997).

We have studied the immune response of mice to different antigens of the hepatitis B virus (HBV). Important antigens of HBV are the hepatitis B surface antigen HBsAg (a 20-30 nm lipoprotein particle composed of 100-150 subunits of the 226 residue p24/gp27 small HBsAg or surface S protein) and the hepatitis B core antigen HBcAg (a 28 nm protein particle composed of 180 subunits of the 185 residue p21 core protein). A single intramuscular or subcutaneous injection of either 100 μg non-packaged plasmid DNA encoding HBsAg (pCI/S), or a single intradermal injection of 1μg particle-coated pCI/S plasmid DNA primed serum antibody responses of similar magnitude and longevity but strikingly different isotype profiles. The i.m. injection of 100 μg pCI/S DNA stimulated long-lasting IgG2a serum antibody and potent MHC-I-restricted CTL responses. In contrast, priming mice with an intradermal injection of a low dose of pCI/S DNA (0.1-1 μg/mouse) stimulated long-lasting IgG1 serum antibody but no CTL response. This was confirmed by the cytokine expression profile of T cells primed *in vivo* by the two alternative DNA delivery strategies: interferon-γ (IFN-γ)-producing T cells were preferentially primed by the injection of 100 μg pCI/S plasmid DNA, but IL-4-, IL-5- and IL-10-producing T cells predominated after intradermal delivery of 100 ng or 1 μg pCI/S plasmid DNA with the gene gun. The H-2 haplotype or the genetic background of the immunized mice had no major influence on priming these alternative phenotypes of the immune response to HBsAg by the two different DNA vaccination protocols (R.S., unpublished data). A similar polarization of immune responses elicited by the two alternative techniques of DNA-based vaccination has been reported (Feltquate *et al.*, 1997). CTL priming to HBsAg by DNA vaccination is CD4[+] T cell-dependent (Wild *et al.*, 1999). This is unexpected because the immunostimulatory effect of bacterial plasmid DNA facilitates CD4[+] T cell-independent priming of naïve CD8[+] CTL precursors. The CD4[+] T cell-dependence of the immune response stimulated by DNA-based vaccination points to a regulatory control that may determine the polarization of the response.

Vaccination using the 'gene gun' delivery of low doses of DNA intradermally preferentially primes a Th2 response and fails to prime CTL. Many factors may contribute to the exclusive Th2 priming in this system, such as e.g.

intrinsic features of this DNA delivery technique, the low dose of DNA injected, the intradermal route of DNA transfer, or the type of antigen used for vaccination. The local skin area in which the gene gun-delivered plasmid DNA is expressed can be conditioned to support priming of Th1 immune reactivity. A single subcutaneous injection of 20-50 μg oligodesoxynucleotide (ODN) at the site of the intradermal DNA inoculation shifts the polarization of the elicited immune response to HBsAg towards the Th1 phenotype. This treatment allows efficient priming of a HBsAg-specific CTL response and shifts the IgG1/IgG2a ratio of the serum antibody response from 80 to <1. To change the polarization of the immune response, the ODN has to be delivered locally at the site of particle injection from 48 h prior to, till 48 h after the gene gun vaccination. In addition to ODN, cytokines (IL-12, IL-18) can change the Th2 into a Th1 response pattern in this system. The condition of the skin patch used for DNA inoculation by the gene gun thus critically influences the polarization of the elicited immune response (Feltquate *et al*, 1997). Conditioning of the skin to support priming of a Th1 response by the gene gun may be of practical interest for the design of CTL-stimulating DNA vaccines against persistent virus infections or cancer.

Boosting an established Th2 response by an intramuscular injection of 100 μg pCI/S DNA shifts the response towards a Th1 phenotype. This prime/ boost protocol efficiently elicits a HBsAg-specific CTL response and shifts the IgG1/IgG2a ratio from 100 to <1. A similar shift in the response pattern might operate when a vaccine-induced Th2 response is boosted by the relevant natural virus infection. The instability of a Th2 response is in striking contrast to the stability of an established Th1 response. Boosting an established Th1 response by e.g. intradermal injection of low doses of pCI/S plasmid DNA with the gene gun enhances HBsAg-specific serum antibody titers, does not change the serum antibody isotype profile, and does not suppress CTL reactivity to HBsAg. The stability of established Th1 or Th2 polarizations of the murine immune response to HBsAg thus differs: it is easy to shift a Th2 into a Th1 response, it is difficult to shift an established Th1 into a Th2 response (Schirmbeck and Reimann, 2001).

Neonatal mice primed within 24 h after birth by a single i.m. injection of 100 μg pCI/S DNA develop a specific CTL response and IgG1 antibody response (IgG1/IgG2a ratio >50) to HBsAg. This Th2 response is detectable for at least 4 months after a single neonatal DNA injection. This confirms the experience that neonatal animals preferentially generate a Th2 response (Kovarik and Siegrist, 1998; Hogan *et al.*, 1998). Interestingly, CTL were efficiently primed neonatally in this Th2 immune response to HBsAg.

CO-DELIVERING OF INTRINSIC ADJUVANT ACTIVITY WITH DNA VACCINES

In contrast to the intradermal vaccination with pCI/S DNA (that primes a Th2 immune response), the intradermal vaccination with HBcAg-encoding pCI/C plasmid DNA elicits a Th1 response. Intrinsic properties of an antigen are known to have a decisive influence on the type of specific immunity they elicit. Recombinant DNA technology makes it easy to construct chimeric proteins that contain different antigenic domains and intrinsic immune enhancing and/or modulating domains. A recently reported example is particularly informative for the potential usefulness of this concept. Mice were vaccinated with DNA constructs that encoded the same immunogenic domain fused to two alternative, immunomodulating domains binding either to the L-selectin-binding receptor on high endothelial cells (to target the antigen to lymph nodes), or to costimulator molecules on APC (CD80/86) (Boyle *et al.*, 1998). Both targeting strategies enhanced the immune response to the antigenic domains but resulted in strikingly different polarization profiles of the immune response against the same antigenic determinant. This indicated that chimeric antigens can be designed to preferentially prime a Th1 or Th2 immune response.

Co-delivery of cytokines (GM-CSF, IFN-I, IL2, IL4, IL6, IL10, IL12, IL15, TNF) (Xiang and Ertl, 1995; Bueler and Mulligan, 1996; Kwak *et al.*, 1996; Mahvi *et al.*, 1996; Rakhmilevich *et al.*, 1996; Chow *et al.*, 1997; Geissler *et al.*, 1997; Iwasaki *et al.*, 1997; Kim *et al.*, 1997a, 1997c, 1998b; Maecker *et al.*, 1997; Okada *et al.*, 1997; Tsuji *et al.*, 1997a; Larsen *et al.*, 1998; Sin *et al.*, 1998, 1999; Kimura *et al.*, 1999; Kipps and Mendoza, 1999; Lu *et al.*, 1999; Okubo *et al.*, 1999; Barouch *et al.*, 2000; Chow *et al.*, 2000; Kusakabe *et al.*, 2000; Noisakran and Carr, 2000; Harle *et al.*, 2001), chemokines (Kipps and Mendoza, 1999; Lu *et al.*, 1999; Youssef *et al.*, 1999 and 2000; Eo *et al.*, 2001) or ligand-binding domains of costimulator (CD80, CD86, CD40L, LFA-3) molecules (Bueler and Mulligan, 1996; He *et al.*, 1996a; Iwasaki *et al.*, 1997; Kim *et al.*, 1997b; Tsuji *et al.*, 1997b; Gurunathan *et al.*, 1998; Horspool *et al.*, 1998; Kim *et al.*, 1998a; Santra *et al.*, 2000; Sin *et al.*, 2000) with antigens can enhance and/or modulate their immunogenicity. DNA vaccination protocols have been reported in which these enhancing or modulating factors are either delivered as expression constructs mixed with antigen-encoding DNA, or coexpressed with antigen as fusion constructs or in polycistronic vector systems, or coated onto particles for gene gun delivery together with the antigen-encoding DNA.

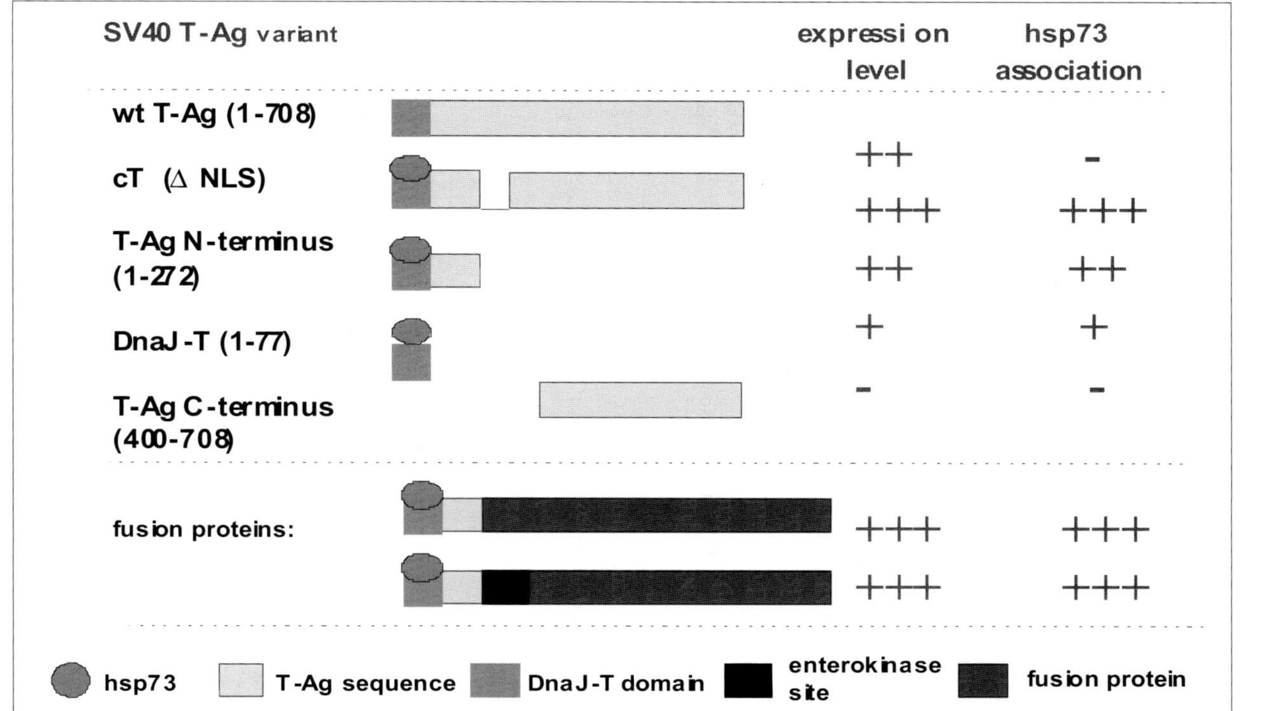

Figure 1. Hsp 70 binds to the N-terminus of mutant SV40 Ag. Wild-type (wt) SV40 large T (tumor) antigen (T-Ag) is readily expressed as a nucleoprotein in mammalian cells; the expressed protein is not stably associated with the cytosolic stress protein hsp73. Mutant T-Ag, *e.g.* the cytosolic cT-Ag mutant and the T1-272 or T1-77 N-terminal fragments are readily expressed and their expression shows stable association with hsp73. C-terminal T-Ag fragments are not expressed. Expression vectors were developed that allow expression of 30-800 aa residue chimeric protein cloned behind the hsp73-binding T-Ag fragments.

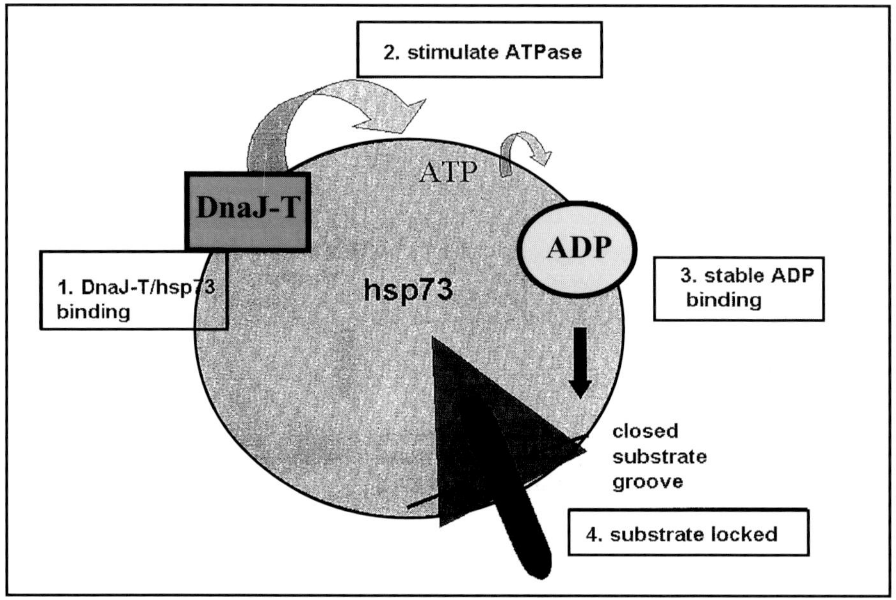

Figure 2. Transfected cells express mutant T-Ag or T-fusion proteins. The DnaJ-T structure on these newly synthesized molecules interacts with cellular hsp73 and stimulates the hsp73 intrinsic ATPase activity. This generates stable ADP bound hsp73/DnaJ-T complexes. The DnaJ-T also contained an hsp73 substrate binding site that might be involved in the long-term stability of the complexes.

STRESS PROTEIN-FACILITATED PRIMING OF THE IMMUNE RESPONSE BY CHIMERIC DNA VACCINES

We have developed a technology to express stress protein-bound chimeric antigens as DNA vaccines. Chimeric proteins (containing domains or epitopes of different antigens) are difficult to express. Expression of such polyepitope vaccines was facilitated by non-covalently associating the chimeric antigen with heat shock protein (hsp). This provided intrinsic 'natural' adjuvant activity to the antigen and enhanced their immunogenicity.

This expression system was developed during work in the simian virus 40 (SV40) large T antigen (T-Ag) system. Unexpectedly, we found stable expression of mutant T-Ag variants with an intact N-terminus in eukaryotic cells. The stable association of a cytosolic heat shock protein (hsp) of the hsp70 family, i.e. hsp73, with mutant or truncated cytoplasmic proteins has been demonstrated in SV40 T-Ag-transformed cells, i.e., hsp73 stably binds to mutant but not a wild-type polyomavirus T-Ag (Grussenmeyer *et al.*, 1985;

Hsp73-regulated Expression of Chimeric Antigens with an 77aa DnaJ-T Domain

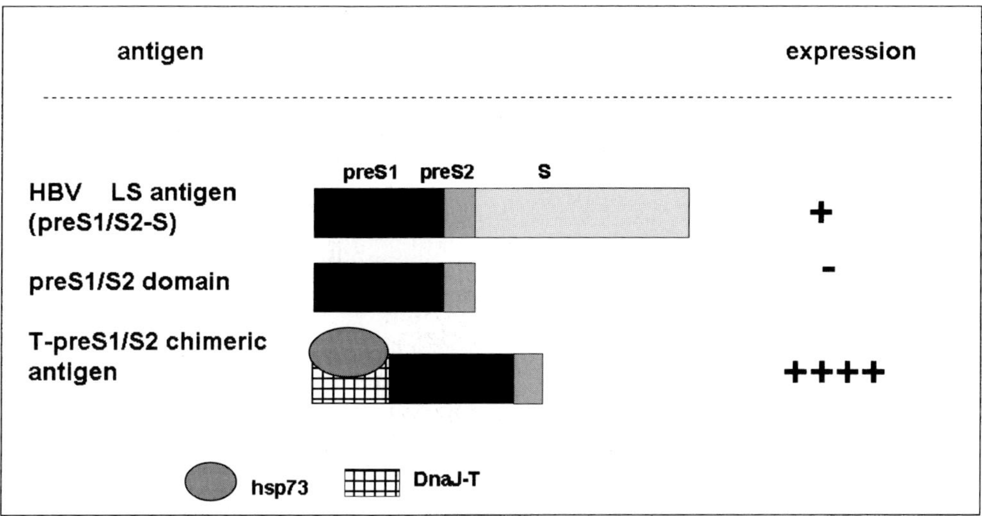

Figure 3. Hsp73-regulated expression of chimeric antigens with a 77 aa DnaJ-T domain. A unique advantage of the hsp73- mediated expression system is that even protein domains could be produced that could not be expressed using conventional vector constructs (*e.g.* the HBV preS1-preS2- domain).

Walter *et al.*, 1987; Sawai and Butel, 1989). We have demonstrated that mutant T-Ag accumulates within cells in tight association with the constitutively expressed, cytoplasmic hsp73 (Figure 1) (Schirmbeck and Reimann, 1994). The N-terminal 77 amino acid sequence of the SV40 T-Ag (with strong DnaJ homology) is required for the strong, non-covalent binding to hsp73, and is essential for the intracellular stability of the mutant proteins. Because of its DnaJ homology, this N-terminal sequence of the nucleoprotein of papovaviruses has a docking site to hsp73, binds to a regulatory site of hsp73 (that facilitates conversion of ATP to ADP), and binds as a substrate to hsp73 (to its substrate-binding site that has increased substrate binding avidity after ATP-to-ADP conversion) (Figure 2). Hence, the N-terminal 77 aa can mediate docking to, regulating of, and substrate binding to constitutively expressed, cytosolic hsp73 molecules.

Expression vectors were developed from these observations that allow expression of up to 800 residue chimeric proteins cloned behind the hsp73-binding (DnaJ-homologuous) T-Ag N-terminus (Figure 1). More than 30 different viral antigens (containing antibody- and CTL-defined epitopes) have been successfully expressed in this system. A unique advantage of this system is that even protein domains could be produced that could not be expressed using conventional vectors (e.g. the HBV preS domain) (Figure 3), or were toxic for the producer cell lines (e.g. HBV X-protein)

MULTIPLE EFFECTS OF STRESS PROTEINS ON THE IMMUNOGENICITY OF PROTEINS AND PEPTIDES

Proteins of the hsp70/90 family are immunodominant antigens of many bacterial and parasite infections (reviewed in Young and Elliott, 1989; Kaufmann *et al.*, 1991; Murray and Young, 1992; Sanchez *et al.*, 2001). Furthermore, hsp molecules are potent 'natural' adjuvants (Suzue and Young, 1996; Roman and Moreno, 1997; Birk *et al.*, 1999; Breloer *et al.*, 1999; Todryk *et al.*, 1999). Hsp molecules bind to surface receptors (Arnold *et al.*, 1999; Singh *et al.*, 2000b; Sondermann *et al.*, 2000) that seem to include CD91 (α2 macroglobulin receptor) (Binder *et al.*, 2000b; Basu *et al.*, 2001; Binder *et al.*, 2001), TLR2/4 (Vabulas *et al.*, 2001) and/or CD14 (Asea *et al.*, 2000). Hsp70/90 molecules activate antigen-presenting cells (APC) including macrophages and dendritic cells (DC) (Tabona *et al.*, 1998; Byrd *et al.*, 1999; Kol *et al.*, 1999; Todryk *et al.*, 1999; Singh *et al.*, 2000a; Yoo *et al.*, 2000; Cho *et al.*, 2000), trigger DC migration to lymph nodes (Binder *et al.*, 2000a), and stimulate their cytokine/chemokine release (IL6, TNF, IL1 β, IL12, IL15, IFNγ, β-chemokines) (Tabona *et al.*, 1998; Todryk *et al.*, 1999; Paul *et al.*, 2000). Hsp/antigen complexes are involved in MHC class II (Lakey *et al.*, 1987; Michalek *et al.*, 1992; Niebling and Pierce, 1993; Pepin et al., 1996) and class I (see below) antigen processing and presentation. Hsp molecules support CD4[+] T helper-independent priming of a CTL response when delivered as an exogenous complex with antigens at low doses without additional adjuvants (Chen *et al.*, 2000; Cho *et al.*, 2000). These data indicate a striking 'innate adjuvant effect' of hsp70/90 molecules on APC recruitment, traffic, maturation, processing, presentation and cytokine/chemokine production.

HSP FACILITATES CTL PRIMING

The most striking adjuvant effect of stress proteins is on priming a MHC class I-restricted CTL response. Hsp73 binds peptides in an extended conformation by hydrogen-bonding, hydrophobic contacts and salt bridges presumably through its putative α-helical channel structure or groove

(Hightower *et al.*, 1994). Preferred substrates for hsp70 chaperones are hydrophobic residues that may include some basic but no acidic residues. Hsp73 seems to distinguish between the folded and the unfolded forms of the same protein, binding only to the latter. Hsp70 molecules probably do not show the exquisite length and motif restrictions of peptide binding characteristic for MHC molecules. Heat shock proteins apparently transfer peptides during antigen processing and CTL priming (Srivastava *et al.*, 1994). This became first evident when hsp70-associated peptides could be shown to elicit specific cancer immunity (Udono and Srivastava, 1993). Later it became clear that hsp molecules of the 70 and 90 kDa class can mediate this effect (Udono and Srivastava, 1994; Feldweg and Srivastava, 1995; Lammert *et al.*, 1996; Nieland *et al.*, 1996), and that peptides derived from tumor antigens, minor H antigens or viruses can be delivered into the MHC class I presentation pathway by hsp molecules (Udono and Srivastava, 1994; Arnold *et al.*, 1995; Feldweg and Srivastava, 1995; Nieland *et al.*, 1996; Roman and Moreno, 1996; Blachere *et al.*, 1997; Heikema *et al.*, 1997; Ciupitu *et al.*, 1998; Ishii *et al.*, 1999). In addition to the adjuvant effects described in the previous section, the hsp/peptide complexes play a more specific role in delivering peptides for MHC class I-restricted presentation as exogenous antigen/carrier complexes. The biochemical details involved in this pathway are not yet understood (Suto and Srivastava, 1995). These complexes may furthermore play a role in cross-priming the CTL response (Todryk *et al.*, 1999; Thery *et al.*, 1999; Kumaraguru *et al.*, 2000; Thery *et al.*, 2001). These observations are of interest for the rational design of CTL-stimulating vaccines against cancer and virus infections.

STRESS PROTEIN-CONTAINING CTL-STIMULATING VACCINES

Two systems have been used to deliver hsp-associated antigens as vaccines. These include:

1. The loading of purified hsp70 or 90 molecules with antigenic peptides *in vitro* (using synthetic, antigenic peptides) or *in vivo* (by isolating 'loaded' hsp70/90 from tumor or virus-infected cells). This technique was pioneered by P.K. Srivastava *et al.* (Udono and Srivastava, 1993; and 1994; Srivastava *et al.*, 1994; Feldweg and Srivastava, 1995; Blachere *et al.*, 1997; Chandawarkar *et al.*, 1999; Ishii *et al.*, 1999), and is summarized in two excellent reviews (Srivastava *et al.*, 1998; Srivastava, 2000). The basic observation has been confirmed in different systems

using hsp from different sources and peptides derived from different antigens (Arnold *et al.*, 1995; Nieland *et al.*, 1996; Roman and Moreno, 1996; Lammert *et al.*, 1997; Roman and Moreno, 1997; Ciupitu *et al.*, 1998; Moroi *et al.*, 2000). A method was developed for the preparative isolation of hsp/peptide complexes from cells to produce a vaccine (Peng *et al.*, 1997; Arnold *et al.*, 2000; Srivastava, 2000; Srivastava and Jaikaria, 2001).

2. An alternative approach used fusion proteins containing an N-terminal antigenic domain and a C-terminal hsp70-encoding sequence (Suzue *et al.*, 1997; Chen *et al.*, 2000; Cho *et al.*, 2000; Huang *et al.*, 2000; Liu *et al.*, 2000; Cheng *et al.*, 2001). The chimeric construct (i.e. a hsp molecule fused to a polypeptide containing a CTL epitope) stimulates CD4[+] T cell-independent CTL responses to the respective epitopes. Hsp fusion proteins with fusion partners of widely differing lengths and sequences elicit CD8[+] CTL to peptides from the fusion partners without requiring exogenous adjuvants or the participation of CD4[+] T cells.

We have chosen a third approach: the expression of chimeric antigens containing an N-terminal viral (DnaJ-homologous) domain with intrinsic hsp73-binding activity, and C-terminal antigen-encoding sequences because (i) it is easier to express, and (ii) it has a strikingly enhanced potential to express even large protein antigens in association with hsp73 (Schirmbeck and Reimann, 1994; Schirmbeck *et al.*, 1997, 1999).

EXPRESSING LARGE FUSION ANTIGENS WITH A DnaJ-HOMOLOGUOUS N-TERMINUS NON-COVALENTLY BOUND TO HSP73

We have demonstrated that the processing of endogenous, mutant T-Ag independently of the transporter assiated with peptide translocation (TAP) correlates with the association of mutant but not wtT-Ag to hsp73, i.e. the truncated cT-Ag or N-terminal T-Ag fragment but not the wtT-Ag are stably associated with the constitutively expressed, cytosolic hsp73 chaperone (Schirmbeck and Reimann, 1994). This was confirmed in studies in which expression plasmids encoding either wtT-Ag, or various truncated or chimeric variants of T-Ag were transfected into different TAP-competent or TAP-deficient cell lines (Schirmbeck *et al.*, 1997 and 1999). Lysosomes are a major site of acid degradation of proteins delivered by many different pathways. The potent proteolytic activities in lysosomes are mediated by endopeptidases (cathepsin B, D, E, H, L, M, N, S, T) and exopeptidases (cathepsin A, B2, C, III; dipeptidyl aminopeptidase II; carboxypeptidase C). Endocytosis of extracellular or membrane-bound proteins, diversion of proteins travelling through the exocytic pathway, and non-selective processes (e.g. constitutive microautophagy or stimulated macroautophagy) deliver proteins to lysosomes. Hsp73-associated cytosolic proteins can directly cross the membrane bilayer to enter lysosomes (reviewed in Dice *et al.*, 1994; Dice and Terlecky, 1994; Hayes and Dice, 1996). This lysosomal polypeptide import resembles the chaperone-assisted transport of proteins into other organelles and does not involve a vesicular pathway. Transport of cytosolic proteins into lysosomes by this pathway is stimulated in cells deprived of nutrients or growth factors (Chiang *et al.*, 1989; Terlecky *et al.*, 1992; Cuervo *et al.*, 1995). Uptake of hsp73-associated proteins into lysosomes is stimulated by ATP, involves the lysosomal membrane glycoprotein LGP96 (identified as a receptor for the import of proteins into lysosomes (Cuervo and Dice, 1996)), is selective and saturable. Our data indicate that this protein degradation pathway can generate peptides that bind to MHC-I molecules in the endolysosomes.

Further studies in this system revealed three findings that are of potential value for vaccine designs and interesting tools to study hsp-facilitated antigen processing (reviewed in Reimann and Schirmbeck, 1999):

- high level expression of mutant or chimeric endogenous antigens
- TAP-independent processing of endogenous antigen for MHC-I-restricted peptide presentation
- priming of an antibody response to endogenous antigen following DNA vaccination.

We have demonstrated that this system supports the design of DNA vaccines that cross-prime TAP-independent and T helper-independent CTL responses due to the co-delivery of intrinsic (natural) adjuvanticity.

We have furthermore used this eukaryotic expression of recombinant chimeric proteins for the production of recombinant proteins and/or bioactive molecules. The expression and production of these recombinant protein-based vaccines containing hsp/antigen complexes is an exciting way to construct a new generation of hsp-based vaccines that contain a greatly extended range of immunogenic information.

UNIQUE ADVANTAGES OF DNA VACCINATION

Exciting new experimental approaches have become accessible through DNA vaccination. We list some points to illustrate the broad potential of this novel technology.

1. *Identification of antigens (or their immunogenic domains or epitopes) by expression library immunization (ELI)* (Barry *et al.*, 1995; Lai *et al.*, 1995; Piedrafita *et al.*, 1999). DNA vaccination can be used to identify antibody-defined domains and T cell-defined epitopes of complex pathogens by immunizing hosts with expression libraries, and identifying the specificity of the immune response obtained.

2. *Construction of polyvalent, chimeric vaccines.* Polyvalent vaccines containing immunodominant domains from different antigens and/or different pathogens can be fused to construct chimeric, polyvalent vaccines.

3. *Generation of immunological probes (monoclonal antibodies, T cell clones) to define immunogenic domains or epitopes of antigens.* DNA vaccination offers an attractive way to generate specific probes (monoclonal antibodies or restricted T cell lines) for antigenic determinants (Martinon *et al.*, 1993; Watanabe *et al.*, 1993; Barry *et al.*, 1994; Hawkins *et al.*, 1994; Shiver *et al.*, 1995; Krasemann *et al.*, 1996).

4. *Overriding low responder status.* DNA vaccination can override low responder status in preclinical animal models because it is more effective than conventional approaches in revealing a CTL response (Schirmbeck *et al.*, 1995). This offers the chance to reduce the fraction of non-responders to the vaccine in a population, the complete protection of which is the goal of the intervention.

5. *Eliciting an immune response in neonates.* Priming an anti-viral T cell response in neonatal animals has been successful with DNA vaccines (reviewed in Siegrist and Lambert, 1997; Siegrist, 1997; Kovarik and Siegrist, 1998). For early protection in life, this vaccine may have advantages that are difficult to obtain with more conventional approaches.

6. *Efficient CTL priming.* Because DNA vaccination is a potent way to prime CTL to internal (non-variant) viral antigens (such as nucleocapsid, matrix or polymerase proteins), it is easier to obtain cross-strain protection

against pathogenic viruses with DNA vaccines than with conventional vaccines that rely on the induction of a neutralizing antibody response against variant envelope proteins of a virus. A case that strikingly illustrates this point is the vaccination against influenza virus.

CONCLUSIONS

Only a few years have passed since its first description in 1992, but many experimental DNA vaccines have moved from preclinical animal models into clinical trials. DNA vaccination involves risks that are difficult to evaluate critically. These include (i) *insertional mutagenesis* (integration of plasmid DNA into coding or regulatory sequences of the eukaryotic genome); *(ii) (low zone) tolerance* (induced by exposure of the immune system to suboptimal doses of antigen); (iii) *induction of an autoimmune response* (e.g. autoantibodies against cytokines); and (iv) *extensive immune-mediated destruction* of tissue transfected *in vivo*. Despite these risks (that are dificult to assess critically at the current stage of our experience with this novel technology), its potential to face new challenges in vaccinology are largely unexplored. A main factor that contributes to the success of a DNA vaccine is the easy design of plasmid vectors, molecular clones of many antigens of interest, and the co-delivery of immuno-modulators. The major challenge is to find efficient techniques for the inoculation, the packaging of the DNA vaccine, and the use of low dose DNA vaccines. These problems are largely unresolved and will decide on the eventual success of this vaccination strategy.

REFERENCES

An, L.L. and Whitton, J.L. 1997. A multivalent minigene vaccine, containing B-cell, cytotoxic T-lymphocyte, and Th epitopes from several microbes, induces appropriate responses *in vivo* and confers protection against more than one pathogen. J. Virol. 71: 2292-2302.

Arnold, D., Faath, S., Rammensee, H.G., and Schild, H. 1995. Cross-priming of minor histocompatibility antigen-specific cytotoxic T cells upon immunization with the heat shock protein gp96. J. Exp. Med. 182: 885-889.

Arnold, S.D., Hanau, D., Spehner, D., Schmid, C., Rammensee, H.G., de la Salle, H., and Schild, H. 1999. Receptor-mediated endocytosis of heat shock proteins by professional antigen-presenting cells. J. Immunol. 162: 3757-3760.

Arnold, S.D., Kleist, C., Welschof, M., Opelz, G., Rammensee, H.G., Schild, H., and Terness, P. 2000. One-step single-chain Fv recombinant antibody-based purification of gp96 for vaccine development. Cancer Res. 60: 4175-4178.

Asea, A., Kraeft, S.K., Kurt-Jones, E.A., Stevenson, M.A., Chen, L.B., Finberg, R.W., Koo, G.C., and Calderwood, S.K. 2000. HSP70 stimulates cytokine production through a CD14-dependant pathway, demonstrating its dual role as a chaperone and cytokine. Nat. Med. 6: 435-442.

Bagarazzi, M.L., Boyer, J.D., Javadian, M.A., Chattergoon, M., Dang, K., Kim, G., Shah, J., Wang, B., and Weiner, D.B. 1997. Safety and immunogenicity of intramuscular and intravaginal delivery of HIV-1 DNA constructs to infant chimpanzees. J. Med. Primatol. 26: 27-33.

Ban, E.M., Van, G.F., Simecka, J.W., Kiyono, H., Robinson, H.L., and McGhee, J.R. 1997. Mucosal immunization with DNA encoding influenza hemagglutinin. Vaccine 15: 811-813.

Barouch, D.H., Craiu, A., Kuroda, M.J., Schmitz, J.E., Zheng, X.X., Santra, S., Frost, J.D., Krivulka, G.R., Lifton, M.A., Crabbs, C.L., Heidecker, G., Perry, H.C., Davies, M.E., Xie, H., Nickerson, C.E., Steenbeke, T.D., Lord, C.I., Montefiori, D.C., Strom, T.B., Shiver, J.W., Lewis, M.G., and Letvin, N.L. 2000. Augmentation of immune responses to HIV-1 and simian immunodeficiency virus DNA vaccines by IL-2/Ig plasmid administration in rhesus monkeys. Proc. Natl. Acad. Sci. USA. 97: 4192-4197.

Barry, M.A., Barry, M.E., and Johnston, S.A. 1994. Production of monoclonal antibodies by genetic immunization. Biotechniques 16: 616-8, 620.

Barry, M.A., Lai, W.C., and Johnston, S.A. 1995. Protection against *Mycoplasma* infection using expression-library immunization. Nature 377: 632-635.

Basu, S., Binder, R.J., Ramalingam, T., and Srivastava, P.K. 2001. CD91 is a common receptor for heat shock proteins gp96, hsp90, hsp70, and calreticulin. Immunity. 14: 303-313.

Binder, R.J., Anderson, K.M., Basu, S., and Srivastava, P.K. 2000a. Heat shock protein gp96 induces maturation and migration of CD11c$^+$ cells *in vivo*. J. Immunol. 165: 6029-6035.

Binder, R.J., Han, D.K., and Srivastava, P.K. 2000b. CD91: a receptor for heat shock protein gp96. Nat. Immunol. 1: 151-155.

Binder, R.J., Karimeddini, D., and Srivastava, P.K. 2001. Adjuvanticity of α2-Macroglobulin, an Independent Ligand for the Heat Shock Protein Receptor CD91. J. Immunol. 166: 4968-4972.

Birk, O.S., Gur, S.L., Elias, D., Margalit, R., Mor, F., Carmi, P., Bockova, J., Altmann, D.M., and Cohen, I.R. 1999. The 60-kDa heat shock protein modulates allograft rejection. Proc. Natl. Acad. Sci. USA. 96: 5159-5163.

Blachere, N.E., Li, Z., Chandawarkar, R.Y., Suto, R., Jaikaria, N.S., Basu, S., Udono, H., and Srivastava, P.K. 1997. Heat shock protein-peptide complexes, reconstituted *in vitro*, elicit peptide-specific cytotoxic T lymphocyte response and tumor immunity. J. Exp. Med. 186: 1315-1322.

Boczkowski, D., Nair, S.K., Snyder, D., and Gilboa, E. 1996. Dendritic cells pulsed with RNA are potent antigen-presenting cells *in vitro* and *in vivo*. J. Exp. Med. 184: 465-472.

Boyle, J.S., Brady, J.L., and Lew, A.M. 1998. Enhanced responses to a DNA vaccine encoding a fusion antigen that is directed to sites of immune induction. Nature 392: 408-411.

Breloer, M., Fleischer, B., and Von Bonin, A. 1999. *In vivo* and *in vitro* activation of T cells after administration of Ag-negative heat shock proteins. J. Immunol. 162: 3141-3147.

Bueler, H. and Mulligan, R.C. 1996. Induction of antigen-specific tumor immunity by genetic and cellular vaccines against MAGE: enhanced tumor protection by coexpression of granulocyte-macrophage colony-stimulating factor and B7-1. Mol. Med. 2: 545-555.

Byrd, C.A., Bornmann, W., Erdjument, B.H., Tempst, P., Pavletich, N., Rosen, N., Nathan, C.F., and Ding, A. 1999. Heat shock protein 90 mediates macrophage activation by Taxol and bacterial lipopolysaccharide. Proc. Natl. Acad. Sci. USA. 96: 5645-5650.

Chandawarkar, R.Y., Wagh, M.S., and Srivastava, P.K. 1999. The dual nature of specific immunological activity of tumor-derived gp96 preparations. J. Exp. Med. 189: 1437-1442.

Chen, C.H., Wang, T.L., Hung, C.F., Yang, Y., Young, R.A., Pardoll, D.M., and Wu, T.C. 2000. Enhancement of DNA vaccine potency by linkage of antigen gene to an HSP70 gene. Cancer Res. 60: 1035-1042.

Chen, S.C., Jones, D.H., Fynan, E.F., Farrar, G.H., Clegg, J.C., Greenberg, H.B., and Herrmann, J.E. 1998. Protective immunity induced by oral immunization with a rotavirus DNA vaccine encapsulated in microparticles. J. Virol. 72: 5757-5761.

Cheng, W.F., Hung, C.F., Chai, C.Y., Hsu, K.F., He, L., Rice, C.M., Ling, M., and Wu, T.C. 2001. Enhancement of sindbis virus self-replicating RNA vaccine potency by linkage of *Mycobacterium tuberculosis* heat shock protein 70 gene to an antigen gene. J. Immunol. 166: 6218-6226.

Chiang, H.-L., Terlecky, S.R., Plant, C.P., and Dice, J.F. 1989. A role for a 70-kilodalton heat shock protein in lysosomal degradation of intracellular proteins. Science 246: 382-385.

Cho, B.K., Palliser, D., Guillen, E., Wisniewski, J., Young, R.A., Chen, J., and Eisen, H.N. 2000. A proposed mechanism for the induction of cytotoxic T lymphocyte production by heat shock fusion proteins. Immunity 12: 263-272.

Choi, A.H., Knowlton, D.R., McNeal, M.M., and Ward, R.L. 1997. Particle bombardment-mediated DNA vaccination with rotavirus VP6 induces high levels of serum rotavirus IgG but fails to protect mice against challenge. Vir 232: 129-138.

Chow, Y.H., Chiang, B.L., Lee, Y.C., Chi, W.K., Lin, W.C., Chen, Y.T., and Tao, M.H. 2000. Development of Th1 and Th2 populations and the nature of immune responses to hepatitis B virus DNA vaccines can be modulated by codelivery of various cytokine genes. J. Immunol. 160: 1320-1329.

Chow, Y.H., Huang, W.L., Chi, W.K., Chu, Y.D., and Tao, M.H. 1997. Improvement of hepatitis B virus DNA vaccines by plasmids coexpressing hepatitis B surface antigen and interleukin-2. J. Virol. 71: 169-178.

Ciupitu, A.M., Petersson, M., O'Donnell, C.L., Williams, K., Jindal, S., Kiessling, R., and Welsh, R.M. 1998. Immunization with a lymphocytic choriomeningitis virus peptide mixed with heat shock protein 70 results in protective antiviral immunity and specific cytotoxic T lymphocytes. J. Exp. Med. 187: 685-691.

Clarke, N.J., Hissey, P., Buchan, K., and Harris, S. 1997. pPV: a novel IRES-containing vector to facilitate plasmid immunization and antibody response characterization. Immunotechnology. 3: 145-153.

Conry, R.M., LoBuglio, A.F., Wright, M., Sumerel, L., Pike, M.J., Johanning, F., Benjamin, R.J., Lu, D., and Curiel, D.T. 1995. Characterization of a messenger RNA polynucleotide vaccine vector. Cancer Res. 55: 1397-1400.

Corr, M., Lee, D.J., Carson, D.A., and Tighe, H. 1996. Gene vaccination with naked plasmid DNA: mechanism of CTL priming. J. Exp. Med. 184: 1555-1560.

Corr, M., Tighe, H., Lee, D., Dudler, J., Trieu, M., Brinson, D.C., and Carson, D.A. 1997. Costimulation provided by DNA immunization enhances antitumor immunity. J. Immunol. 159: 4999-5004.

Cuervo, A.M. and Dice, J.F. 1996. A receptor for the selective uptake and degradation of proteins by lysosomes. Science 273: 501-503.

Cuervo, A.M., Knecht, E., Terlecky, S.R., and Dice, J.F. 1995. Activation of a selective pathway of lysosomal proteolysis in rat liver by prolonged starvation. Am. J. Physiol. 269: C1200-8.

Davis, H.L., Whalen, R.G., and Demeneix, B.A. 1993. Direct gene transfer into skeletal muscle *in vivo*: factors affecting efficiency of transfer and stability of expression. Hum. Gene Ther. 4: 151-159.

Dice, J.F., Agarraberes, F., Kirven-Brooks, M., Terlecky, L.J., and Terlecky, S.R. 1994. Heat shock 70-kD proteins and lysosomal proteolysis. In: The Biology of Heat Shock Proteins and Molecular Chaperones. R.I. Morimoto, A. Tissieres, and C. Georgopoulos, eds. Cold Spring Harbor Laboratory Press, Cold Spring Harbor, New York. p. 137-151.

Dice, J.F. and Terlecky, S.R. 1994. Selective degradation of cytosolic proteins by lysosomes. In: Cellular Proteolytic Systems. A.J. Ciechanover and A.L. Schwartz, eds. Wiley-Liss, New York-Toronto, p. 55-64.

Dirks, W., Wirth, M., and Hauser, H. 1993. Dicistronic transcription units for gene expression in mammalian cells. Gene 128: 247-249.

Doe, B., Selby, M., Barnett, S., Baenziger, J., and Walker, C.M. 1996. Induction of cytotoxic T lymphocytes by intramuscular immunization with plasmid DNA is facilitated by bone marrow- derived cells. Proc. Natl. Acad. Sci. USA. 93: 8578-8583.

Dow, S.W., Fradkin, L.G., Liggitt, D.H., Willson, A.P., Heath, T.D., and Potter, T.A. 1999. Lipid-DNA complexes induce potent activation of innate immune responses and antitumor activity when administered intravenously. J. Immunol. 163: 1552-1561.

Eisenbraun, M.D., Fuller, D.H., and Haynes, J.R. 1993. Examination of parameters affecting the elicitation of humoral immune responses by particle bombardment-mediated genetic immunization. DNA Cell Biol. 12: 791-797.

Eo, S.K., Lee, S., Chun, S., and Rouse, B.T. 2001. Modulation of immunity against herpes simplex virus infection via mucosal genetic transfer of plasmid DNA encoding chemokines. J. Virol. 75: 569-578.

Etchart, N., Buckland, R., Liu, M.A., Wild, T.F., and Kaiserlian, D. 1997. Class I-restricted CTL induction by mucosal immunization with naked DNA encoding measles virus haemagglutinin. J. Gen. Virol. 78: 1577-1580.

Feldweg, A.M. and Srivastava, P.K. 1995. Molecular heterogeneity of tumor rejection antigen/heat shock protein GP96. Int. J. Cancer 63: 310-314.

Feltquate, D.M., Heaney, S., Webster, R.G., and Robinson, H.L. 1997. Different T helper cell types and antibody isotypes generated by saline and gene gun DNA immunization. J. Immunol. 158: 2278-2284.

Fuller, D.H., Murphey, C.M., Clements, J., Barnett, S., and Haynes, J.R. 1996. Induction of immunodeficiency virus-specific immune responses in rhesus monkeys following gene gun-mediated DNA vaccination. J. Med. Primatol. 25: 236-241.

Fuller, J.T., Fuller, D.H., McCabe, D., Haynes, J.R., and Widera, G. 1995. Immune responses to hepatitis B virus surface and core antigens in mice, monkeys, and pigs after Accell particle-mediated DNA immunization. Ann. NY Acad. Sci. 772: 282-284.

Fynan, E.F., Webster, R.G., Fuller, D.H., Haynes, J.R., Santoro, J.C., and Robinson, H.L. 1993. DNA Vaccines: protective immunizations by parenteral, mucosal, and gene-gun inoculations. Proc. Natl. Acad. Sci. USA. 90: 11478-11482.

Geissler, M., Gesien, A., Tokushige, K., and Wands, J.R. 1997. Enhancement of cellular and humoral immune responses to hepatitis C virus core protein using DNA-based vaccines augmented with cytokine-expressing plasmids. J. Immunol. 158: 1231-1237.

Goldman, C.K., Soroceanu, L., Smith, N., Gillespie, G.Y., Shaw, W., Burgess, S., Bilbao, G., and Curiel, D.T. 1997. *In vitro* and *in vivo* gene delivery mediated by a synthetic polycationic amino polymer. Nat. Biotechnol. 15: 462-466.

Grussenmeyer, J., Scheidtmann, K.H., Hutchinson, M.A., Eckhart, W., and Walter, G. 1985. Complexes of polyoma virus medium T antigen and cellular proteins. Proc. Natl. Acad. Sci. USA. 82: 7952-7954.

Gurunathan, S., Irvine, K.R., Wu, C.Y., Cohen, J.I., Thomas, E., Prussin, C., Restifo, N.P., and Seder, R.A. 1998. CD40 ligand/trimer DNA enhances both humoral and cellular immune responses and induces protective immunity to infectious and tumor challenge. J. Immunol. 161: 4563-4571.

Harle, P., Noisakran, S., and Carr, D.J. 2001. The application of a plasmid DNA encoding IFN-α1 postinfection enhances cumulative survival of herpes simplex virus type 2 vaginally infected mice. J. Immunol. 166: 1803-1812.

Harrison, G.S., Wang, Y., Tomczak, J., Hogan, C., Shpall, E.J., Curiel, T.J., and Felgner, P.L. 1995. Optimization of gene transfer using cationic lipids in cell lines and primary human CD4+ and CD34+ hematopoietic cells. Biotechniques 19: 816-823.

Hawkins, R.E., Zhu, D., Ovecka, M., Winter, G., Hamblin, T.J., Long, A., and Stevenson, F.K. 1994. Idiotypic vaccination against human B-cell lymphoma. Rescue of variable region gene sequences from biopsy material for assembly as single-chain Fv personal vaccines. Blood 83: 3279-3288.

Hayes, S.A. and Dice, J.F. 1996. Roles of molecular chaperones in protein degradation. J. Cell Biol. 132: 255-258.

Haynes, J.R., McCabe, D.E., Swain, W.F., Widera, G., and Fuller, J.T. 1996. Particle-mediated nucleic acid immunization. J. Biotechnol. 44: 37-42.

He, X.S., Chen, H.S., Chu, K., Rivkina, M., and Robinson, W.S. 1996a. Costimulatory protein B7-1 enhances the cytotoxic T cell response and antibody response to hepatitis B surface antigen. Proc. Natl. Acad. Sci. USA. 93: 7274-7278.

He, X.S., Rivkina, M., and Robinson, W.S. 1996b. Construction of adenoviral and retroviral vectors coexpressing the genes encoding the hepatitis B surface antigen and B7-1 protein. Gene 175: 121-125.

Heikema, A., Agsteribbe, E., Wilschut, J., and Huckriede, A. 1997. Generation of heat shock protein-based vaccines by intracellular loading of gp96 with antigenic peptides. Immunol. Lett. 57: 69-74.

Hightower, L.E., Sadis, S.E., and Takenaka, I.M. 1994. Interaction of vertebrate hsc70 and hsp70 with unfolded proteins and peptides. In: The Biology of Heat Shock Proteins and Molecular Chaperones. R.I. Morimoto, A. Tissieres, and C. Georgopoulos, eds. Cold Spring Harbor Laboratory Press, Cold Spring Harbor, New York. p. 179-207.

Hoerr, I., Obst, R., Rammensee, H.G., and Jung, G. 2000. *In vivo* application of RNA leads to induction of specific cytotoxic T lymphocytes and antibodies. Eur. J. Immunol. 30: 1-7.

Hogan, S.P., Foster, P.S., Charlton, B., and Slattery, R.M. 1998. Prevention of Th2-mediated murine allergic airways disease by soluble antigen administration in the neonate. Proc. Natl. Acad. Sci. USA. 95: 2441-2445.

Horspool, J.H., Perrin, P.J., Woodcock, J.B., Cox, J.H., King, C.L., June, C.H., Harlan, D.M., St, and Lee, K.P. 1998. Nucleic acid vaccine-induced immune responses require CD28 costimulation and are regulated by CTLA4. J. Immunol. 160: 2706-2714.

Huang, H.V. 1996. Sindbis virus vectors for expression in animal cells. Curr. Opin. Biotechnol. 7: 531-535.

Huang, Q., Richmond, J.F., Suzue, K., Eisen, H.N., and Young, R.A. 2000. *In vivo* cytotoxic T lymphocyte elicitation by mycobacterial heat shock protein 70 fusion proteins maps to a discrete domain and is CD4(+) T cell independent. J. Exp. Med. 191: 403-408.

Ishii, N., Fukushima, J., Kaneko, T., Okada, E., Tani, K., Tanaka, S.I., Hamajima, K., Xin, K.Q., Kawamoto, S., Koff, W., Nishioka, K., Yasuda, T., and Okuda, K. 1997. Cationic liposomes are a strong adjuvant for a DNA vaccine of human immunodeficiency virus type 1. AIDS Res. Hum. Retroviruses 13: 1421-1428.

Ishii, T., Udono, H., Yamano, T., Ohta, H., Uenaka, A., Ono, T., Hizuta, A., Tanaka, N., Srivastava, P.K., and Nakayama, E. 1999. Isolation of MHC class I-restricted tumor antigen peptide and its precursors associated with heat shock proteins hsp70, hsp90, and gp96. J. Immunol. 162: 1303-1309.

Iwasaki, A., Stiernholm, B.J., Chan, A.K., Berinstein, N.L., and Barber, B.H. 1997. Enhanced CTL responses mediated by plasmid DNA immunogens encoding costimulatory molecules and cytokines. J. Immunol. 158: 4591-4601.

Jenkins, M., Kerr, D., Fayer, R., and Wall, R. 1995. Serum and colostrum antibody responses induced by jet-injection of sheep with DNA encoding a Cryptosporidium parvum antigen. Vaccine 13: 1658-1664.

Jiao, S., Williams, P., Berg, R.K., Hodgeman, B.A., Liu, L.M., Repetto, G., and Wolff, J.A. 1992. Direct gene transfer into nonhuman primate myofibers *in vivo*. Hum. Gene Ther. 3: 21-33.

Johanning, F.W., Conry, R.M., LoBuglio, A.F., Wright, M., Sumerel, L.A., Pike, M.J., and Curiel, D.T. 1995. A Sindbis virus mRNA polynucleotide vector achieves prolonged and high level heterologous gene expression *in vivo*. Nucleic Acids Res. 23: 1495-1501.

Johnston, S.A. and Tang, D.C. 1994. Gene gun transfection of animal cells and genetic immunization. Methods Cell Biol. 43 Pt A: 353-365.

Kaufmann, S.H.E., Schoel, B., van Embden, J.D., Koga, T., Wand Wurttenberger, A., Munk, M.E., and Steinhoff, U. 1991. Heat-shock protein 60: implications for pathogenesis of and protection against bacterial infections. Immunol. Rev. 121: 67-90.

Keller, E.T., Burkholder, J.K., Shi, F., Pugh, T.D., McCabe, D., Malter, J.S., MacEwen, E.G., Yang, N.S., and Ershler, W.B. 1996. *In vivo* particle-mediated cytokine gene transfer into canine oral mucosa and epidermis. Cancer Gene Ther. 3: 186-191.

Kim, J.J., Ayyavoo, V., Bagarazzi, M.L., Chattergoon, M.A., Dang, K., Wang, B., Boyer, J.D., and Weiner, D.B. 1997a. *In vivo* engineering of a cellular immune response by coadministration of IL-12 expression vector with a DNA immunogen. J. Immunol. 158: 816-826.

Kim, J.J., Bagarazzi, M.L., Trivedi, N., Hu, Y., Kazahaya, K., Wilson, D.M., Ciccarelli, R., Chattergoon, M.A., Dang, K., Mahalingam, S., Chalian, A.A., Agadjanyan, M.G., Boyer, J.D., Wang, B., and Weiner, D.B. 1997b. Engineering of *in vivo* immune responses to DNA immunization via codelivery of costimulatory molecule genes. Nat. Biotechnol. 15: 641-646.

Kim, J.J., Nottingham, L.K., Wilson, D.M., Bagarazzi, M.L., Tsai, A., Morrison, L.D., Javadian, A., Chalian, A.A., Agadjanyan, M.G., and Weiner, D.B. 1998a. Engineering DNA vaccines via co-delivery of co-stimulatory molecule genes. Vaccine 16: 1828-1835.

Kim, J.J., Trivedi, N.N., Nottingham, L.K., Morrison, L., Tsai, A., Hu, Y., Mahalingam, S., Dang, K., Ahn, L., Doyle, N.K., Wilson, D.M., Chattergoon, M.A., Chalian, A.A., Boyer, J.D., Agadjanyan, M.G., and Weiner, D.B. 1998b. Modulation of amplitude and direction of *in vivo* immune responses by co-administration of cytokine gene expression cassettes with DNA immunogens. Eur. J. Immunol. 28: 1089-1103.

Kim, T.S., DeKruyff, R.H., Rupper, R., Maecker, H.T., Levy, S., and Umetsu, D.T. 1997c. An ovalbumin-IL-12 fusion protein is more effective than ovalbumin plus free recombinant IL-12 in inducing a T helper cell type 1-dominated immune response and inhibiting antigen-specific IgE production. J. Immunol. 158: 4137-4144.

Kimura, K., Nishimura, H., Hirose, K., Matsuguchi, T., Nimura, Y., and Yoshikai, Y. 1999. Immunogene therapy of murine fibrosarcoma using IL-15 gene with high translation efficiency. Eur. J. Immunol. 29: 1532-1542.

Kipps, T. and Mendoza, R. 1999. Extending genetic vaccines with chemokines. Nat. Biotechnol. 17: 226-227.

Klavinskis, L.S., Barnfield, C., Gao, L., and Parker, S. 1999. Intranasal immunization with plasmid DNA-lipid complexes elicits mucosal immunity in the female genital and rectal tracts. J. Immunol. 162: 254-262.

Kol, A., Bourcier, T., Lichtman, A.H., and Libby, P. 1999. Chlamydial and human heat shock protein 60s activate human vascular endothelium, smooth muscle cells, and macrophages. J. Clin. Invest. 103: 571-577.

Kovarik, J. and Siegrist, C.A. 1998. Immunity in early life. Immunol. Today 19: 150-152.

Krasemann, S., Groschup, M., Hunsmann, G., and Bodemer, W. 1996. Induction of antibodies against human prion proteins (PrP) by DNA-mediated immunization of PrP0/0 mice. J. Immunol. Methods 199: 109-118.

Kuklin, N., Daheshia, M., Karem, K., Manickan, E., and Rouse, B.T. 1997. Induction of mucosal immunity against herpes simplex virus by plasmid DNA immunization. J. Virol. 71: 3138-3145.

Kumaraguru, U., Rouse, R.J., Nair, S.K., Bruce, B.D., and Rouse, B.T. 2000. Involvement of an ATP-dependent peptide chaperone in cross-presentation after DNA immunization. J. Immunol. 165: 750-759.

Kusakabe, K., Xin, K.Q., Katoh, H., Sumino, K., Hagiwara, E., Kawamoto, S., Okuda, K., Miyagi, Y., Aoki, I., Nishioka, K., and Klinman, D.M. 2000. The timing of GM-CSF expression plasmid administration influences the Th1/Th2 response induced by an HIV-1-specific DNA vaccine. J. Immunol. 164: 3102-3111.

Kwak, L.W., Young, H.A., Pennington, R.W., and Weeks, S.D. 1996. Vaccination with syngeneic, lymphoma-derived immunoglobulin idiotype combined with granulocyte/macrophage colony-stimulating factor primes mice for a protective T-cell response. Proc. Natl. Acad. Sci. USA. 93: 10972-10977.

Kwissa, M., Unsinger, J., Schirmbeck, R., Hauser, H., and Reimann, J. 2000. Polyvalent DNA vaccines with bidirectional promoters. J. Mol. Med. 78: 495-506.

Kwoh, D.Y., Coffin, C.C., Lollo, C.P., Jovenal, J., Banaszczyk, M.G., Mullen, P., Phillips, A., Amini, A., Fabrycki, J., Bartholomew, R.M., Brostoff, S.W., and Carlo, D.J. 1999. Stabilization of poly-L-lysine/DNA polyplexes for *in vivo* gene delivery to the liver. Biochim. Biophys. Acta 1444: 171-190.

Lai, W.C., Bennett, M., Johnston, S.A., Barry, M.A., and Pakes, S.P. 1995. Protection against *Mycoplasma pulmonis* infection by genetic vaccination. DNA Cell Biol. 14: 643-651.

Lakey, E.K., Margoliash, E., and Pierce, S.K. 1987. Identification of a peptide-binding protein having a role in antigen presentation. Proc. Natl. Acad. Sci. USA. 84: 1659.

Lammert, E., Arnold, D., Nijenhuis, M., Momburg, F., Hammerling, G.J., Brunner, J., Stevanovic, S., Rammensee, H.G., and Schild, H. 1997. The endoplasmic reticulum-resident stress protein gp96 binds peptides translocated by TAP. Eur. J. Immunol. 27: 923-927.

Lammert, E., Arnold, D., Rammensee, H.G., and Schild, H. 1996. Expression levels of stress protein gp96 are not limiting for major histocompatibility complex class I-restricted antigen presentation. Eur. J. Immunol. 26: 875-879.

Larsen, D.L., Dybdahl, S.N., McGregor, M.W., Drape, R., Neumann, V., Swain, W.F., Lunn, D.P., and Olsen, C.W. 1998. Coadministration of DNA encoding interleukin-6 and hemagglutinin confers protection from influenza virus challenge in mice. J. Virol. 72: 1704-1708.

Leitner, W.W., Seguin, M.C., Ballou, W.R., Seitz, J.P., Schultz, A.M., Sheehy, M.J., and Lyon, J.A. 1997. Immune responses induced by intramuscular or gene gun injection of protective deoxyribonucleic acid vaccines that express the circumsporozoite protein from *Plasmodium berghei* malaria parasites. J. Immunol. 159: 6112-6119.

Liu, D.W., Tsao, Y.P., Kung, J.T., Ding, Y.A., Sytwu, H.K., Xiao, X., and Chen, S.L. 2000. Recombinant adeno-associated virus expressing human papillomavirus type 16 E7 peptide DNA fused with heat shock protein DNA as a potential vaccine for cervical cancer. J. Virol. 74: 2888-2894.

Liu, Y., Mounkes, L.C., Liggitt, H.D., Brown, C.S., Solodin, I., Heath, T.D., and Debs, R.J. 1997. Factors influencing the efficiency of cationic liposome-mediated intravenous gene delivery. Nat. Biotechnol. 15: 167-173.

Livingston, J.B., Lu, S., Robinson, H.L., and Anderson, D.J. 1998. Immunization of the female genital tract with a DNA-based vaccine. Infect. Immun. 66: 322-329.

Lu, Y., Xin, K.Q., Hamajima, K., Tsuji, T., Aoki, I., Yang, J., Sasaki, S., Fukushima, J., Yoshimura, T., Toda, S., Okada, E., and Okuda, K. 1999.

Macrophage inflammatory protein-1alpha (MIP-1alpha) expression plasmid enhances DNA vaccine-induced immune response against HIV-1. Clin. Exp. Immunol. 115: 335-341.

Macklin, M.D., McCabe, D., McGregor, M.W., Neumann, V., Meyer, T., Callan, R., Hinshaw, V.S., and Swain, W.F. 1998. Immunization of pigs with a particle-mediated DNA vaccine to influenza A virus protects against challenge with homologous virus. J. Virol. 72: 1491-1496.

Maecker, H.T., Umetsu, D.T., DeKruyff, R.H., and Levy, S. 1997. DNA vaccination with cytokine fusion constructs biases the immune response to ovalbumin. Vaccine 15: 1687-1696.

Mahvi, D.M., Burkholder, J.K., Turner, J., Culp, J., Malter, J.S., Sondel, P.M., and Yang, N.S. 1996. Particle-mediated gene transfer of granulocyte-macrophage colony- stimulating factor cDNA to tumor cells: implications for a clinically relevant tumor vaccine. Hum. Gene Ther. 7: 1535-1543.

Martinon, F., Krishnan, S., Lenzen, G., Magné, R., Gomard, E., Guillet, J.-G., Lévy, J.-P., and Meulien, P. 1993. Induction of virus-specific cytotoxic T lymphocytes *in vivo* by liposome-entrapped mRNA. Eur. J. Immunol. 23: 1719-1722.

Michalek, M.T., Benacerraf, B., and Rock, K.L. 1992. The class II MHC-restricted presentation of endogenously synthesized ovalbumin displays clonal variation, requires endosomal/lysosomal processing, and is upregulated by heat shock. J. Immunol. 148: 1016-1024.

Michel, M.-L., Davis, H.L., Schleef, M., Mancini, M., Tiollais, P., and Whalen, R.G. 1995. DNA-mediated immunization to the hepatitis B surface antigen in mice: aspects of the humoral response mimic hepatitis B viral infection in humans. Proc. Natl. Acad. Sci. USA. 92: 5307-5311.

Moroi, Y., Mayhew, M., Trcka, J., Hoe, M.H., Takechi, Y., Hartl, F.U., Rothman, J.E., and Houghton, A.N. 2000. Induction of cellular immunity by immunization with novel hybrid peptides complexed to heat shock protein 70. Proc. Natl. Acad. Sci. USA. 97: 3485-3490.

Murray, P.J. and Young, R. 1992. Stress and immunological recognition in host-pathogen interactions. J. Bacteriol. 174: 4193-4196.

Nabel, E.G., Gordon, D., Yang, Z.Y., Xu, L., San, H., Plautz, G.E., Wu, B.Y., Gao, X., Huang, L., and Nabel, G.J. 1992. Gene transfer *in vivo* with DNA-liposome complexes: lack of autoimmunity and gonadal localization. Hum. Gene Ther. 3: 649-656.

Niebling, W.L. and Pierce, S.K. 1993. Antigen entry into early endosomes is insufficient for MHC class II processing. J. Immunol. 150: 2687-2697.

Nieland, T.J.F., Tan, M.C.A., van Muijen, M.M., Koning, F., Kruisbeek, A.M., and van Bleek, G.M. 1996. Isolation of an immunodominant viral peptide that is endogenously bound to the stress protein GP96/GRP94. Proc. Natl. Acad. Sci. USA. 93: 6135-6139.

Noisakran, S. and Carr, D.J. 2000. Plasmid DNA encoding IFN-α1 antagonizes herpes simplex virus type 1 ocular infection through CD4[+] and CD8[+] T lymphocytes. J. Immunol. 164: 6435-6443.

Okada, E., Sasaki, S., Ishii, N., Aoki, I., Yasuda, T., Nishioka, K., Fukushima, J., Miyazaki, J., Wahren, B., and Okuda, K. 1997. Intranasal immunization of a DNA vaccine with IL-12- and granulocyte-macrophage colony-stimulating factor (GM-CSF)-expressing plasmids in liposomes induces strong mucosal and cell-mediated immune responses against HIV-1 antigens. J. Immunol. 159: 3638-3647.

Okubo, T., Hagiwara, E., Ohno, S., Tsuji, T., Ihata, A., Ueda, A., Shirai, A., Aoki, I., Okuda, K., Miyazaki, J., and Ishigatsubo, Y. 1999. Administration of an IL-12-encoding DNA plasmid prevents the development of chronic graft-versus-host disease (GVHD). J. Immunol. 162: 4013-4017.

Paul, A.G., van Kooten, P.J., van Eden, W., and van der, Z.R. 2000. Highly autoproliferative T cells specific for 60-kDa heat shock protein produce IL-4/IL-10 and IFN-γ and are protective in adjuvant arthritis. J. Immunol. 165: 7270-7277.

Peng, P., Menoret, A., and Srivastava, P.K. 1997. Purification of immunogenic heat shock protein 70-peptide complexes by ADP-affinity chromatography. J. Immunol. Methods 204: 13-21.

Pepin, E., Villiers, C.L., Gabert, F.M., Serra, V.A., Marche, P.N., and Colomb, M.G. 1996. Heat shock increases antigenic peptide generation but decreases antigen presentation. Eur. J. Immunol. 26: 2939-2943.

Pertmer, T.M., Eisenbraun, M.D., McCabe, D., Prayaga, S.K., Fuller, D.H., and Haynes, J.R. 1995. Gene gun-based nucleic acid immunization: elicitation of humoral and cytotoxic T lymphocyte responses following epidermal delivery of nanogram quantities of DNA. Vaccine 13: 1427-1430.

Piedrafita, D., Xu, D., Hunter, D., Harrison, R.A., and Liew, F.Y. 1999. Protective immune responses induced by vaccination with an expression genomic library of *Leishmania major*. J. Immunol. 163: 1467-1472.

Plautz, G.E., Nabel, E.G., Fox, B., Yang, Z.Y., Jaffe, M., Gordon, D., Chang, A., and Nabel, G.J. 1994. Direct gene transfer for the understanding and treatment of human disease. Ann. NY Acad. Sci. 716: 144-153.

Porgador, A., Irvine, K.R., Iwasaki, A., Barber, B.H., Restifo, N.P., and Germain, R.N. 1998. Predominant role for directly transfected dendritic cells in antigen presentation to CD8+ T cells after gene gun immunization. J. Exp. Med. 188: 1075-1082.

Prayaga, S.K., Ford, M.J., and Haynes, J.R. 1997. Manipulation of HIV-1 gp120-specific immune responses elicited via gene gun-based DNA immunization. Vaccine 15: 1349-1352.

Qiu, P., Ziegelhoffer, P., Sun, J., and Yang, N.S. 1996. Gene gun delivery of mRNA *in situ* results in efficient transgene expression and genetic immunization. Gene Ther. 3: 262-268.

Rakhmilevich, A.L., Turner, J., Ford, M.J., McCabe, D., Sun, W.H., Sondel, P.M., Grota, K., and Yang, N.S. 1996. Gene gun-mediated skin transfection with interleukin 12 gene results in regression of established primary and metastatic murine tumors. Proc. Natl. Acad. Sci. USA. 93: 6291-6296.

Raz, E., Carson, D.A., Parker, S.E., Parr, T.B., Abai, A.M., Aichinger, G., Gromkowski, S.H., Singh, M., Lew, D., Yankauckas, M.A., *et al.* 1994. Intradermal gene immunization: the possible role of DNA uptake in the induction of cellular immunity to viruses. Proc. Natl. Acad. Sci. USA. 91: 9519-9523.

Reimann, J. and Schirmbeck, R. 1999. Alternative pathways for processing exogenous and endogenous antigens that can generate peptides for MHC class I-restricted presentation. Immunol. Rev. 172: 131-152.

Roman, E. and Moreno, C. 1996. Synthetic peptides non-covalently bound to bacterial hsp70 elicit peptide-specific T-cell responses *in vivo*. imm 88: 487-492.

Roman, E. and Moreno, C. 1997. Delayed-type hypersensitivity elicited by synthetic peptides complexed with *Mycobacterium tuberculosis* hsp 70. Immunol. 90: 52-56.

Sanchez, G.I., Sedegah, M., Rogers, W.O., Jones, T.R., Sacci, J., Witney, A., Carucci, D.J., Kumar, N., and Hoffman, S.L. 2001. Immunogenicity and protective efficacy of a *Plasmodium yoelii* Hsp60 DNA vaccine in BALB/c mice. Infect. Immun. 69: 3897-3905.

Santra, S., Barouch, D.H., Jackson, S.S., Kuroda, M.J., Schmitz, J.E., Lifton, M.A., Sharpe, A.H., and Letvin, N.L. 2000. Functional equivalency of B7-1 and B7-2 for costimulating plasmid DNA vaccine-elicited CTL responses. J. Immunol. 165: 6791-6795.

Sasaki, S., Hamajima, K., Fukushima, J., Ihata, A., Ishii, N., Gorai, I., Hirahara, F., Mohri, H., and Okuda, K. 1998a. Comparison of intranasal and intramuscular immunization against human immunodeficiency virus type 1 with a DNA-monophosphoryl lipid A adjuvant vaccine. Infect. Immun. 66: 823-826.

Sasaki, S., Sumino, K., Hamajima, K., Fukushima, J., Ishii, N., Kawamoto, S., Mohri, H., Kensil, C.R., and Okuda, K. 1998b. Induction of systemic and mucosal immune responses to human immunodeficiency virus type 1 by a DNA vaccine formulated with QS-21 saponin adjuvant via intramuscular and intranasal routes. J. Virol. 72: 4931-4939.

Sawai, E.T. and Butel, J.S. 1989. Association of heat shock proteins with the SV40 large T antigen. J. Virol. 63: 3961-3973.

Schirmbeck, R., B^hm, W., Ando, K.-I., Chisari, F.V., and Reimann, J. 1995. Nucleic acid vaccination primes hepatitis B surface antigen-specific cytotoxic T lymphocytes in nonresponder mice. J. Virol. 69: 5929-5934.

Schirmbeck, R., B^hm, W., and Reimann, J. 1997. Stress protein (hsp73)-mediated, TAP-independent processing of endogenous, truncated SV40 large T antigen for Db-restricted peptide presentation. Eur. J. Immunol. 27: 2016-2023.

Schirmbeck, R., Gerstner, O., and Reimann, J. 1999. Truncated or chimeric endogenous protein antigens gain immunogenicity for B cells by stress protein-facilitated expression. Eur. J. Immunol. 29: 1740-1749.

Schirmbeck, R. and Reimann, J. 1994. Peptide transporter-independent, stress protein-mediated endosomal processing of endogenous protein antigens for major histocompatibility complex class I presentation. Eur. J. Immunol. 24: 1478-1486.

Schirmbeck,R. and Reimann,J. 2001. Modulation of Gene-Gun-Mediated Th2 Immunity to Hepatitis B Surface Antigen by Bacterial CpG Motifs or IL-12. Intervirology 44: 115-123.

Shiver, J.W., Perry, H.C., Davies, M.E., Freed, D.C., and Liu, M.A. 1995. Cytotoxic T lymphocyte and helper T cell responses following HIV polynucleotide vaccination. Ann. NY Acad. Sci. 772: 198-208.

Siegrist, C.A. 1997. Vaccination strategies for children with specific medical conditions: a paediatrician's viewpoint. Eur. J. Pediatr. 156: 899-904.

Siegrist, C.A. and Lambert, P.H. 1997. Immunization with DNA vaccines in early life: advantages and limitations as compared to conventional vaccines. Springer Semin. Immunopathol. 19: 233-243.

Simon, M.M., Gern, L., Hauser, P., Zhong, W., Nielsen, P.J., Kramer, M.D., Brenner, C., and Wallich, R. 1996. Protective immunization with plasmid DNA containing the outer surface lipoprotein A gene of *Borrelia burgdorferi* is independent of an eukaryotic promoter. Eur. J. Immunol. 26: 2831-2840.

Sin, J.I., Kim, J., Dang, K., Lee, D., Patchuk, C., Satishchandran, C., and Weiner, D.B. 2000. LFA-3 plasmid DNA enhances Ag-specific humoral- and cellular-mediated protective immunity against herpes simplex virus-2 *in vivo*: involvement of CD4+ T cells in protection. Cell Immunol. 203: 19-28.

Sin, J.I., Kim, J.J., Arnold, R.L., Shroff, K.E., McCallus, D., Pachuk, C., McElhiney, S.P., Wolf, M.W., Pompa-de, B.S., Higgins, T.J., Ciccarelli, R.B., and Weiner, D.B. 1999. IL-12 gene as a DNA vaccine adjuvant in a herpes mouse model: IL-12 enhances Th1-type CD4+ T cell-mediated protective immunity against herpes simplex virus-2 challenge. J. Immunol. 162: 2912-2921.

Sin, J.I., Kim, J.J., Ugen, K.E., Ciccarelli, R.B., Higgins, T.J., and Weiner, D.B. 1998. Enhancement of protective humoral (Th2) and cell-mediated (Th1) immune responses against herpes simplex virus-2 through co-delivery of granulocyte-macrophage colony-stimulating factor expression cassettes. Eur. J. Immunol. 28: 3530-3540.

Singh, J.H., Scherer, H.U., Hilf, N., Arnold, S.D., Rammensee, H.G., Toes, R.E., and Schild, H. 2000a. The heat shock protein gp96 induces maturation of dendritic cells and down-regulation of its receptor. Eur. J. Immunol. 30: 2211-2215.

Singh, J.H., Toes, R.E., Spee, P., Munz, C., Hilf, N., Schoenberger, S.P., Ricciardi, C.P., Neefjes, J., Rammensee, H.G., Arnold, S.D., and Schild, H. 2000b. Cross-presentation of glycoprotein 96-associated antigens on major histocompatibility complex class I molecules requires receptor-mediated endocytosis. J. Exp. Med. 191: 1965-1974.

Sondermann, H., Becker, T., Mayhew, M., Wieland, F., and Hartl, F.U. 2000. Characterization of a receptor for heat shock protein 70 on macrophages and monocytes. Biol. Chem. 381: 1165-1174.

Srivastava, P.K. 2000. Immunotherapy of human cancer: lessons from mice. Nat. Immunol. 1: 363-366.

Srivastava, P.K. and Jaikaria, N.S. 2001. Methods of purification of heat shock protein-peptide complexes for use as vaccines against cancers and infectious diseases. Methods Mol. Biol. 156: 175-186.

Srivastava, P.K., Menoret, A., Basu, S., Binder, R.J., and McQuade, K.L. 1998. Heat shock proteins come of age: primitive functions acquire new roles in an adaptive world. Immunity. 8: 657-665.

Srivastava, P.K., Udono, H., Blachere, N.E., and Li, Z. 1994. Heat shock proteins transfer peptides during antigen processing and CTL priming. Immgen 39: 93-98.

Sun, W.H., Burkholder, J.K., Sun, J., Culp, J., Turner, J., Lu, X.G., Pugh, T.D., Ershler, W.B., and Yang, N.S. 1995. *In vivo* cytokine gene transfer by gene gun reduces tumor growth in mice. Proc. Natl. Acad. Sci. USA. 92: 2889-2893.

Suto, R. and Srivastava, P.K. 1995. A mechanism for the specific immunogenicity of heat shock protein-chaperoned peptides. Science 269: 1585-1588.

Suzue, K. and Young, R. 1996. Adjuvant-free hsp70 fusion protein system elicits humoral and cellular immune responses to HIV-1 p24. J. Immunol. 156: 873-879.

Suzue, K., Zhou, X., Eisen, H.N., and Young, R. 1997. Heat shock fusion proteins as vehicles for antigen delivery into the major histocompatibility complex class I presentation pathway. Proc. Natl. Acad. Sci. USA. 94: 13146-13151.

Tabona, P., Reddi, K., Khan, S., Nair, S.P., Crean, S.J., Meghji, S., Wilson, M., Preuss, M., Miller, A.D., Poole, S., Carne, S., and Henderson, B. 1998. Homogeneous *Escherichia coli* chaperonin 60 induces IL-1β and IL-6 gene expression in human monocytes by a mechanism independent of protein conformation. J. Immunol. 161: 1414-1421.

Tanelian, D.L., Barry, M.A., Johnston, S.A., Le, T., and Smith, G. 1997. Controlled gene gun delivery and expression of DNA within the cornea. Biotechniques 23: 484-488.

Tang, D.C., DeVit, M., and Johnston, S.A. 1992. Genetic immunization is a simple method for eliciting an immune response. Nature 356: 152-154.

Terlecky, S.R., Chiang, H.-L., Olson, T.S., and Dice, J.F. 1992. Protein and peptide binding and stimulation of *in vitro* lysosomal proteolysis by the 73-kDa heat shock cognate protein. J. Biol. Chem. 267: 9202.

Thery, C., Boussac, M., Veron, P., Ricciardi-Castagnoli, P., Raposo, G., Garin, J., and Amigorena, S. 2001. Proteomic analysis of dendritic cell-derived exosomes: a secreted subcellular compartment distinct from apoptotic vesicles. J. Immunol. 166: 7309-7318.

Thery, C., Regnault, A., Garin, J., Wolfers, J., Zitvogel, L., Ricciardi-Castagnoli, P., Raposo, G., and Amigorena, S. 1999. Molecular characterization of dendritic cell-derived exosomes. Selective accumulation of the heat shock protein hsc73. J. Cell Biol. 147: 599-610.

Thomson, S.A., Elliott, S.L., Sherritt, M.A., Sproat, K.W., Coupar, B.E., Scalzo, A.A., Forbes, C.A., Ladhams, A.M., Mo, X.Y., TRipp, R.A., Doherty, P.C., Moss, D.J., and Suhrbier, A. 1996. Recombinant polyepitope vaccines for the delivery of multiple CD8 cytotoxic T cell epitopes. J. Immunol. 157: 822-826.

Toda, S., Ishii, N., Okada, E., Kusakabe, K.I., Arai, H., Hamajima, K., Gorai, I., Nishioka, K., and Okuda, K. 1997. HIV-1-specific cell-mediated immune responses induced by DNA vaccination were enhanced by mannan-coated liposomes and inhibited by anti-interferon–γ antibody. imm 92: 111-117.

Todryk, S., Melcher, A.A., Hardwick, N., Linardakis, E., Bateman, A., Colombo, M.P., Stoppacciaro, A., and Vile, R.G. 1999. Heat shock protein

70 induced during tumor cell killing induces Th1 cytokines and targets immature dendritic cell precursors to enhance antigen uptake. J. Immunol. 163: 1398-1408.

Torres, C.A., Iwasaki, A., Barber, B.H., and Robinson, H.L. 1997. Differential dependence on target site tissue for gene gun and intramuscular DNA immunizations. J. Immunol. 158: 4529-4532.

Tsuji, T., Hamajima, K., Fukushima, J., Xin, K.Q., Ishii, N., Aoki, I., Ishigatsubo, Y., Tani, K., Kawamoto, S., Nitta, Y., Miyazaki, J., Koff, W.C., Okubo, T., and Okuda, K. 1997a. Enhancement of cell-mediated immunity against HIV-1 induced by coinoculation of plasmid-encoded HIV-1 antigen with plasmid expressing IL-12. J. Immunol. 158: 4008-4013.

Tsuji, T., Hamajima, K., Ishii, N., Aoki, I., Fukushima, J., Xin, K.Q., Kawamoto, S., Sasaki, S., Matsunaga, K., Ishigatsubo, Y., Tani, K., Okubo, T., and Okuda, K. 1997b. Immunomodulatory effects of a plasmid expressing B7-2 on human immunodeficiency virus-1-specific cell-mediated immunity induced by a plasmid encoding the viral antigen. Eur. J. Immunol. 27: 782-787.

Udono, H. and Srivastava, P.K. 1993. Heat shock protein 70-associated peptides elicit specific cancer immunity. J. Exp. Med. 178: 1391-1396.

Udono, H. and Srivastava, P.K. 1994. Comparison of tumor-specific immunogenicity of stress-induced protein gp96, hsp90, and hsp70. J. Immunol. 152: 5398-5403.

Ulmer, J.B., Deck, R.R., DeWitt, C.M., Donnhly, J.I., and Liu, M.A. 1996. Generation of MHC class I-restricted cytotoxic T lymphocytes by expression of a viral protein in muscle cells: antigen presentation by non-muscle cells. imm 89: 59-67.

Ulmer, J.B., Donnelly, J.J., Parker, S.E., Rhodes, G.H., Felgner, P.L., Dwarki, V.J., Gromkowski, S.H., Deck, R.R., DeWitt, C.M., Friedman, A., *et al.* 1993. Heterologous protection against influenza by injection of DNA encoding a viral protein. Science 259: 1745-1749.

Vabulas, R.M., Ahmad-Nejad, P., da Costa, C., Miethke, T., Kirschning, C.J., Hacker, H., and Wagner, H. 2001. Endocytosed heat shock protein 60s use TLR2 and TLR4 to activate the toll/interleukin-1 receptor signaling pathway in innate immune cells. J. Biol. Chem. 276: 31332-31339.

Vahlsing, H.L., Yankauckas, M.A., Sawdey, M., Gromkowski, S.H., and Manthorpe, M. 1994. Immunization with plasmid DNA using a pneumatic gun. J. Immunol. Methods 175: 11-22.

Walter, G., Carbone, A., and Welch, W.J. 1987. Medium tumor antigen of polyoma virus transformation-defective mutant NG59 is associated with 73-kilodalton heat shock protein. J. Virol. 61: 405-410.

Wang, B., Dang, K., Agadjanyan, M.G., Srikantan, V., Li, F., Ugen, K.E., Boyer, J., Merva, M., Williams, W.V., and Weiner, D.B. 1997. Mucosal immunization with a DNA vaccine induces immune responses against HIV-1 at a mucosal site. Vaccine 15: 821-825.

Watanabe, A., Raz, E., Kohsaka, H., Tighe, H., Baird, S.M., Kipps, T.J., and Carson, D.A. 1993. Induction of antibodies to a kappa V region by gene immunization. J. Immunol. 151: 2871-2876.

Wild, J., Grusby, M.J., Schirmbeck, R., and Reimann, J. 1999. Priming MHC-I-restricted, cytotoxic T lymphocyte responses to exogenous hepatitis B surface antigen is CD4$^+$ T cell-dependent. J. Immunol. 163: 1880-1887.

Wild, J., Gr‚ner, B., Metzger, K., Kuhrˆber, A., Pudollek, H.-P., Hauser, H., Schirmbeck, R., and Reimann, J. 1998. Polyvalent vaccination against hepatitis B surface and core antigen using dicistronic expression plasmids. Vaccine 16: 353-360.

Williams, R.S., Johnston, S.A., Riedy, M., DeVit, M.J., McElligott, S.G., and Sanford, J.C. 1991. Introduction of foreign genes into tissues of living mice by DNA-coated microprojectiles. Proc. Natl. Acad. Sci. USA. 88: 2726-2730.

Wolff, J.A., Ludtke, J.J., Acsadi, G., Williams, P., and Jani, A. 1992. Long-term persistence of plasmid DNA and foreign gene expression in mouse muscle. Hum. Mol. Genet. 1: 363-369.

Xiang, Z.Q. and Ertl, H.C.J. 1995. Manipulation of the immune response to a plasmid-encoded viral antigen by coinoculation with plasmids expressing cytokines. Immunity 2: 129-135.

Yang, N.S. and Sun, W.H. 1995. Gene gun and other non-viral approaches for cancer gene therapy. Nature Med. 1: 481-483.

Yokoyama, M., Zhang, J., and Whitton, J.L. 1996. DNA immunization: effects of vehicle and route of administration on the induction of protective antiviral immunity. FEMS Immunol. Med. Microbiol. 14: 221-230.

Yoo, C.G., Lee, S., Lee, C.T., Kim, Y.W., Han, S.K., and Shim, Y.S. 2000. Anti-inflammatory effect of heat shock protein induction is related to stabilization of I kappa B alpha through preventing I kappa B kinase activation in respiratory epithelial cells. J. Immunol. 164: 5416-5423.

Young, R. and Elliott, T.J. 1989. Stress proteins, infection, and immune surveillance. Cell 59: 5-8.

Youssef, S., Maor, G., Wildbaum, G., Grabie, N., Gour, L.A., and Karin, N. 2000. C-C chemokine-encoding DNA vaccines enhance breakdown of tolerance to their gene products and treat ongoing adjuvant arthritis. J. Clin. Invest 106: 361-371.

Youssef, S., Wildbaum, G., and Karin, N. 1999. Prevention of experimental autoimmune encephalomyelitis by MIP-1α and MCP-1 naked DNA vaccines. J. Autoimmun. 13: 21-29.

Zarozinski, C.C., Fynan, E.F., Selin, L.K., Robinson, H.L., and Welsh, R.M. 1995. Protective CTL-dependent immunity and enhanced immunopathology in mice immunized by particle bombardment with DNA encoding an internal virion protein. J. Immunol. 154: 4010-4017.

Zhou, X., Berglund, P., Zhao, H., Liljestrom, P., and Jondal, M. 1995. Generation of cytotoxic and humoral immune responses by nonreplicative recombinant Semliki Forest virus. Proc. Natl. Acad. Sci. USA. 92: 3009-3013.

From: *Vaccine Delivery Strategies*
Edited by: Guido Dietrich and Werner Goebel

Chapter 6

CpG Motifs in Vaccination

Stefan Zimmermann and Klaus Heeg

ABSTRACT

Bacterial DNA has been recognized as pathogen associated molecular pattern (PAMP) that activates innate immune cells. Bacterial DNA differs from mammalian DNA due to the abundance of unmethylated CpG dinucleotides. This difference is sensed by innate immune cells via Toll-like receptor 9. Synthetic oligonucleotides comprising a certain DNA motif (CpG motif) mimic bacterial DNA and are immunostimulatory *in vitro* and *in vivo*. These CpG oligonucleotides are potent agents that could be used as an adjuvant to aid humoral as well as cellular immune responses. Due to its marked ability to induce interleukin (IL)-12 and IL-18, CpG DNA directs the immune response to a Th1 phenotype. Moreover, synthetic oligonucleotides are chemically and structurally well defined and can be manufactured with high quality. These features of CpG DNA characterize it as a universal and versatile adjuvants in combination with various antigens and delivery systems.

INTRODUCTION

The innate limb of the immune system has evolved to recognize pathogen associated molecular patterns (PAMPs) in order to signal infectious danger and to elicit immunological effector functions (Medzhitov and Janeway, 1997). Both properties are viewed as obligatory for the induction of an adaptive immune response (Bendelac and Fearon, 1997). Accordingly, besides antigen delivery strategies, successful vaccination protocols require strong auxiliary signals which signal infection and thus initiate the adaptive immune system's response. The last decade has witnessed the molecular and functional definition of a large array of PAMPs capable to act as an adjuvants during vaccination. One of these PAMPs, the CpG DNA, has gained particular interest due to its strong adjuvants and modulatory properties (Krieg and Wagner, 2000).

THE DISCOVERY OF THE IMMUNOSTIMULATORY PROPERTIES OF BACTERIAL DNA

Almost three decades ago, it was recognized that certain mycobacterial strains could be used as an immunostimulatory adjuvants to combat cancer (Shimada *et al.*, 1985). It was entirely unexpected when Tokunaga and colleagues identified the DNA-rich fraction as the active component of mycobacteria. This fraction caused tumor regression as well as activation of natural killer (NK) cells. Importantly, it was noticed that mammalian DNA was totally ineffective (Yamamoto *et al.*, 1992a). To further elucidate the structural requirements for this effect, oligonucleotides were synthesized from genomic mycobacterial sequences (Kataoka *et al.*, 1992; Tokunaga *et al.*, 1999). This approach led to the identification of an immunostimulatory DNA motif that induced immune cell activation and cytokine secretion (Kuramoto *et al.*, 1992). The minimal immunostimulatory motif turned out to be a 6-mer palindromic DNA sequence which was effective when the central bases consisted of a cytosine and a guanosine linked via a phosphodiester bond (CpG-motif) (Yamamoto *et al.*, 1992b).

Two further approaches led as well to the characterization of the CpG motif. In analyzing the immune response of patients suffering from systemic lupus erythematodes, the group of Pisetsky reported that bacterial but not mammalian DNA could be detected in immune complexes. This DNA was capable to induce proliferation and IgM secretion from B cells (Pisetsky and

Reich, 1993). Furthermore, these authors were the first to show that methylation of the bacterial DNA abolished its immunostimulatory activity (Pisetsky, 1996). In parallel, when analyzing the efficacy of anti-sense DNA as a means to inhibit genomic translation, several groups recognized unforeseen side effects even with control sense oligonucleotides (Branda *et al.*, 1996; Pisetsky and Reich, 1994). These effects included B cell activation and polyclonal antibody secretion. It was the group of A. Krieg that succeeded in defining the structural DNA base sequence requirements for these immunostimulatory effects as a hexameric motif: two purins at the 5' end centered by a CpG dinucleotide and two pyrimidines at the 3' end (CpG motif) (Krieg *et al.*, 1995). Oligonucleotides containing this motif were immunostimulatory for B cells.

CpG Motifs And Immunostimulation

CpG motifs are abandoned in bacterial, viral and eukaryotic genomes. While most bacterial genomes contain CpG dinucleotides at the expected statistical frequency of 1/16, the overall frequency of CpG dinucleotides in the mammalian genome is reduced (Bird, 1980). This phenomenon was recognized long before and was termed "CG suppression". In addition, most CpG dinucleotides in mammalian genomes are located in so called CpG islands and are supposed to be involved in gene regulatory functions. These regulatory properties are in part due to excessive methylation of cytosine bases which rarely if at all occurs in bacteria. Thus, bacterial DNA contains large amounts of "free" CpG dinucleotides compared to mammalian. DNA, a feature that allows CpG motifs to be recognized as a pathogen associated molecular pattern (Krieg and Wagner, 2000).

CpG dinucleotides are necessary and represent the minimal requirement for immunostimulation by DNA. However, the intrinsic activity of CpG DNA is controlled by the 5' and 3' flanking regions of the CpG nucleotides (Lipford *et al.*, 1997a). Although plentiful of different oligonucleotides have been synthesized and analyzed, the rules to predict optimal flanking sequences have not been elucidated so far. In addition, empirical approaches have resulted in categorization of species-specific immunostimulatory sequences: while the classical CpG motif seems to be most effective only in rodents, innate immune cells of primates seem to recognize multiple CpG motifs in the context of a degenerated flanking region (Figure 1) (Bauer *et al.*, 1999, 2001; Hartmann *et al.*, 2000). These structural requirements seem to be directly correlated to the species-specificity of the receptors involved in CpG

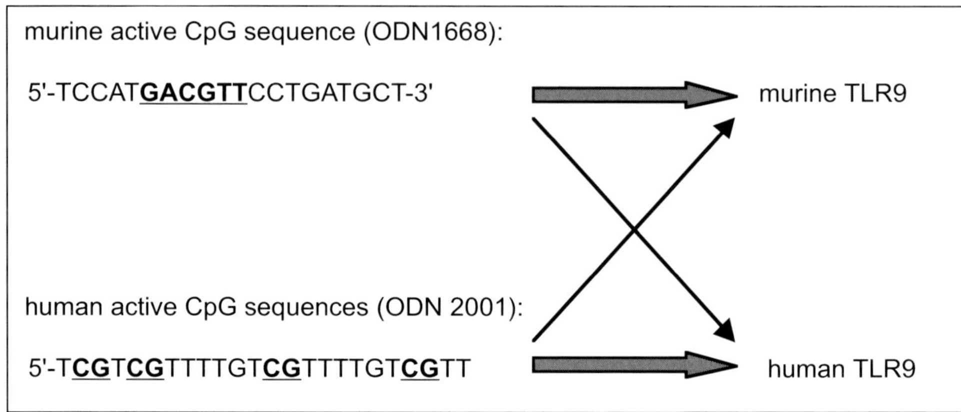

Figure 1. Species specificity of CpG DNA. ODN: oligonucleotide

recognition. It was shown that transfection with the human receptor (human Toll-like receptor 9, hTLR9) conveyed responsiveness to CpG in the context of "human" flanking sequences, while transfection with the murine counterpart (mTLR9) rendered cells reactive to CpG with "murine" flanking regions (Bauer *et al.*, 2001).

Flanking regions not only play an important role in enhancing immunostimulative properties of oligonucleotides, but may also lead to inhibitory oligonucleotides. Indeed, CpG oligonucleotides derived from adenoviral genomic sequences have been found that are able to antagonize the immunostimulatory effects of CpG oligonucleotides (Krieg *et al.*, 1998a). The mechanisms underlying this antagonism are not fully understood, yet might have important consequences for the understanding of the role of CpG DNA during infection. Moreover, flanking regions also might be critical to target CpG DNA to distinct cellular subsets. Recently, CpG oligonucleotides were described that contain G-rich flanking regions. These oligonucleotides failed to activate macrophages yet were active on NK cells (Ballas *et al.*, 1996; Iho *et al.*, 1999). Thus, flanking regions control CpG DNA's effectiveness as well as its cellular selectivity (Verthelyi *et al.*, 2001).

UPTAKE, RECEPTORS AND SIGNALING INDUCED BY CPG DNA

Compelling evidence suggests that in macrophages and dendritic cells (DC), bacterial DNA and CpG oligonucleotides meet their receptors within the endosome. This conclusion is mainly based on studies using inhibitors of endosomal maturation like bafilomycin or chloroquine (Macfarlane and Manzel, 1998; Yi and Krieg, 1998). Only some effects on human B cells might be triggered by a surface receptor. Detailed mechanisms of uptake of CpG DNA are still under debate: multiple receptor systems, e.g. the scavenger receptors or integrins, seem to be involved. However, studies in gene deleted cell lines or mice suggest that multiple mechanisms for uptake exist (Butler *et al.*, 2000; Liang *et al.*, 2000; Zhu *et al.*, 2001). In addition, the pharmaceutical composition of oligonucleotides strongly influences cellular uptake (*vide infra*).

After cellular uptake, signal cascades of the Toll-like receptor/IL-1 receptor signal transduction system are activated within minutes. These include translocation of NFκB and activation of MAP kinases (Häcker *et al.*, 1998, 1999; Yi and Krieg, 1998). The response to CpG DNA is strictly dependent on intracellular adaptor proteins like MyD88 and TRAF6 (Hacker *et al.*, 2000; Schnare *et al.*, 2000). Other adaptors could be involved in addition (Chu *et al.*, 2000). Accordingly, it was concluded that CpG DNA might be recognized in dependence on Toll-like receptors (TLR). Using a knock out approach, Akira and colleagues identified the receptor involved in recognition of CpG DNA as TLR9 (Hemmi *et al.*, 2000). Thus, CpG DNA is a member of PAMPs like endotoxin or bacterial lipoproteins which are recognized by the innate Toll-like receptor family (Akira *et al.*, 2001). Although a direct interaction of CpG DNA with TLR9 has not been shown so far, the cellular expression of TLR9 correlates with sensitivity to CpG DNA. In mice, TLR9 is primarily expressed by macrophages, DC and B cells. In humans, expression of TLR9 seems to be more restricted: lymphocytic DC express high levels of TLR9 while monocyte derived DC lack TLR9 expression and fail to respond to CpG DNA (Bauer *et al.*, 2001). Interestingly, recent evidence suggests that TLR9 molecules can be found in the endosome but not on the cell surface (Zimmermann and Heeg, unpublished observations), corroborating the functional data on cellular uptake and endosomal action of CpG DNA.

CpG DNA: Cellular Profiles

CpG DNA activates a variety of different cell types and cellular functions either directly and/or indirectly (Figure 2) (Lipford *et al.*, 1998; Wagner, 1999). The broad range of induced activities include mitogenic effects on B-lymphocytes (Krieg *et al.*, 1995; Liang *et al.*, 1996), induction of polyclonal Ig secretion, activation of macrophages, macrophage function (Sparwasser

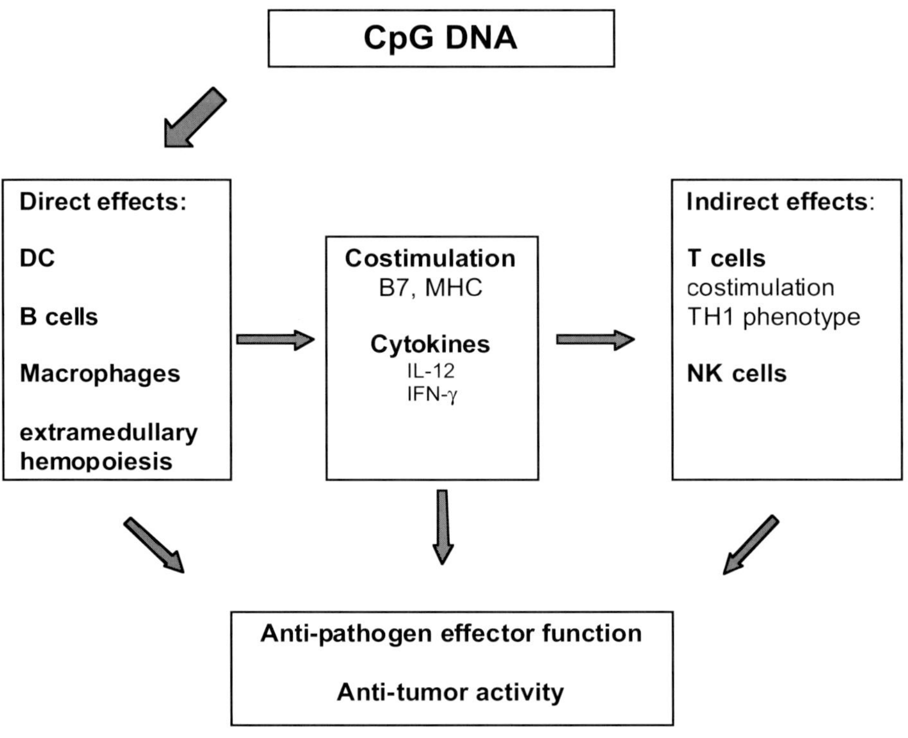

Figure 2. Effects of CpG DNA

et al., 1997a; Stacey *et al.*, 1996), differentiation of DC (Sparwasser *et al.*, 1998), augmentation of antigen processing and presentation (Ban *et al.*, 2000), activation of NK and T cells and finally induction of extramedullary hemopoiesis (Lipford *et al.*, 2000a; Sparwasser *et al.*, 1999). The effects on T cells and NK cells are most likely due to indirect stimulation via IL-12 and type I interferons (Sun *et al.*, 1998) produced by other innate immune cells upon CpG DNA stimulation (Halpern *et al.*, 1996; Heeg, 2000; Kranzer *et al.*, 2000). Although all cellular effects contribute to the activity of CpG DNA *in vivo*, with regard to vaccination the action of CpG DNA on macrophages and DC is most important.

Recognition of CpG DNA by immature DC leads to maturation and induction of immune functions like cytokine secretion, up-regulation of MHC and costimulatory molecules, resulting in an enhancement of their immunostimulatory potency towards adaptive immune cells (Hartmann *et al.*, 1999). Induced cytokines include IL-12, IL-18, IL-6, TNF and Interferons (Bohle *et al.*, 1999; Sparwasser *et al.*, 1998). Of particular importance is the propensity of CpG DNA to induce large amounts of IL-12 and IL-18 (Lipford *et al.*, 1997a). This is in contrast to the lower potency to induce IL-12 of endotoxin which is recognized in association with TLR4 (Cowdery *et al.*, 1999). Other PAMPs like lipoteichoic acid (TLR2 dependent) even fail to induce IL-12 at all (Lehner *et al.*, 2001). The molecular basis of the strong IL-12 induction by CpG DNA is not known.

One important and compared to other PAMPs unique hallmark of CpG DNA is its ability to induce a Th1 phenotype *in vivo* and *in vitro* (Heeg and Zimmermann, 2000). The cytokines IL-12, IL-18 and IFN-gamma play a pivotal role during imprintment of the T helper cell phenotype. T helper cells induced in the presence of CpG DNA predominantly produce IFN-gamma and not IL-4. Thus, CpG DNA is extremely helpful in balancing an immune response towards a Th1 type of reactivity.

CPG DNA: *IN VIVO* EFFECTS

At very high doses, CpG DNA administered *in vivo* might induce a lethal shock syndrome. This is due to an uncontrolled and dys-regulated production of pro-inflammatory cytokines which in turn induce systemic inflammation and cardiovascular pathophysiology. Ultimately, this may lead to a lethal cytokine syndrome (Sparwasser *et al.*, 1997a and 1997b). However, when CpG DNA is used to support immune responses in a proper dosage, these systemic effects could be neglected.

In vivo injection of CpG DNA strongly supports the induction of innate and adaptive immune responses. Macrophages and DCs are activated and effector functions like intracellular bactericidal functions are induced. NK cells are activated and produce IFN-gamma due to macrophage derived IL-12 (Halpern *et al.*, 1996). Thus, CpG DNA alerts innate immune cells and generates initial anti-pathogen directed effector functions. Accordingly, the first line of defense is strengthened (Klinman *et al.*, 1999). In parallel, the innate immune system is enabled to communicate with the adaptive immune system to induce a strong specific immune response. Key players are cytokines and antigen presented by innate immune cells (antigen presenting cells, APC). In addition, a cytokine milieu is induced which favors the induction of cellular responses of Th1 phenotype (Lipford *et al.*, 1997b).

CpG DNA As Adjuvants

These features qualify CpG DNA as an vaccine adjuvants. Indeed, when administered together with an antigen, CpG DNA strongly supports the induction of B- and T cell responses (Krieg, 1999; Lipford *et al.*, 1997b). In addition, CpG DNA was even active as an adjuvants in mucosal immunizations (Horner *et al.*, 1998; McCluskie and Davis, 1999). Titers of antigen specific immunoglobulins are enhanced and clearly are associated with the production of IgG2a antibodies indicating a predominant Th1 response (Roman *et al.*, 1997). CpG DNA is highly efficient as adjuvant and requires less immunizations when compared to other adjuvants (Weeratna *et al.*, 2000).

Besides its impressive effects on induction of adaptive immune responses, CpG DNA also strengthens the effector function of the innate immune system. This effect in itself contributes to an enhanced clearance of infectious pathogens. Moreover, innate defense mechanisms are triggered that are long lasting (Gao *et al.*, 1999; Klinman *et al.*, 1999; Krieg *et al.*, 1998b). It was shown that injection of CpG DNA alone rendered mice resistant to otherwise lethal infections with *Listeria* (Krieg *et al.*, 1998b; Wagner *et al.*, 2000) or *Leishmania* (Zimmermann *et al.*, 1998). Therefore, CpG DNA assists the innate immune system to combat infections. Accordingly, CpG DNA could be used as a solitary agent or in combination with an antigen in therapeutic vaccinations during ongoing infections. In addition, CpG DNA could also serve as adjuvants and immunomodulator in vaccination strategies aiming to induce an anti-cancer immune response (Weiner, 2000).

A further distinctive feature of CpG DNA as adjuvants is its ability to provide a costimulative milieu that favors activation of T lymphocytes. Those include CD4+ T helper cells as well as CD8+ T cells (Lipford *et al.*, 1997b). CD4 cells induced predominately express the Th1 phenotype. A characteristic quality of CpG DNA is its ability to support the generation of CD8 cytotoxic T cells (Lipford *et al.*, 1997b; Tascon *et al.*, 2000; Warren *et al.*, 2000). This implies that antigen is delivered via the MHC class I presentation pathway and that the CpG induced cytokine and costimulatory milieu is sufficient for the induction of CD8 T cells. CpG DNA induced adjuvanticity is so strong and efficient that CD4/CD8 T cell collaboration is not required for induction of CD8 T cells. Accordingly, MHC class II deficient mice still elicit a cytotoxic T cell response when immunized with antigen and CpG DNA. Furthermore, CpG DNA allows immunization of CD8 T cells with peptide fragments of antigen *in vivo* (Vabulas *et al.*, 2000). Thus, CpG DNA broadens

Table 1. CpG DNA as adjuvants in animal models

Antigen	Reference
Ovalbumin	Lipford *et al.*, 1997b
Hepatitis B surface antigen	Brazolot Millan *et al.*, 1998; Davis *et al.*, 2000; Davis *et al.*, 1998; McCluskie *et al.*, 1998
Influenza virus	Moldoveanu *et al.*, 1998
Respiratory Syncitial Virus	Hancock *et al.*, 2001
Simian/Human Immunodeficiency Virus	Cafaro *et al.*, 2001
Herpes Simplex Virus-2	Gallichan *et al.*, 2001
Human Immunodeficiency Virus	Moss *et al.*, 1999
Mycobacteria	Freidag *et al.*, 2000
Hib Polysaccharide	von Hunolstein *et al.*, 2000
Listeria	Elkins *et al.*, 1999; Krieg *et al.*, 1998b; Wagner *et al.*, 2000
Brucella	Al Mariri *et al.*, 2001
Leishmania	Stacey and Blackwell, 1999; Zimmermann *et al.*, 1998
Plasmodium	Jones *et al.*, 1999
Trypanosoma	Corral *et al.*, 2000
Schistosoma	Chiaramonte *et al.*, 2000
Neuroblastoma	Carpentier *et al.*, 1999
Glioma	Carpentier *et al.*, 2000
Fibrosarcoma	Hafner *et al.*, 2001
Allergy	Magone *et al.*, 2000
Ragweed amb a1	Tighe *et al.*, 2000a
Pollen bet v1	Jahn-Schmid *et al.*, 1999
Asthma	Broide and Raz, 1999; Broide *et al.*, 1998; Kline *et al.*, 1998; Metzger and Nyce, 1999

the adaptive immune cell types which can be targeted by an adjuvants. Hence, several lines of evidence support the concept that CpG DNA can be utilized as an universal adjuvants which improves efficacy of vaccines for B cell as well as for T cell responses. Indeed, a wide variety of different antigens have been tested with CpG DNA as adjuvants (Table 1) and thus proved the versatility of CpG DNA.

CpG motifs in vectors used for DNA vaccination might also be important for the efficacy of a DNA vaccine (Klinman *et al.*, 1997; Krieg *et al.*, 1998c). It was reported that CpG motifs within the vector's sequence enhance immunogenicity as well as induction of Th1-related immunoglobulin isotypes (Sato *et al.*, 1996). However, CpG related effects are dose dependent and seem to be minor in gene gun immunizations where the amount of vector DNA delivered is rather low. In addition, CpG DNA is recognized in the endosomal compartment and presumably not within the cytosol or nucleus. Moreover, endosomal plasmids are degraded by nucleases and thus loose immunostimulatory potency. Therefore, complementation of vectors with CpG motifs might be less effective compared to simultaneous administration of vectors and nuclease resistant CpG oligonucleotides (Fensterle *et al.*, 1999).

CpG DNA And Th1/Th2 Regulation

Since CpG DNA harbors the unique propensity to induce Th1 instructing cytokines, it was used in various experimental protocols to instruct or to redirect T helper cell responses. First it was recognized that CpG DNA skewed the immunoglobulin isotypes induced after immunization to a Th1-dependent pattern (Brazolot Millan *et al.*, 1998; Carson and Raz, 1997; Chu *et al.*, 1997; Heeg and Zimmermann, 2000), including up-regulation of IgG2a and down-regulation of IgG1. In murine leishmaniasis, a model for a lethal Th2 dominated infectious disease, CpG DNA prevented the induction of undesired Th2 responses and thus protected mice from uncontrolled infection (Mody *et al.*, 1999; Walker *et al.*, 1999; Zimmermann *et al.*, 1998). Moreover, in the presence of CpG DNA, a lasting and efficient Th1 memory response was induced (Zimmermann *et al.*, 1998). So far, other adjuvants failed to elicit similar protective responses in this model. Analogous results were obtained when murine models of allergic asthma were examined. Again, CpG DNA strongly favored the induction of Th1 responses and suppressed the development of pathogenic Th2 cells. Thus CpG DNA seems to be a favorable adjuvants when used in vaccination strategies aiming to prevent the induction of Th2 dominated allergic diseases (Broide *et al.*, 2000; Van Uden and Raz, 1999).

Even more encouraging are the actions of CpG DNA on already established Th2 dominated immune responses. In murine leishmaniasis, treatment with CpG oligonucleotides was capable to cure an established disease up to 3 weeks after infection. So far, no compound was equally efficient. Interestingly, the T cell phenotype of cured mice was Th1, indicating that CpG DNA can re-direct an existing Th2 immune phenotype to a Th1 type of reactivity. Similar results have been obtained in the murine asthma model (Broide *et al.*, 1998; Kline *et al.*, 1998; Serebrisky *et al.*, 2000). Hence, CpG DNA has good chances to become a favorable adjuvants in prevention and therapy of allergic diseases.

CpG DNA: Pharmaceutical Compositions

CpG DNA is advantageous to other PAMPs since synthetic oligonucleotides mimic the effect of bacterial DNA. Therefore, well defined pharmaceutical compositions can be manufactured with controlled purity. Synthetic oligonucleotides were shown to not only replace bacterial DNA in its activity but also to harbor some features which are superior to bacterial DNA. First, short (~20 bases) synthetic oligonucleotides are sufficient to exert immunostimulatory activity. Second, oligonucleotides with specific and optimized DNA sequences can be synthesized with defined quality and purity. Third, synthetic oligonucleotides are chemical compounds that can be modified or chemically altered and finally synthetic oligonucleotides can be protected from the attack of nucleases by introducing several backbone modifications.

The latter feature of oligonucleotides is of special advantage. Bacterial DNA as well as phosphodiester (PO) oligonucleotides are degraded and thus act as an adjuvants only for a limited period of time. In contrast, phosphothioate (PTO) modifications protect oligonucleotides from nucleases and thus guarantee a sustained activity. However, prolonged activity also might have its price and might cause severe side effects. In mice, a long lasting swelling of the local lymph nodes, increased cellularity and a concomitant cytokine production was observed (Baek *et al.*, 2001; Lipford *et al.*, 2000b). During the duration of the lymphadenopathy, proteins injected at the local site induced a cytolytic T cell response without the aid of further adjuvants (Lipford *et al.*, 2000b). CpG DNA induced arthritis when injected directly (Deng *et al.*,

1999) and was able to activate T cell clones in models of experimental autoimmune encephalitis (EAE) (Segal *et al.*, 2000; Tsunoda *et al.*, 1999). Whether these observations might indicate a general capacity of CpG DNA to induce autoreactive responses can not be excluded yet.

Phosphothioate modification of oligonucleotides alters their biological properties. Although protection from nucleases is a desired effect, PTO oligonucleotides show unspecific binding to proteins which might restrict their distribution and cellular uptake (Britigan *et al.*, 2001). PTO modification enhances uptake into endocytic active cells, yet this effect is independent of the oligonucleotide's sequence (Iversen *et al.*, 1992). In contrast, PTO modification alters the sterical shape of the central CpG region. Some effects of CpG DNA thus require an unprotected CpG core motif within the oligonucleotide, while other effects seem to be independent of the backbone modification (Zhao and Agrawal, 1999). Clearly optimized oligonucleotides with defined sequences and appropriate backbone modifications have still to be developed.

It would be advantageous to target CpG oligonucleotides and antigen to the same antigen presenting cell. Although most antigens and oligonucleotides are endocytosed and can be found within endosomes, a direct coupling of antigen to oligonucleotides could enhance the efficacy of adjuvanticity. Indeed, chemical linkage of antigens (including allergens) to CpG oligonucleotides enhanced their efficacy (Shirota *et al.*, 2001; Tighe *et al.*, 2000a and 2000b). This approach allowed a reduction of the doses of oligonucleotide needed for effective vaccination by a factor of 100 (Shirota *et al.*, 2000; Tighe *et al.*, 2000a and 2000b). In addition, pharmaceutical compositions targeting CpG oligonucleotides directly to APC via antibody coated liposomes or ligand coupling might further enhance their efficacy and thus reduce potential side effects.

CpG DNA: Prospects

Delineation of the immunostimulatory function of bacterial DNA has led to a new class of synthetic well defined adjuvants: CpG oligonucleotides (Krieg *et al.*, 2000). There is no doubt that CpG DNA can be used as an universal adjuvants in combination with many different antigen preparations. One important and unique feature of CpG DNA is its profound ability to induce Th1 dominated immune responses, including induction of cytolytic CD8+ T cells. The synthetic chemical composition allows multiple modifications in structure and sequence and simplifies combinatorial compositions with antigen or various delivery systems. However, immunostimulatory sequences used were deduced empirically, leaving the possibility that synthetic oligonucleotides can still be optimized in their functional activity. The identification of TLR9 as receptor involved in recognition of CpG DNA will allow to definitively determine the structure-function relationship between CpG DNA and its receptor and thus will lead to structurally defined new immunostimulatory oligonucleotides.

REFERENCES

Akira, S., Takeda, K., and Kaisho, T. 2001. Toll-like receptors: critical proteins linking innate and acquired immunity. Nat. Immunol. 2: 675-680.

Al Mariri, A., Tibor, A., Mertens, P., De, B., Michel, P., Godefroid, J., Walravens, K., and Letesson, J.J. 2001. Protection of BALB/c mice against *Brucella abortus* 544 challenge by vaccination with bacterioferritin or P39 recombinant proteins with CpG oligodeoxynucleotides as adjuvant. Infect. Immun. 69: 4816-4822.

Baek, K.H., Ha, S.J., and Sung, Y.C. 2001. A novel function of phosphorothioate oligodeoxynucleotides as chemoattractants for primary macrophages. J. Immunol. 167: 2847-2854.

Ballas, Z.K., Rasmussen, W.L., and Krieg, A.M. 1996. Induction of NK activity in murine and human cells by CpG motifs in oligodeoxynucleotides and bacterial DNA. J. Immunol. 157: 1840-1845.

Ban, E., Dupre, L., Hermann, E., Rohn, W., Vendeville, C., Quatannens, B., Ricciardi-Castagnoli, P., Capron, A., and Riveau, G. 2000. CpG motifs induce Langerhans cell migration *in vivo*. Int. Immunol. 12: 737-745.

Bauer, M., Heeg, K., Wagner, H., and Lipford, G.B. 1999. DNA activates human immune cells through a CpG sequence dependent manner. Immunology 97: 699-705.

Bauer, S., Kirschning, C.J., Hacker, H., Redecke, V., Hausmann, S., Akira, S., Wagner, H., and Lipford, G.B. 2001. Human TLR9 confers responsiveness to bacterial DNA via species-specific CpG motif recognition. Proc. Natl. Acad. Sci.USA. 98: 9237-9242.

Bendelac, A., and Fearon, D.T. 1997. Innate immunity; innate pathways that control acquired immunity. Curr. Opin. Immunol. 9: 1-3.

Bird, A.P. 1980. DNA methylation and the frequency of CpG in animal DNA. Nucleic. Acids. Res. 8: 1499-1504.

Bohle, B., Jahn-Schmid, B., Maurer, D., Kraft, D., and Ebner, C. 1999. Oligodeoxynucleotides containing CpG motifs induce IL-12, IL-18 and

IFN- gamma production in cells from allergic individuals and inhibit IgE synthesis *in vitro*. Eur. J. Immunol. 29: 2344-2353.

Branda, R.F., Moore, A.L., Lafayette, A.R., Mathews, L., Hong, R., Zon, G., Brown, T., and McCormack, J.J. 1996. Amplification of antibody production by phosphorothioate oligodeoxynucleotides. J. Lab. Clin. Med. 128: 329-338.

Brazolot Millan, C.L., Weeratna, R., Krieg, A.M., Siegrist, C.A., and Davis, H.L. 1998. CpG DNA can induce strong Th1 humoral and cell-mediated immune responses against hepatitis B surface antigen in young mice. Proc. Natl. Acad. Sci.USA. 95: 15553-15558.

Britigan, B.E., Lewis, T.S., Waldschmidt, M., McCormick, M.L., and Krieg, A.M. 2001. Lactoferrin binds CpG-containing oligonucleotides and inhibits their immunostimulatory effects on human B cells. J. Immunol. 167: 2921-2928.

Broide, D., Cho, J.Y., Miller, M., Nayar, J., Stachnick, G., Castaneda, D., Roman, M., and Raz, E. 2000. Modulation of asthmatic response by immunostimulatory DNA sequences. Springer Semin. Immunopathol. 22: 117-124.

Broide, D., and Raz, E. 1999. DNA-Based Immunization for Asthma. Int. Arch. Allergy Immunol. 118: 453-456.

Broide, D., Schwarze, J., Tighe, H., Gifford, T., Nguyen, M.D., Malek, S., Van Uden, J., Martin-Orozco, E., Gelfand, E.W., and Raz, E. 1998. Immunostimulatory DNA sequences inhibit IL-5, eosinophilic inflammation, and airway hyperresponsiveness in mice. J. Immunol. 161: 7054-7062.

Butler, M., Crooke, R.M., Graham, M.J., Lemonidis, K.M., Lougheed, M., Murray, S.F., Witchell, D., Steinbrecher, U., and Bennett, C.F. 2000. Phosphorothioate oligodeoxynucleotides distribute similarly in class A scavenger receptor knockout and wild-type mice. J. Pharmacol. Exp. Ther. 292: 489-496.

Cafaro, A., Titti, F., Fracasso, C., Maggiorella, M.T., Baroncelli, S., Caputo, A., Goletti, D., Borsetti, A., Pace, M., Fanales-Belasio, E., Ridolfi, B., Negri, D.R., Sernicola, L., Belli, R., Corrias, F., Macchia, I., Leone, P., Michelini, Z., ten Haaft, P., Butto, S., Verani, P., and Ensoli, B. 2001. Vaccination with DNA containing tat coding sequences and unmethylated CpG motifs protects cynomolgus monkeys upon infection with simian/ human immunodeficiency virus (SHIV89.6P). Vaccine 19: 2862-2877.

Carpentier, A.F., Chen, L., Maltonti, F., and Delattre, J.Y. 1999. Oligodeoxynucleotides containing CpG motifs can induce rejection of a neuroblastoma in mice. Cancer Res. 59: 5429-5432.

Carpentier, A.F., Xie, J., Mokhtari, K., and Delattre, J.Y. 2000. Successful treatment of intracranial gliomas in rat by oligodeoxynucleotides containing CpG motifs. Clin. Cancer Res. 6: 2469-2473.

Carson, D.A., and Raz, E. 1997. Oligonucleotide adjuvants for T helper 1 (Th1)-specific vaccination. J. Exp. Med. 186: 1621-1622.

Chiaramonte, M.G., Hesse, M., Cheever, A.W., and Wynn, T.A. 2000. CpG oligonucleotides can prophylactically immunize against Th2-mediated schistosome egg-induced pathology by an IL-12-independent mechanism. J. Immunol. 164: 973-985.

Chu, R.S., Targoni, O.S., Krieg, A.M., Lehmann, P.V., and Harding, C.V. 1997. CpG oligodeoxynucleotides act as adjuvants that switch on T helper 1 (Th1) immunity. J. Exp. Med. 186: 1623-1631.

Chu, W., Gong, X., Li, Z., Takabayashi, K., Ouyang, H., Chen, Y., Lois, A., Chen, D.J., Li, G.C., Karin, M., and Raz, E. 2000. DNA-PKcs is required for activation of innate immunity by immunostimulatory DNA. Cell 103: 909-918.

Corral, R.S. and Petray, P.B. 2000. CpG DNA as a Th1-promoting adjuvant in immunization against *Trypanosoma cruzi*. Vaccine 19: 234-242.

Cowdery, J.S., Boerth, N.J., Norian, L.A., Myung, P.S., and Koretzky, G.A. 1999. Differential regulation of the IL-12 p40 promoter and of p40 secretion by CpG DNA and lipopolysaccharide. J. Immunol. 162: 6770-6775.

Davis, H.L., Suparto, I.I., Weeratna, R.R., Jumintarto, Iskandriati, D.D., Chamzah, S.S., Ma'ruf, A.A., Nente, C.C., Pawitri, D.D., Krieg, A.M., Heriyanto, Smits, W., and Sajuthi, D.D. 2000. CpG DNA overcomes hyporesponsiveness to hepatitis B vaccine in orangutans. Vaccine 18: 1920-1924.

Davis, H.L., Weeranta, R., Waldschmidt, T.J., Tygrett, L., Schorr, J., and Krieg, A.M. 1998. CpG DNA is a potent enhancer of specific immunity in mice immunized with recombinant Hepatitis B surface antigen. J. Immunol. 160: 870-876.

Deng, G.M., Nilsson, I.M., Verdrengh, M., Collins, L.V., and Tarkowski, A. 1999. Intra-articulary localized bacterial DNA containig CpG motifs induces arthritis. Nature Med. 5: 702-705.

Elkins, K.L., Rhinehart-Jones, T.R., Stibitz, S., Conover, J.S., and Klinman, D.M. 1999. Bacterial DNA containing CpG motifs stimulates lymphocyte-dependent protection of mice against lethal infection with intracellular bacteria. J. Immunol 162: 2291-2298.

Fensterle, J., Grode, L., Hess, J., and Kaufmann, S.H. 1999. Effective DNA vaccination against listeriosis by Prime/Boost inoculation. J. Immunol. 163: 4510-4518.

Freidag, B.L., Melton, G.B., Collins, F., Klinman, D.M., Cheever, A., Stobie, L., Suen, W., and Seder, R.A. 2000. CpG oligodeoxynucleotides and interleukin-12 improve the efficacy of *Mycobacterium bovis* BCG vaccination in mice challenged with *M. tuberculosis*. Infect. Immun. 68: 2948-2953.

Gallichan, W.S., Woolstencroft, R.N., Guarasci, T., McCluskie, M.J., Davis, H.L., and Rosenthal, K.L. 2001. Intranasal Immunization with CpG oligodeoxynucleotides as an adjuvant dramatically increases IgA and protection against Herpes Simplex Virus-2 in the genital tract. J. Immunol. 166: 3451-3457.

Gao, J.J., Zuvanich, E.G., Xue, Q., Horn, D.L., Silverstein, R., and Morrison, D.C. 1999. Cutting edge: bacterial DNA and LPS act in synergy in inducing nitric oxide production in RAW 264.7 macrophages. J. Immunol. 163: 4095-4099.

Hacker, H., Vabulas, R.M., Takeuchi, O., Hoshino, K., Akira, S., and Wagner, H. 2000. Immune cell activation by bacterial CpG-DNA through myeloid differentiation marker 88 and tumor necrosis factor receptor-associated factor (TRAF)6. J. Exp. Med. 192: 595-600.

Hafner, M., Zawatzky, R., Hirtreiter, C., Buurman, W.A., Echtenacher, B., Hehlgans, T., and Mannel, D.N. 2001. Antimetastatic effect of CpG DNA mediated by type I IFN. Cancer Res. 61: 5523-5528.

Halpern, M.D., Kurlander, R.J., and Pisetsky, D.S. 1996. Bacterial DNA induces murine interferon-gamma production by stimulation of interleukin 12 and tumor necrosis factor-alpha. Cell. Immunol. 167: 72-78.

Hancock, G.E., Heers, K.M., Smith, J.D., Scheuer, C.A., Ibraghimov, A.R., and Pryharski, K.S. 2001. CpG containing oligodeoxynucleotides are potent adjuvants for parenteral vaccination with the fusion (F) protein of respiratory syncytial virus (RSV). Vaccine 19: 4874-4882.

Hartmann, G., Weeratna, R.D., Ballas, Z.K., Payette, P., Blackwell, S., Suparto, I., Rasmussen, W.L., Waldschmidt, M., Sajuthi, D., Purcell, R.H., Davis, H.L., and Krieg, A.M. 2000. Delineation of a CpG phosphorothioate oligodeoxynucleotide for activating primate immune responses *in vitro* and *in vivo*. J. Immunol. 164: 1617-1624.

Hartmann, G., Weiner, G.J., and Krieg, A.M. 1999. CpG DNA: A potent signal for growth, activation, and maturation of human dendritic cells. Proc. Natl. Acad. Sci. USA. 96: 9305-9310.

Häcker, H., Mischak, H., Häcker, G., Eser, S., Prenzel, N., Ullrich, A., and Wagner, H. 1999. Cell type-specific activation of mitogen-activated protein kinases by CpG-DNA controls interleukin-12 release from antigen- presenting cells. EMBO J. 18: 6973-6982.

Häcker, H., Mischak, H., Miethke, T., Liptay, S., Schmid, R., Sparwasser, T., Heeg, K., Lipford, G.B., and Wagner, H. 1998. CpG-DNA specific activation of antigen presenting cells requires stress kinase activity and is proceeded by non-specific endocytosis and endosomal maturation. EMBO J. 17: 6230-6240.

Heeg, K. 2000. CpG-DNA costimulates antigen reactive T cells. Curr. Top. Microbiol. Immunol. 247: 93-105.

Heeg, K., and Zimmermann, S. 2000. CpG DNA as a Th1 trigger. Int. Arch. Allergy Immunol. 121: 87-97.

Hemmi, H., Takeuchi, O., Kawai, T., Kaisho, T., Sato, S., Sanjo, H., Matsumoto, M., Hoshino, K., Wagner, H., Takeda, K., and Akira, S. 2000. A Toll-like receptor recognizes bacterial DNA.[In Process Citation]. Nature 408: 740-745.

Horner, A.A., Ronaghy, A., Cheng, P.M., Nguyen, M.D., Cho, H.J., Broide, D., and Raz, E. 1998. Immunostimulatory DNA is a potent mucosal adjuvant. Cell. Immunol. 190: 77-82.

Iho, S., Yamamoto, T., Takahashi, T., and Yamamoto, S. 1999. Oligodeoxynucleotides containing palindrome sequences with internal 5'-CpG-3' act directly on human NK and activated T cells to induce IFN-gamma production *In vitro*. J. Immunol. 163: 3642-3652.

Iversen, P.L., Zhu, S., Meyer, A., and Zon, G. 1992. Cellular uptake and subcellular distribution of phosphorothioate oligonucleotides into cultured cells. Antisense Res. Dev. 2: 211-222.

Jahn-Schmid, B., Wiedermann, U., Bohle, B., Repa, A., Kraft, D., and Ebner, C. 1999. Oligodeoxynucleotides containing CpG motifs modulate the allergic TH2 response of BALB/c mice to bet v 1, the major birch pollen allergen. J. Allergy Clin. Immunol. 104: 1015-1023.

Jones, T.R., Obaldia, N.3., Gramzinski, R.A., Charoenvit, Y., Kolodny, N., Kitov, S., Davis, H.L., Krieg, A.M., and Hoffman, S.L. 1999. Synthetic oligodeoxynucleotides containing CpG motifs enhance immunogenicity of a peptide malaria vaccine in Aotus monkeys. Vaccine 17: 3065-3071.

Kataoka, T., Yamamoto, S., Yamamoto, T., Kuramoto, E., Kimura, Y., Yano, O., and Tokunaga, T. 1992. Antitumor activity of synthetic oligonucleotides with sequences from cDNA encoding proteins of *Mycobacterium bovis* BCG. Jpn.J.Cancer Res. 83: 244-247.

Kline, J.N., Waldschmidt, T.J., Businga, T.R., Lemish, J.E., Weinstock, J.V., Thorne, P.S., and Krieg, A.M. 1998. Modulation of airway inflammation by CpG oligodesoxynucleotides in a murine model of asthma. J. Immunol. 160: 2555-2559.

Klinman, D.M., Conover, J., and Coban, C. 1999. Repeated administration of synthetic oligodeoxynucleotides expressing CpG motifs provides long-term protection against bacterial infection. Infect. Immun. 67: 5658-5663.

Klinman, D.M., Yamshchikov, G., and Ishigatsubo, Y. 1997. Contribution of CpG motifs to the immunogenicity of DNA vaccines. J. Immunol. 158: 3635-3639.

Kranzer, K., Bauer, M., Lipford, G.B., Heeg, K., Wagner, H., and Lang, R. 2000. CpG oligodeoxynucleotides enhance T cell receptor-triggered IFN-gamma production and up-regulation of CD69 via induction of antigen-presenting cell-derived interferon type I and IL-12. Immunology 99: 170-178.

Krieg, A.M. 1999. CpG DNA: a novel immunomodulator. Trends Microbiol. 7: 64-65.

Krieg, A.M., Love-Homan, L., Yi, A.K., and Harty, J.T. 1998b. CpG DNA induces sustained IL-12 expression *in vivo* and resistance to *Listeria monocytogenes* challenge. J. Immunol. 161: 2428-2434.

Krieg, A.M., and Wagner, H. 2000. Causing a commotion in the blood: immunotherapy progresses from bacteria to bacterial DNA. Immunol. Today 21: 521-526.

Krieg, A.M., Wu, T., Weeratna, R., Efler, S.M., Love-Homan, L., Yang, L., Yi, A.K., Short, D., and Davis, H.L. 1998a. Sequence motifs in adenoviral DNA block immune activation by stimulatory CpG motifs. Proc. Natl. Acad. Sci. USA. 95: 12631-12636.

Krieg, A.M., Yi, A.K., Matson, S., Waldschmidt, T.J., Bishop, G.A., Teasdale, R., Koretzky, G.A., and Klinman, D.M. 1995. CpG motifs in bacterial DNA trigger direct B-cell activation. Nature 374: 546-549.

Krieg, A.M., Yi, A.K., Schorr, J., and Davis, H. 1998c. The role of CpG oligonucleotides in DNA vaccines. Trends Microbiol. 6: 23-27.

Kuramoto, E., Yano, O., Kimura, Y., Baba, M., Makino, T., Yamamoto, S., Yamamoto, T., Kataoka, T., and Tokunaga, T. 1992. Oligonucleotide sequences required for natural killer cell activation. Jpn. J. Cancer Res. 83: 1128-1131.

Lehner, M.D., Morath, S., Michelsen, K.S., Schumann, R.R., and Hartung, T. 2001. Induction of cross-tolerance by lipopolysaccharide and highly purified lipoteichoic acid via different Toll-Like Receptors independent of paracrine mediators. J. Immunol. 166: 5161-5167.

Liang, H., Nishioka, Y., Reich, C.F., Pisetsky, D.S., and Lipsky, P.E. 1996. Activation of human B cells by phosphorothioate oligonucleotides. J. Clin. Invest. 98: 1119-1129.

Liang, H., Reich, C.F., Pisetsky, D.S., and Lipsky, P.E. 2000. The role of cell surface receptors in the activation of human B cells by phosphorothioate oligonucleotides. J. Immunol. 165: 1438-1445.

Lipford, G.B., Bauer, M., Blank, C., Reiter, R., Wagner, H., and Heeg, K. 1997b. CpG-containing synthetic oligonucleotides promote B and cytotoxic T cell responses to protein antigen: a new class of vaccine adjuvants. Eur. J. Immunol. 27: 2340-2344.

Lipford, G.B., Heeg, K., and Wagner, H. 1998. Bacterial DNA as immune cell activator. Trends Microbiol. 6: 496-500.

Lipford, G.B., and Sparwasser, T. 2000a. Hematopoietic remodeling triggered by CpG DNA. Curr. Top. Microbiol. Immunol. 247:119-29: 119-129.

Lipford, G.B., Sparwasser, T., Bauer, M., Zimmermann, S., Koch, E.S., Heeg, K., and Wagner, H. 1997a. Immunostimulatory DNA: sequence dependent production of potentially harmful or useful cytokines. Eur. J. Immunol. 27: 3420-3426.

Lipford, G.B., Sparwasser, T., Zimmermann, S., Heeg, K., and Wagner, H. 2000b. CpG-DNA mediated transient lymphoadenopathy is associated with a state of Th1 predisposition to antige driven responses. J. Immunol. 165: 1228-1235.

Macfarlane, D.E., and Manzel, L. 1998. Antagonism of immunostimulatory CpG-Oligodeoxynucleotides by quinacrine, chloroquine, and structurally related compounds. J. Immunol. 160: 1122-1131.

Magone, M.T., Chan, C.C., Beck, L., Whitcup, S.M., and Raz, E. 2000. Systemic or mucosal administration of immunostimulatory DNA inhibits early and late phases of murine allergic conjunctivitis. Eur. J. Immunol. 30: 1841-1850.

McCluskie, M.J. and Davis, H.L. 1998. CpG DNA is a potent enhancer of systemic and mucosal immune responses against hepatitis B surface antigen with intranasal administration to mice. J. Immunol. 161: 4463-4466.

McCluskie, M.J., and Davis, H.L. 1999. CpG DNA as mucosal adjuvant. Vaccine 18: 231-237.

Medzhitov, R., and Janeway, C.A. 1997. Innate immunity: impact on the adaptive immune response. Curr. Opin. Immunol. 9: 4-9.

Metzger, W.J. and Nyce, J.W. 1999. Oligonucleotide therapy of allergic asthma. J. Allergy Clin. Immunol. 104: 260-266.

Mody, C.H., Wood, C.J., Syme, R.M., and Spurrell, J.C. 1999. The cell wall and membrane of *Cryptococcus neoformans* possess a mitogen for human T lymphocytes. Infect. Immun. 67: 936-941.

Moldoveanu, Z., Love-Homan, L., Huang, W.Q., and Krieg, A.M. 1998. CpG DNA, a novel immune enhancer for systemic and mucosal immunization with influenza virus. Vaccine 16: 1216-1224.

Moss, R.B., Diveley, J., Jensen, F., and Carlo, D.J. 1999. *In vitro* immune function after vaccination with an inactivated, gp120-depleted HIV-1 antigen with immunostimulatory oligodeoxynucleotides. Vaccine 18: 1081-1087.

Pisetsky, D.S. 1996. Immune activation by bacterial DNA: a new genetic code. Immunity 5: 303-310.

Pisetsky, D.S., and Reich, C. 1993. Stimulation of *in vitro* proliferation of murine lymphocytes by synthetic oligonucleotides. Mol. Biol. Rep. 18: 217-221.

Pisetsky, D.S., and Reich, C.F. 1994. Stimulation of murine lymphocyte proliferation by a phosphorothioate oligonucleotide with antisense activity for herpes simplex virus. Life Sci. 54: 101-107.

Roman, M., Martin-Orozco, E., Goodman, J.S., Nguyen, M.-D., Sato, Y., Ronaghy, A., Kornbluth, R.S., Richman, D.D., Carson, D.A., and Raz, E. 1997. Immunostimulatory DNA sequences function as T helper-1-promoting adjuvants. Nature Med. 3: 849-854.

Sato, Y., Roman, M., Tighe, H., Lee, D., Corr, M., Nguyen, M.D., Silverman, G.J., Lotz, M., Carson, D.A., and Raz, E. 1996. Immunostimulatory DNA sequences necessary for effective intradermal gene immunization. Science 273: 352-354.

Schnare, M., Holt, A.C., Takeda, K., Akira, S., and Medzhitov, R. 2000. Recognition of CpG DNA is mediated by signaling pathways dependent on the adaptor protein MyD88. Curr. Biol. 10: 1139-1142.

Segal, B.M., Chang, J.T., and Shevach, E.M. 2000. CpG oligonucleotides are potent adjuvants for the activation of autoreactive encephalitogenic T cells *in vivo*. J. Immunol. 164: 5683-5688.

Serebrisky, D., Teper, A.A., Huang, C.K., Lee, S.Y., Zhang, T.F., Schofield, B.H., Kattan, M., Sampson, H.A., and Li, X.M. 2000. CpG oligodeoxynucleotides can reverse Th2-associated allergic airway responses and alter the B7.1/B7.2 expression in a murine model of asthma. J. Immunol. 165: 5906-5912.

Shimada, S., Yano, O., Inoue, H., Kuramoto, E., Fukuda, T., Yamamoto, H., Kataoka, T., and Tokunaga, T. 1985. Antitumor activity of the DNA fraction from Mycobacterium bovis BCG. II. Effects on various syngeneic mouse tumors. J. Natl. Cancer Inst. 74: 681-688.

Shirota, H., Sano, K., Kikuchi, T., Tamura, G., and Shirato, K. 2000. Regulation of murine airway eosinophilia and Th2 cells by antigen-conjugated CpG oligodeoxynucleotides as a novel antigen-specific immunomodulator. J. Immunol. 164: 5575-5582.

Shirota, H., Sano, K., Hirasawa, N., Terui, T., Ohuchi, K., Hattori, T., Shirato, K., and Tamura, G. 2001. Novel Roles of CpG oligodeoxynucleotides as a leader for the sampling and presentation of CpG-tagged antigen by dendritic cells. J. Immunol. 167: 66-74.

Sparwasser, T., Hültner, L., Koch, E.S., Luz, A., Lipford, G.B., and Wagner, H. 1999. Immunostimulatory CpG-oligodeoxynucleotides cause extramedullary murine hemopoiesis. J. Immunol. 162: 2368-2374.

Sparwasser, T., Koch, E.S., Vabulas, R.M., Heeg, K., Lipford, G.B., Ellwart, J., and Wagner, H. 1998. Bacterial DNA and immunostimulating CpG oligonucleotides trigger maturation and activation of murine dendritic cells. Eur. J. Immunol. 28: 2045-2054.

Sparwasser, T., Miethke, T., Lipford, G.B., Borschert, K., Häcker, H., Heeg, K., and Wagner, H. 1997b. Bacterial DNA cause septic shock. Nature 386: 336-337.

Sparwasser, T., Miethke, T., Lipford, G.B., Erdmann, A., Häcker, H., Heeg, K., and Wagner, H. 1997a. Macrophages sense pathogens via DNA motifs: Induction of TNF-alpha mediated shock. Eur. J. Immunol. 27: 1671-1679.

Stacey, K.J., and Blackwell, J.M. 1999. Immunostimulatory DNA as an adjuvant in vaccination against *Leishmania major*. Infect. Immun. 67: 3719-3726.

Stacey, K.J., Sweet, M.J., and Hume, D.A. 1996. Macrophages ingest and are activated by bacterial DNA. J. Immunol. 157: 2116-2122.

Sun, S., Zhang, X., Tough, D.F., and Sprent, J. 1998. Type I interferon-mediated stimulation of T cells by CpG DNA. J. Exp. Med. 188: 2335-2342.

Tascon, R.E., Ragno, S., Lowrie, D.B., and Colston, M.J. 2000. Immunostimulatory bacterial DNA sequences activate dendritic cells and promote priming and differentiation of CD8+ T cells. Immunology 99: 1-7.

Tighe, H., Takabayashi, K., Schwartz, D., Marsden, R., Beck, L., Corbeil, J., Richman, D.D., Eiden, J.J., Jr., Spiegelberg, H.L., and Raz, E. 2000b. Conjugation of protein to immunostimulatory DNA results in a rapid, long-lasting and potent induction of cell-mediated and humoral immunity. Eur. J. Immunol. 30: 1939-1947.

Tighe, H., Takabayashi, K., Schwartz, D., Van Nest, G., Tuck, S., Eiden, J.J., Kagey-Sobotka, A., Creticos, P.S., Lichtenstein, L.M., Spiegelberg, H.L., and Raz, E. 2000a. Conjugation of immunostimulatory DNA to the short ragweed allergen amb a 1 enhances its immunogenicity and reduces its allergenicity. J. Allergy Clin. Immunol. 106: 124-134.

Tokunaga, T., Yamamoto, T., and Yamamoto, S. 1999. How BCG led to the discovery of immunostimulatory DNA. Jpn. J. Infect. Dis. 52: 1-11.

Tsunoda, I., Tolley, N.D., Theil, D.J., Whitton, J.L., Kobayashi, H., and Fujinami, R.S. 1999. Exacerbation of viral and autoimmune animal models for multiple sclerosis by bacterial DNA. Brain Pathol. 9: 481-493.

Vabulas, R.M., Pircher, H., Lipford, G.B., Häcker, H., and Wagner, H. 2000. CpG-DNA activates *in vivo* T cell epitope presenting dendritic cells to trigger protective antiviral cytotoxic T cell responses. J. Immunol. 164: 2372-2378.

Van Uden, J., and Raz, E. 1999. Immunostimulatory DNA and applications to allergic disease. J. Allergy Clin. Immunol. 104: 902-910.

Verthelyi, D., Ishii, K.J., Gursel, M., Takeshita, F., and Klinman, D.M. 2001. Human peripheral blood cells differentially recognize and respond to two distinct CpG motifs. J. Immunol. 166: 2372-2377.

von Hunolstein, C., Teloni, R., Mariotti, S., Recchia, S., Orefici, G., and Nisini, R. 2000. Synthetic oligodeoxynucleotide containing CpG motif induces an anti-polysaccharide type 1-like immune response after immunization of mice with *Haemophilus influenzae* type b conjugate vaccine. Int. Immunol. 12: 295-303.

Wagner, H. 1999. Bacterial CpG DNA activates immune cells to signal infectious danger. Adv. Immunol. 73: 329-368.

Wagner, H., Hacker, H., and Lipford, G.B. 2000. Immunostimulatory DNA sequences help to eradicate intracellular pathogens. Springer Semin. Immunopathol. 22: 147-152.

Walker, P.S., Scharton-Kersten, T., Krieg, A.M., Love-Homan, L., Rowton, E.D., Udey, M.C., and Vogel, J.C. 1999. Immunostimulatory oligodeoxynucleotides promote protective immunity and provide systemic therapy for leishmaniasis via IL-12 and IFN-gamma-dependent mechanisms. Proc. Natl. Acad. Sci. USA. 96: 6970-6975.

Warren, T.L., Bhatia, S.K., Acosta, A.M., Dahle, C.E., Ratliff, T.L., Krieg, A.M., and Weiner, G.J. 2000. APC stimulated by CpG oligodeoxynucleotide enhance activation of MHC class I-restricted T cells. J. Immunol. 165: 6244-6251.

Weeratna, R.D., McCluskie, M.J., Xu, Y., and Davis, H.L. 2000. CpG DNA induces stronger immune responses with less toxicity than other adjuvants. Vaccine 18: 1755-1762.

Weiner, G.J. 2000. CpG DNA in cancer immunotherapy. Curr. Top. Microbiol. Immunol. 247:157-70: 157-170.

Yamamoto, S., Yamamoto, T., Kataoka, T., Kuramoto, E., Yano, O., and Tokunaga, T. 1992b. Unique palindromic sequences in synthetic oligonucleotides A required to induce IFN and augment IFN-mediated natural killer activity. J. Immunol. 148: 4072-4076.

Yamamoto, S., Yamamoto, T., Shimada, S., Kuramoto, E., Yano, O., Kataoka, T., and Tokunaga, T. 1992a. DNA from bacteria, but not from vertebrates, induces interferons, activates natural killer cells and inhibits tumor growth. Microbiol. Immunol. 36: 983-997.

Yi, A.K., and Krieg, A.M. 1998. Rapid induction of mitogen-activated protein kinases by immune stimulatory CpG DNA. J. Immunol. 161: 4493-4497.

Zhao, Q., Yu, D., and Agrawal, S. 1999. Site of chemical modifications in CpG containing phosphorothioate oligodeoxynucleotide modulates its immunostimulatory activity. Bioorg. Med. Chem. Lett. 9: 3453-3458.

Zhu, F.G., Reich, C.F., III, and Pisetsky, D.S. 2001. The role of the macrophage scavenger receptor in immune stimulation by bacterial DNA and synthetic oligonucleotides. Immunology 103: 226-234.

Zimmermann, S., Egeter, O., Hausmann, S., Lipford, G.B., Röcken, M., Wagner, H., and Heeg, K. 1998. CpG oligodeoxynucleotides trigger protective and curative Th1 responses in lethal murine leishmaniasis. J. Immunol. 160: 3627-3630.

From: *Vaccine Delivery Strategies*
Edited by: Guido Dietrich and Werner Goebel

Chapter 7

Bacterial Ghosts as Carrier and Targeting Systems for Antigen Delivery

W. Jechlinger, W. Haidinger, S. Paukner, P. Mayrhofer, E. Riedmann, J. Marchart, U. Mayr, C. Haller, G. Kohl, P. Walcher, P. Kudela, J. Bizik, D. Felnerova, E.M.B. Denner, A. Indra, A. Haslberger, M. Szostak, S. Resch, F. Eko, T. Schukovskaya, V. Kutyrev, A. Hensel, S. Friederichs, T. Schlapp, and W. Lubitz

ABSTRACT

The application of new strategies to develop effective delivery vehicles is essential in modern vaccine design. The bacterial ghost system is a novel vaccine delivery system endowed with intrinsic adjuvant properties as well as carrier and targeting functions. This new platform technology improves vaccine design by facilitating the efficient delivery of target antigens to promote effective mucosal and systemic immunity. Bacterial ghosts are non-living bacterial cells devoid of cytoplasmic contents while maintaining their cellular morphology and native surface antigenic structures including bioadhesive properties. They are produced by PhiX174 protein E-mediated lysis of Gram-negative bacteria. The retention by ghosts of the morphological characteristics and structural integrity of their living counterparts make them attractive for use as vaccines. The intrinsic adjuvant properties of bacterial ghost preparations enhance immune responses against target antigens, including enhanced T-cell activation and mucosal immunity. Since multiple proteins can be expressed on these ghosts in a deliberately controlled manner, high levels of the antigen or antigens can be presented to the immune system simultaneously to produce effective combination vaccines against multiple agents. This extended bacterial ghost system is an alternative to living bacterial delivery systems and may have an added advantage because of its safety and flexibility. Furthermore, the specificity of ghosts for targeting primary antigen presenting cells, the simplicity of the method of production and its versatility in entrapping and packaging various antigens in different compartments make recombinant ghosts particularly suitable for use as combination vaccines. The endotoxin component of the Gram-negative outer membrane does not limit the use of ghosts as vaccine candidates because of the minimal toxicity of the cell-associated lipopolysaccharide compared to the free soluble form.

INTRODUCTION

The use of killed microorganisms to induce protective immunity to several pathogens has a long tradition in vaccinology. Despite the efficacy of killed bacterial vaccines, there is concern over their safety when administered by injections. Although subunit vaccines composed of purified components can be produced from many microorganisms, they are very often less immunogenic and need additional adjuvants which have to be added in the vaccine formulation. Also for DNA vaccines to reach their full potential, new methods for vaccine delivery need to be developed which primarily can activate mucosal immune responses. The bacterial ghost system is one such delivery system combining targeting of antigen components to mucosal tissues and providing adjuvant activity without the need of other additions.

Bacterial ghosts can be regarded as natural engineered liposomes being composed of two membranes which are separated by a distinct space wherein the rigid peptidoglycan corsette and membrane-derived oligosaccharides are located. The outer membrane contains proteins, lipopolysaccharides (LPS) and pili which are able to recognize receptors on target cells or are recognized themselves by the innate immune system. For the construction of combination vaccines, bacterial ghosts can be equipped with foreign antigens, nucleic acids, or other compounds with numerous applications in human and animal health.

MECHANISM OF BACTERIAL GHOST FORMATION

Gene *E* of phage PhiX174 codes for a membrane protein of 91 amino acids (aa) which is able to fuse inner and outer membranes of Gram-negative bacteria (Witte *et al.*, 1990a and1990b), forming an E-specific lysis tunnel. The border values of the E-specific transmembrane lysis tunnel through which the cytoplasmic content of the bacteria is expelled fluctuate between 40 and 200 nm (Witte *et al.*, 1992). The remaining empty internal space of the bacteria is devoid of nucleic acids, ribosomes or other constituents, whereas the inner and outer membrane structures of the ghosts are well preserved (Witte *et al.*, 1990a and 1993). The inner membrane not involved in tunnel formation remains intact during expulsion of cytoplasmic material. Electron micrographs clearly show a sealed periplasmic space at the border of the lysis tunnel (Witte *et al.*, 1990a and 1992). The protein E-induced occurrence of lysophosphatidylethanol amine in the host cell membrane most probably facilitates the inner and outer membrane fusion (Lubitz *et al.*, 1985). Peptidoglycan sacculi prepared from E-lysed cells remain intact emphasizing that the overall composition of this rigid layer is not changed by the E-mediated lysis process, and that the diameter of the E-specific transmembrane tunnel structure is determined by the mesh size of the surrounding murein (Witte *et al.*, 1998a).

By secondary structure prediction of protein E, the polypeptide can be divided into four domains. A theoretical arrangement of the four domains in the envelope complex of Gram-negative bacteria is represented in Figure 1. The most likely arrangement according to the model of the E-fusion process described below is given in Figure 1b.

The E-specific membrane fusion process can be divided into three phases (Schön *et al.*, 1995). Phase 1 is characterised by integration of protein E into the inner membrane with its C-terminal part facing the cytoplasmic side (Figure 1a), followed by a conformational change of protein E transferring its C-terminus across the inner membrane and assembling into multimers at potential cell division sites (Phase 2). The mechanism for the conformational change is most probably a *cis-trans* isomerisation of the proline 21 residue

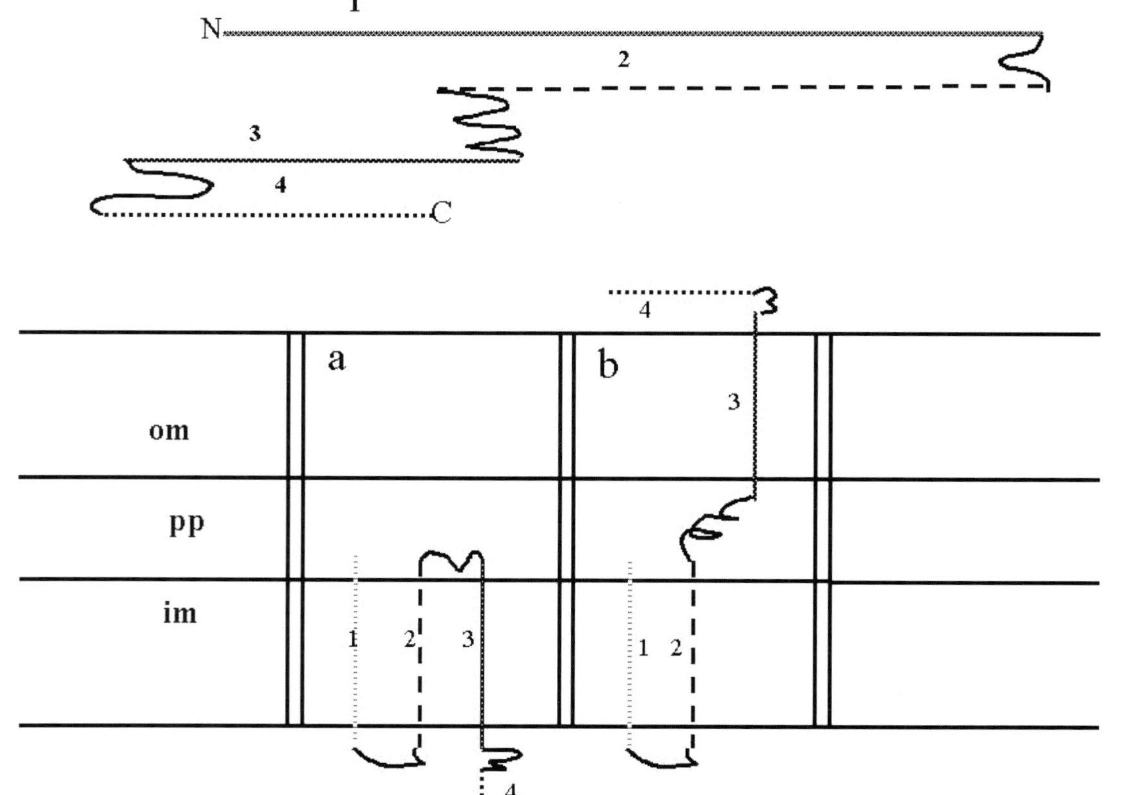

Figure 1. Arrangements of E-specific domains in the envelope complex of Gram-negative bacteria. Protein E integrates cotranslationally into the inner membrane of Gram-negative bacteria (a) and fuses the inner and outer membranes (b). om, outer membrane; pp, periplasmic space; im, inner membrane; 1 – 4, different domains of protein E from N- to C-terminus.

within the first membrane-embedded α-helix of protein E (Witte *et al.*, 1997). In Phase 3, a local fusion of the inner and outer membranes is achieved by a transfer of the C-terminal domain of protein E towards the surface of the outer membrane of the bacterium (Figure 1b). The very C-terminal end of protein E, domain 4 (aa 85-91), which is highly hydrophilic is not essential, but contributes to a better efficiency of the bacterial lysis process (Schüller *et al.*, 1985).

Electron microscopic studies emphasize that the protein E-specific transmembrane tunnel structure, which permeabilizes the bacterium, is not randomly distributed over the cell envelope but is restricted to areas of potential division sites, predominantly in the middle of the cell or at polar sites (Witte *et al.*, 1990a; Witte *et al.* 1992). Analysis of E-mediated lysis in bacterial mutant strains with defects in cell division suggest that initiation of cell division rather than specific functions of the septosome plays an essential role in protein E-mediated lysis (Witte *et al.*, 1993 and 1998a).

In a modified E-lysis procedure for bacteria, high concentrations of $MgSO_4$ can be used to lower the fluidity of the outer membrane by forming ion bridges between the negativly charged 3-deoxy-D-manno-2-octulosonic acid (KDO) units of the LPS and thus inhibiting the E-specific transmembrane tunnel formation. Bacteria already primed for E-mediated lysis can be harvested by centrifugation and resuspension of the cell pellet either in water or low ionic strength buffers results in immediate lysis of the cells. Electron micrographs of bacteria lysed by this alternative procedure (Resch *et al.*, 1998) show holes in the cell envelopes large enough to release polyhydroxybutyrate (PHB) granules as given schematically in Figure 2. Such ghosts with large holes can be used as empty bags into which bulky substances like DNA-complexing polymers or larger protein particles can be filled and packaged.

E-mediated lysis has been achieved in various Gram-negative bacteria, including *Escherichia coli* K12 strain*s*, Enterohaemorrhagic *E. coli* (EHEC*)*, *Salmonella typhimurium*, *Salmonella enteritidis*, *Klebsiella pneumoniae*, *Bordetella bronchiseptica*, *Vibrio cholerae*, *Actinobacillus pleuropneumoniae*, *Mannheimia haemolytica*, *Pasteurella multocida*, *Pseudomonas putida*, *Ralstonia eutropha* and *Erwinia cypripedii*. This broad spectrum of bacteria shows that E-mediated lysis most probably works in every Gram-negative bacterium, provided that the E lysis cassette can be introduced into the new recipient by an appropriate vector allowing tight repression and induction control of lethal gene *E*.

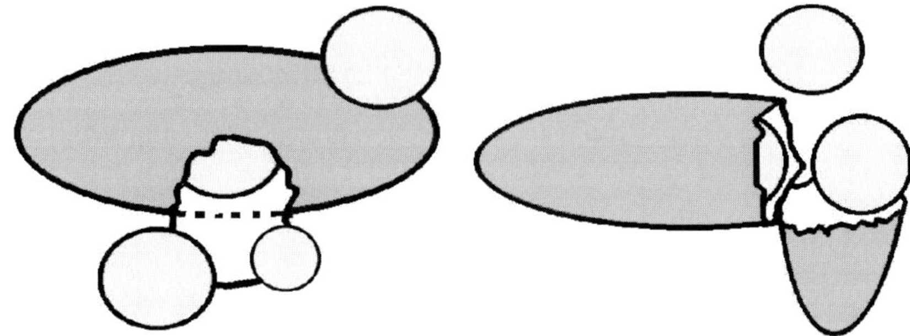

Figure 2. Modified E-lysis procedure of bacteria. Schematic drawing according to electron micrographs presented in reference 11. Larger cell openings in the envelope complex are produced by the modified E-lysis either in the middle of the bacteria or at polar sides releasing particles with a diameter of roughly 500 nm.

GENETIC CONTROL OF GENE *E* EXPRESSION

Expression of lysis gene *E* can be placed under transcriptional control of either the thermosensitive λpL/pR-cI857, or under the lac PO -lacI^q promoter repressor systems, or the tol expression system (Szostak *et al.*, 1996; Ronchel *et al.*, 1998, Kloos *et al.*, 1994). A major breakthrough in temperature control of E-mediated lysis has been achieved by mutating the λpR gene expression regulation circuit extending the heat stability of the λpR promoter/cI857 repressor system. The mutated λpR promoter/operator region (Jechlinger *et al.*, 1999) resulted in new expression systems which stably repress gene *E* expression at temperatures of up to 37°C, but still allow induction of cell lysis at a temperature range of 39 - 42°C (Figure 3).

Alternatively, a cold-sensitive system for ghost formation by lowering the growth temperature of the bacteria from 37°C or higher to 28°C or lower could be obtained by combining the λpR promoter/cI repressor system with the lacI/lacPO for control of gene *E* expression (Figure 4). At 37°C, the temperature-sensitive cI857 repressor is inactivated and therefore the λp$_R$ promoter-driven expression of the *lacI* gene results in a high amount of Lac repressor molecules which bind to the corresponding *lacZpo* site, repressing the expression of lysis gene *E*. At 28°C, the functional cI857 repressor prevents the expression of Lac repressor molecules from the λp$_R$ promoter. As the *lac* promoter is no longer repressed, gene *E* expression and thus lysis of bacteria takes place (Jechlinger *et al.*, 1998).

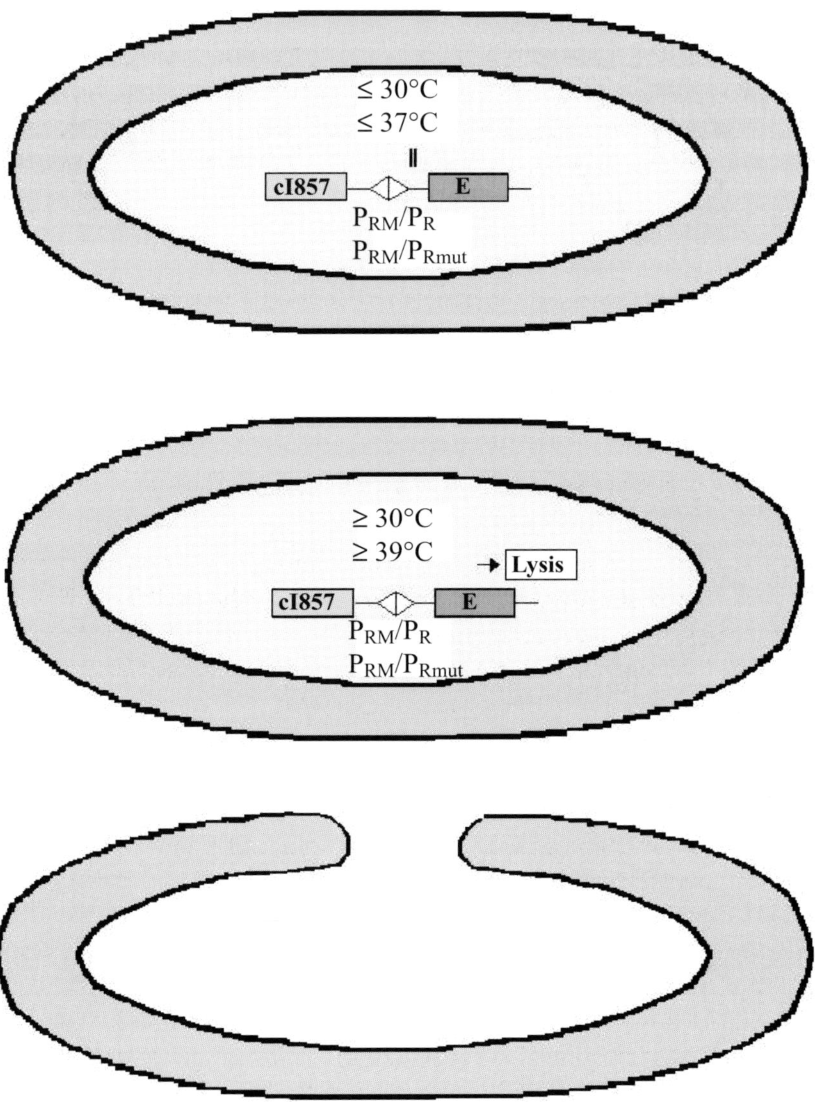

Figure 3. Production of bacterial ghosts by E-mediated lysis. The PhiX174 lysis gene *E* is under transcriptional control of the temperature-sensitive cI857 repressor and either a mutated (P_Rmut; induction of gene *E* expression at 39°C or higher) or the wildtype rightward λp_R promoter (PR; induction of gene *E* expression at 30°C or higher). As result of gene *E* expression, a transmembrane tunnel structure is formed by fusion of the inner and outer membranes through which the cytoplasm is expelled. cI857, λcI857 temperature sensitive repressor gene; λp_R/p_RM, P_Rmut promoters of phage Lambda. E, PhiX174 lysis gene *E*.

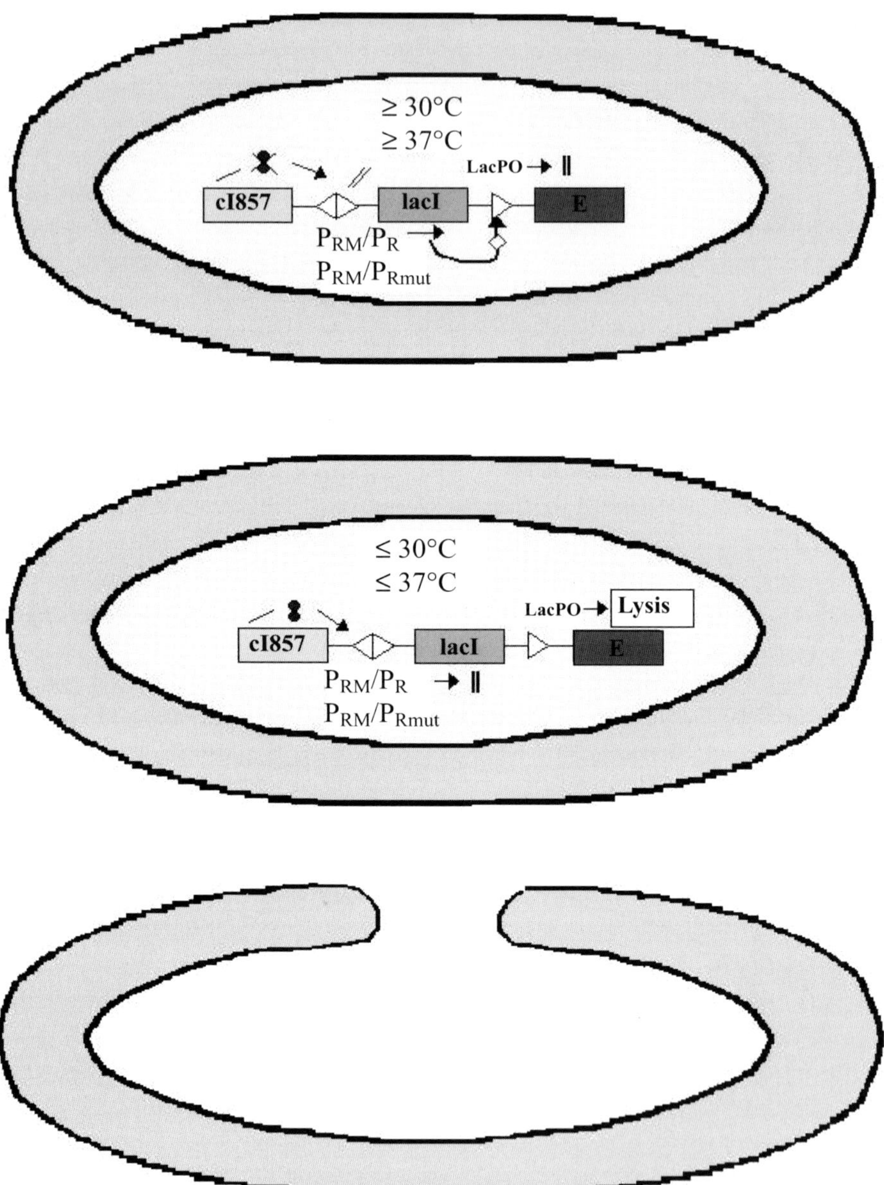

Figure 4. Cold-sensitive E-mediated lysis system of Gram-negative bacteria. The *lacI* gene is under transcriptional control of the temperature-sensitive cI857 repressor and either a mutated (P_{Rmut}) or the wildtype (PR) rightward λp_R promoter, whereas gene *E* is under control of the *lacZpo* promoter. cI857, λcI857 temperature sensitive repressor gene: $\lambda p_R/p_{RM}$, promoters of phage Lambda. E, PhiX174 lysis gene *E*. lacI- repressor gene *lacI*; lacZpo, lacZ promoter-operator region.

PARENTERAL IMMUNIZATION WITH BACTERIAL GHOSTS

Pasteurella ghosts were used for immunization of rabbits and mice. Rabbits immunized s. c. with either *P. multocida-* or *M. haemolytica*-ghosts developed antibodies reacting with the homologous strain, as well as with heterologous *Pasteurella* strains. The number of proteins in whole cell protein extracts recognized by the sera constantly increased during the observation period of 50 days. In addition, dose-dependent protection against homologous challenge was observed in mice immunized with *P. multocida* ghosts. Animals which received 3 times 10^8 ghosts per immunization and a challenge dose of up to 60 cfu/dose, showed 100% protection (Marchart *et al.*, unpublished data).

M. haemolytica is a cattle pathogen of significant economic impact. An effective vaccine against bovine pneumonic pasteurellosis is therefore of high importance. Apart from economic concerns, pasteurellosis caused by *M. haemolytica* is a serious disease leading to death in cattle if it remains untreated. With *M. haemolytica* ghosts, cattle immunization studies were performed based on a cattle challenge model. It was shown that protective immunization of cattle against homologous challenge was induced by alum-adjuvanted *M. haemolytica-* ghosts. In this case, alum was added to the ghost vaccine to compare the antigenicity of the ghosts with a commercially available vaccine (Marchart *et al.*, unpublished data).

Pigs immunized i.m. with *Actinobacillus pleuropneumoniae* (App) ghosts or a formalin-inactivated bacterin were found to be protected against clinical disease in both vaccination groups, whereas colonization of the lungs with *A. pleuropneumoniae* was only prevented in ghost-vaccinated pigs. Immune sera of both groups were tested on whole cell antigen or purified virulence factors including outer membrane protein preparations (OMPs), outer membrane lipoprotein OmlA1, transferrin binding proteins (TfbA1, TfbA7 and TfbB) and Apx toxins (ApxI, II and III). SDS-PAGE and immunoblots revealed no specific antibody response against the single virulence factors tested in any vaccinated animal. The two vaccination groups showed different recognition patterns of whole cell antigen and OMP-enriched preparations. A 100 kDa protein was recognized significantly stronger by ghost-vaccinated pigs than convalescent pigs. This unique antibody population induced by ghosts could play a determining role in the prevention of lung colonization. The same 100 kDa antigen was recognized by ghost-sera in homologous as well as heterologous serotype App protein preparations. Indications for a crossprotective potential in the ghost vaccine were supported by studies on rabbit hyperimmune sera (Huter *et al.*, 2000).

The protective efficacy of immunization in pigs vaccinated twice i.m. with a dose of 5×10^9 App ghosts (GVPs) or formalin-inactivated App bacterins (BVPs) was evaluated by clinical, bacteriological, serological and post-mortem examinations. Bronchoalveolar lavage in pigs was performed during the experiment to obtain lavage samples (BALF) for assessment of local antibodies. Isotype-specific antibody responses in serum and BALF were determined by ELISAs based on whole-cell antigen. Immunization with ghosts did not cause clinical side-effects. After aerosol challenge, the control group of pigs developed fever and pleuropneumonia. GVPs or BVPs were found to be fully protected against clinical disease or lung lesions in both vaccination groups, whereas colonization of the respiratory tract with App was only prevented in GVPs. Specific immunoglobulins against App were not detectable in BALF after immunization. A significant systemic increase of IgM, IgA, IgG(Fc'), or IgG(H+L) antibodies reactive with App was measured in GVPs and BVPs when compared to the non-exposed controls. BVPs reached higher titers of IgG(Fc') and IgG(H+L) than GVP. However, prevention of carrier state in GVPs coincided with a significant increase of serum IgA when compared to BVPs. These results suggest that immunization with ghosts, that bias antibody populations specific to non-denatured surface antigens, may be more efficacious in protecting pigs against colonization and infection than bacterins (Hensel *et al.*, 2000).

Rabbits were immunized s.c./i.m. with ghosts which were prepared from *Vibrio cholerae* strains of O1 or O139 serogroup after growth under culture conditions, which favor or repress the production of toxin-coregulated pili (TCP). Immunoblotting confirmed the TCP status of these *V. cholerae* ghosts (VCG), which retained the cellular morphology and surface component profile of viable bacteria. The resulting sera were assayed for antibodies to lipopolysaccharide (LPS) and to TCP. Regardless of the TCP status of the VCG preparations used for immunization, all animals produced antibodies to LPS as demonstrated in bactericidal assays. These antibodies were probably responsible for the capacity of the antisera to confer passive immunity to challenge with the homologous O139 strain in the infant mouse cholera model (IMCM). Cross protection was seen only after immunization with TCP-positive VCG where antibodies to TCP were generated, as judged by the potential of antisera to mediate protection against a challenge strain of a heterologous serogroup (Eko *et al.*, 2000).

AEROSOL AND ORAL IMMUNIZATIONS WITH BACTERIAL GHOSTS

Inhalation and deposition of bacterial ghosts within the airways are the initial steps preceeding adherence of the vaccine candidates to the respiratory tract. Once the bacterial ghosts are deposited in the lung lining fluids, they do not remain at the location where they first came into contact with the mucus membranes. Lung clearance mechanisms translocate all deposited particles and most of them are swallowed and cleared *via* the gastro-intestinal-tract (Hensel and Lubitz, 1997). Oral, intranasal, intravaginal or rectal immunizations with bacterial ghosts can also target the mucosal immune system.

In order to outline basic concepts for the design of bacterial ghost immunizations, a pig lung infection model with *A. pleuropneumoniae* (App) has been developed (Hensel *et al.*, 1996). Aerosol immunisation with App ghosts is a safe way to induce complete protection against pleuropneumonia in pigs caused by this lung pathogenic bacterium (Katinger *et al.*, 1999). This aerosol infection model with computer-controlled standardized inhalation conditions for the recipient pigs can serve as a model for human aerosol immunization.

In the pig model system, the capability of bacterial ghosts to induce a T cell-mediated immune response was studied focusing on the uptake of App ghosts by primary antigen presenting cells (APC). The specific immune responses were detected after re-stimulation of primed blood T-cells with App ghosts. Maximal stimulation was detected in cultures, where the proportion of the primed T cells to ghosts ranged from 1: 2.5 to 1: 5. The effectiveness of the specific anti-ghosts response increased significantly if the ghosts were presented by APC. Together with the specific T cell response to the antigen processed by the APC, it could be shown that porcine APC have the capacity to stimulate antigen-specific T cells after internalization and processing of the App bacterial ghosts.

As antigen presentation is especially effective in porcine dendritic cells (DC) and even uptake of low amount of antigen is sufficient for an induction of immune responses, we investigated uptake of bacterial ghosts by DC and subsequent DC activation. DC are known to be phagocytic in specific immature stages. For these experiments, bacterial ghosts were conjugated with FITC (fluoresceinisothiocyanate). After exposure of APC to FITC-labelled bacterial ghosts, a remarkable increase of fluorescence was detected in the APC population. Following the internalization and processing of the antigens, increased expression of MHC class II molecules in APC was shown 12 hr after their exposure to bacterial ghosts. The data suggest that bacterial ghosts effectively stimulate monocytes and macrophages for the induction of TH1-type cytokine directed immune responses and that dendritic cells stimulated by bacterial ghosts may serve as a promising vehicle for active immunization and immunotherapy *in situ* (Haslberger *et al.*, 2000).

V. cholerae ghosts which are developed as oral vaccines for humans can be prepared in large quantities by fermentation under culture conditions which favour the expression of toxin-co-regulated pili (TCP). Analysis of immune responses in animal models indicate that *V. cholerae* ghosts induce humoral and cellular immune responses against cell envelope constituents including protective immunity against challenge infections. It should be pointed out that the oral ghost vaccination experiments were carried out with freeze-dried ghosts resuspended in saline for oral route immunizations, without the addition of adjuvants, stabilisers or other substances (Haslberger *et al.* 2000).

Existing oral cholera vaccines either consist of killed whole *V. cholerae* O1 cells in combination with a recombinant B subunit of cholera toxin or of the live, attenuated *V. cholerae* strain CVD 103-HgR. The latter vaccine, however, does not provide protection in populations living in endemic areas and none of both oral vaccines has demonstrated sustained protection in children of less than 2 years of age. Thus, there is an urgent need for new generations of oral cholera vaccines that are also efficient against the different epidemic types of *V. cholerae*, including the O139 strain, and that confer reliable and long-term protection in all age groups (WHO/CDS/CSR/EDC/99.4).

In a recent study the immunological and protective efficacy of *V. cholerae* ghosts expressing TCP (VCG-TCP) from *V. cholerae* serogroups O1 and O139 has been investigated in the reversible intestinal tie adult rabbit diarrhea (RITARD) model. Rabbits were immunized 3 times intragastrically with a mixture of lyophilized VCG-TCP from serogroup O1 and serogroup O139 (total of 4 mg) and were challenged 30 days after the first immunization with 2×10^9 CFU of fully virulent *V. cholerae* O1 and *V. cholerae* O139 strains. Increasing median geometric means of serum vibriocidal antibodies were observed in all immunized animals at levels of more than twenty-fold over baseline. It could also be shown that oral administration of *V. cholerae* ghosts protects adult rabbits against diarrhea and death following intralumen challenge with fully virulent *V. cholerae* serogroups O1 and O139 (Eko *et al.*, unpublished data).

BACTERIAL GHOSTS AS ADJUVANTS

The ability of an antigen to induce an immune response depends not only on the molecular properties of the antigen or on the immunogenic susceptibility of the host, but also on the formulation of the antigen. Adjuvants like tapioca, Alum, Freund's adjuvant, Cholera toxin, *E. coli* heat labile toxin (LT), lectins, muramyl dipeptide, ISCOMS, lipid A and other cell wall constituents as well as microencapsulation with natural or synthetic polymers and liposomes have been used to non-specifically potentiate the immune response to target antigens. Although it is not fully understood how each of the adjuvants acts to enhance the immune response, the activation of macrophages and dendritic cells are major properties of adjuvants. Bacterial ghosts contain some well-known immune stimulating compounds such as LPS and peptidoglycan. Thus, ghosts *per se* or ghosts used as carriers of foreign proteins should enhance the immune response against target antigens. Other adjuvant components of ghosts consist of the specific receptor recognition abilities of the envelope, contributing to effective uptake by macrophages and DC.

To investigate the activation of APC by bacterial ghosts we studied the uptake of bacterial ghosts in DC and RAW macrophages and the induction of inflammatory mediators in the THP-1 human macrophage cell line. The synthesis of inflammatory macrophage mediators such as TNFα in the THP-1 cell line was stimulated by a hundred-fold higher dose of VCG than the corresponding LPS using ELISA-analysis (Haslberger *et al.*, 1997 and 2000). These results confirm *in vivo* experiments in rabbits with i.v. administration of ghosts, in which up to a certain border value no toxic effects of the ghost administration could be detected and the doses used stimulated significant humoral immune responses (Mader *et al.*, 1997). A significant activation of IL-12 by ghosts in DC was observed, indicated by the analysis of IL-12(p70) synthesis and IL-12(p40) mRNA accumulation (40 fold). IL-18 mRNA synthesis was stimulated 14 fold. The cytokine secretion of TNFα and IL-12 was 37 and 18 fold, respectively, increased in DC whereas in PBMC the secretion of TNFα and IL-12 was increased only twofold. These results suggest that bacterial ghosts stimulate the activation of cellular Th1 immune responses. In addition, maturation of DC is a prerequisite for their efficient stimulation of T-cells and exposure of ghosts to DC results in a marked increase in their ability to activate T-cells. Thus, ghosts may serve as promising carrier and adjuvants for target antigens.

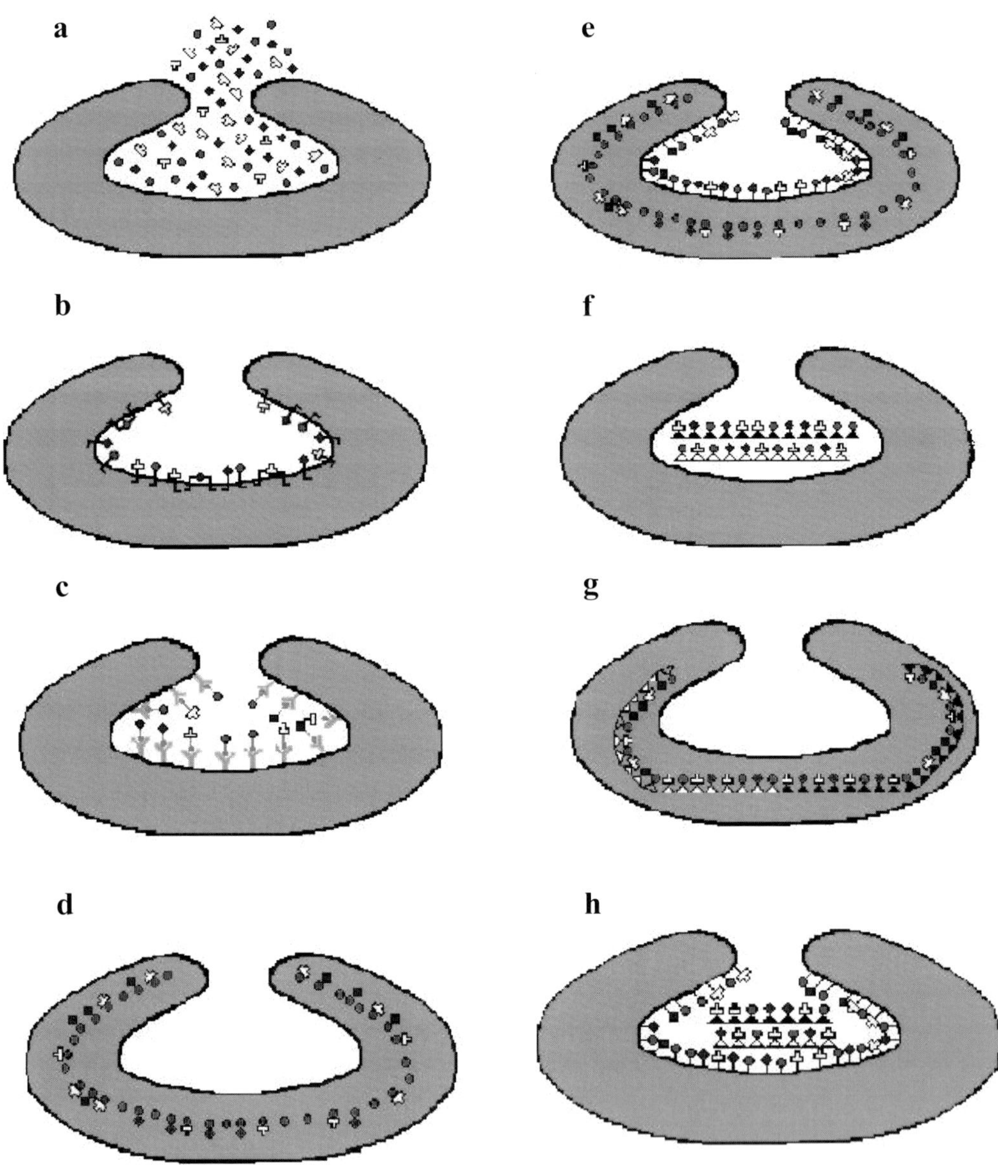

Figure 5. Bacterial ghosts as adjuvant and/or carriers for foreign target antigens. (a) Ghosts are mixed with different antigens and act as carrier and adjuvant. (b) Antigens are attached to the inside of the cytoplasmic membrane via N-terminal-, C-terminal- or N-and C-terminal anchor sequences. (c) Membrane-anchored streptavidin can bind any biotinylated target antigen to the inner membrane. (d) Target antigens can be exported to the periplasmic space (pp). (e) Ghost with a combination of membrane-anchored target antigens and antigens exported to the pp. (f) Recombinant S-layer proteins rSbsA or rSbsB as carriers of foreign antigens filling the cytoplasmic space of ghosts. (g) rSbsA, rSbsB proteins with foreign target antigens exported to the pp. (h) Combination of membrane anchored antigens and rSbsA-, rSbsB- target antigens in the inner lumen of the ghosts.

THE EXTENDED BACTERIAL GHOST SYSTEM AS CARRIER AND ADJUVANT FOR FOREIGN TARGET ANTIGENS

In the extended ghost system (Szostak and Lubitz, 1991), foreign proteins are either mixed with ghosts (Figure 5a) or attached on the inside of the cytoplasmic membrane (Figure 5b), exported into the periplasmic space (Figure 5d), or are expressed as S-layer fusion proteins, which form shell-like self assembly structures filling the cytoplasmic (Figure 5f) or periplasmic space (Figure 5g). If streptavidin is anchored to the inner membrane, biotinylated substances can be attached to such sites (Huter *et al.*, 1999) by resuspending freeze-dried streptavidin ghosts in a solution of biotinylated antigens (Figure 5c).

As the periplasmic space of ghosts is sealed, soluble antigens become part of the ghost envelope when they are exported to the periplasmic space by fused signal sequences prior to E-mediated lysis (Figure 5d). This finding provides the possibility to combine membrane-anchored proteins with other antigens exported to the periplasmic space (Figure 5e).

When heterologous expression of the cloned S-layer genes *sbsA* and *sbsB* in *E. coli* is followed by E-mediated lysis (Kuen *et al.*, 1994; Kuen et al, 1995; Kuen *et al.*, 1997), the S-layer structures are not released to the external medium but are retained within the inner lumen of the cytoplasmic space as they have the ability to self-assemble into crystalline planar arrays (Figure 5f). Site-directed mutagenesis of *sbsA* and *sbsB* and structural/functional analysis of S-layer domains essential for intra- and/or inter-molecular interactions revealed flexible surface loops in both proteins that accept foreign antigen sequences coding for up to 600 aa (Truppe *et al.*, 1997). Such recombinant S-layer fusion proteins consist of several hundred thousand monomers per cell and because of their ability to assemble into a superstructure, they do not form inclusion bodies.

It depends very much on the specific aim, whether the immobilisation of the target antigens within the S-layer has any additional beneficial effect compared to the corresponding antigen carried in a soluble or membrane-anchored form in the ghost envelope.

The intracellular space of bacterial ghosts can be filled either with water soluble subunit antigens (Figure 5a) or emulsions such that the protein antigen of interest or a matrix carrying DNA can be coupled to appropriate anchors on the inside of the cytoplasmic membrane of recombinant ghosts

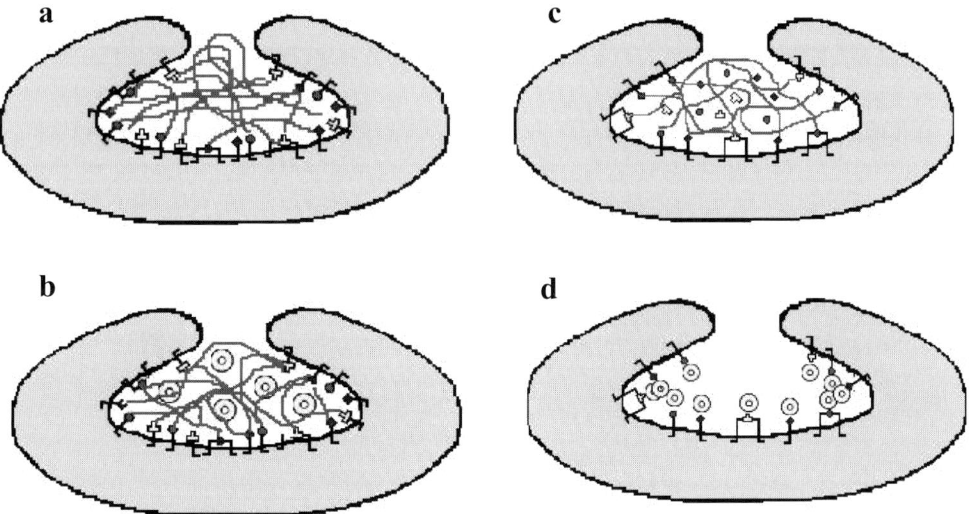

Figure 6. Bacterial ghosts as adjuvant and/or carriers for foreign target antigens. (a) Ghost with membrane-anchored antigens and polymers filling the inner lumen of the ghost. (b) Ghost with membrane-anchored antigens and polymers filling the inner lumen of the ghost entrapping plasmid DNA (circles). (c) Ghost with membrane-anchored antigens and polymers filling the inner lumen of the ghost entrapping soluble antigens. (d) Ghost with membrane-anchored polypeptides binding plasmid DNA.

(Figure 6a-d). Methods for preparing and filling ghosts with various materials are currently under development. For example, ghosts with streptavidin anchored on the inside of the cytoplasmic membrane can be filled by resuspending lyophilised ghosts in solutions carrying the biotinylated antigens (Huter *et al.*, 1999). It has also been shown that nucleic acids either attached to a matrix or alone (Figure 6b,d) can be efficiently packaged into bacterial ghosts. For various purposes, it is advantageous to fill the internal space of the ghost with a substituted matrix which then binds the substance of interest.

Delivery systems of DNA by cationic liposomes, cationic polymers like poly-L-lysins, polyethylenimine, polyamidoamine dendromers, polymeric vesicles or naked DNA alone are less efficient than viral means of gene delivery (Schätzlein and Uchegbu, 2001). As already mentioned above, bacterial ghosts have also been developed as DNA delivery vectors (Figure 6b,d). DNA packed into ghosts produces a high level of gene expression measured by the green fluorescent protein (GFP) when targeted under tissue culture conditions to Caco-2 cells, DC and macrophages (Paukner, Kohl, Lubitz, unpublished data). As the latter two cell types are well known for their high capacity to degrade phagocytosed material it is even more astonishing that

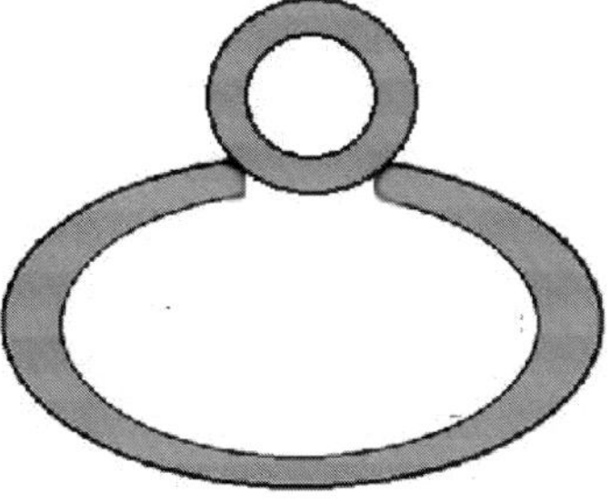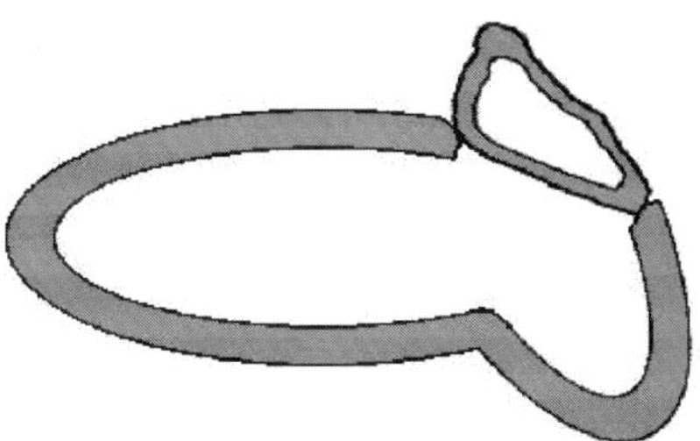

Figure 7. Sealing bacterial ghosts. Ghosts are sealed either with inside-out membrane vesicles (small circle) produced by French pressing bacteria of the same strain or by liposomes (oval colapsed circle) with a lipid content resembling the bacterial cytoplasmic membrane.

GFP plasmids delivered by bacterial ghosts transfer the DNA from the endosome to the nucleus without any help of endosomolytic agents or of nuclear localization signals. This system is under current evaluation for DNA encoded antigens.

Bacterial ghosts can be plugged in order to use ghosts as adjuvant systems for soluble, non-attached, hydrophilic antigens using a vesicle-to-ghost membrane fusion system. The sealing process of ghosts needs inside-out vesicles of the bacterium used to produce ghosts and fuses the vesicles to the inner membrane presented at the edges of the lysis tunnel of the ghost carrier (Figure 7).

Ortho-nitrophenyl-galactoside (ONPG), calcein and fluorescein-labelled DNA were used as reporter substances determining the ratio of resealed ghosts by fluorescence and quenching procedures. At present, the integrity of the resealed ghosts fluctuates between 1 and 20% depending on the methods used. However, the process of closing ghosts is under current improvement and it can be envisaged that new plugged ghost antigen carriers can be obtained in the near future (Paukner, Kohl, Lubitz, unpublished data).

Immune Response To Target Antigens Expressed In The Extended Bacterial Ghost System

V. cholerae ghosts can also be used as carrier for foreign antigens, e.g. to control *Chlamydia trachomatis* infections. An efficacious vaccine is needed to control the morbidity and huge healthcare cost associated with genital infection by *C. trachomatis*. In accordance with the new paradigm for vaccine design, an efficacious anti-chlamydial vaccine should elicit a genital mucosal Th1 response. Despite considerable efforts, the development of reliable chlamydial vaccines using conventional strategies has proven to be elusive. To design a candidate vaccine against *Chlamydia* based on the ghost technology, the gene encoding the major outer membrane protein (MOMP), *omp1*, of *C. trachomatis* serovar D was expressed in *V. cholerae*, as a membrane-anchored protein. Intranasal and intramuscular immunization of naive mice with *V. cholerae* ghosts expressing rMOMP induced a strong Th1 immune response in the genital mucosa. The ability of this vaccine regimen to protect susceptible animals from chlamydial infection will establish it as a potentially efficacious vaccine capable of protecting against human infections. The *V. cholerae* ghost carrier system offers a unique opportunity for designing recombinant subunit vaccines capable of simultaneously presenting multiple chlamydial membrane proteins to the immune system (Eko *et al.*, 2001).

The development and evaluation of oral systems for the delivery of antifertility vaccines for wild-life-control offers a humane and ethical method for the management of brushtail possums in New Zealand. Bacterial ghosts carrying the possum specific *zona pellucida* (ZP) antigen 3 are used to induce immunologically mediated fertility control (Duckworth *et al.*, unpublished data). The ZP is an extracellular coat present around all mammalian eggs and an attractive target for the development of immunocontraceptive vaccines. Antibodies against ZP are ovary-specific and act by preventing sperm from binding and penetrating the ova and/or by disrupting the development of follicles in the ovary (Paterson *et al.*, 2000).

E. coli ghosts carrying membrane-anchored truncated ZP3 in the envelope complex were used for their inherent adjuvant properties to induce specific humoral and cellular immune responses against the ZP3 target components. Oral and nasal immunization routes were used in mice to induce an immune response against possum ZP3. The target antigen was given at a dose of 3x3 μg in a context of ghosts without any other adjuvant or substance added. Serum antibody titers were detectable up to 1: 1000 dilutions and could be detected in most individuals. Antibody titers in the nasally immunized group appeared to be better than for the orally vaccinated group. Membrane anchored ZP3 antigens and ghosts carrying ZP3-S-layer fusion proteins are currently being tested in immunogenicity and fertility trials to develop an oral delivery system for the dissemination of fertility vaccines in the field (Duckworth *et al.*, unpublished data).

CONCLUSIONS

The capacity of all spaces within ghosts, including the periplasm, membranes and the internal lumen to carry antigens, DNA or mediators of the immune response is surprisingly large and can be used to design new vaccine candidates. The formulation of the substances packaged into the ghost envelope structures largely depends on their own nature and it might be of benefit to either loosely package them into the inner space of the envelopes or to firmly attach them to a matrix. It is obvious that different combinations of substances might need different components of the system for appropriate formulation. The extended recombinant ghost system warrants further investigation as it has great strategic potential in the areas of vaccine development and of targeting vehicles.

REFERENCES

Eko, F.O., Mayr, B.U., Attridge, S.R., and Lubitz, W. 2000. Characterization and Immunogenicity of *Vibrio cholerae* ghosts expressing toxin-coregulated pili. J. Biotechnol. 83: 115-123.

Eko, F.O., Lubitz, W. and Igietseme, J.U. 2001. Immunogenicity of a novel recombinant subunit candidate vaccine against *Chlamydia trachomatis*. Abstract book ASM Meeting, Orlando, USA. p. 341.

Haslberger, A.G., Mader, H.J., Schmalnauer, M., Kohl, G., Messner, P., Sleytr, U.B., Wanner, G., Fürst-Ladani, S., and Lubitz, W. 1997. Bacterial cell envelopes (ghosts) and LPS but not bacterial S-layers induce synthesis of immune-mediators in mouse macrophages involving CD14. J. Endotox. Res. 4: 431-441.

Haslberger, A.G., Kohl, G., Felnerova, D., Mayr, B., Fürst-Ladani, S., and Lubitz, W. 2000. Activation, stimulation and uptake of bacterial ghosts in antigen presenting cells. J. Biotechnol. 83: 57-66.

Hensel, A., van Leengoed, L.A.G., Szostak, M.P., Windt, H., Weissenböck, H., Stockhofe-Zurwieden, N., Katinger, A., Stadler, M., Ganter, M., Bunka, S., Pabst, R., and Lubitz, W. 1996. Induction of protective immunity by aerosol or oral application of candidate vaccines in a dose-controlled pig aerosol infection model. J. Biotechnol. 44: 171-181.

Hensel, A., and Lubitz, W. 1997. Vaccination by aerosols, modulation of clearance mechanisms in the lung. Behring Inst. Mitt. 98: 212-219.

Hensel, A., Huter, V., Katinger, A., Raza, P., Strnistschie, C., Roesler, U., Brand, E., and Lubitz, W. 2000. Intramuscular immunization with genetically inactivated (ghosts) *Acinobacillus pleuropneumoniae* serotype 9 protects pigs against homologous aerosol challenge and prevents carrier state. Vaccine 18: 2945-2955.

Huter, V., Szostak, M.P., Gampfer, J., Prethaler, S., Wanner, G., Gabor, F., and Lubitz, W. 1999. Bacterial ghosts as drug carrier and targeting vehicles. J. Controll. Release 61: 51-63.

Huter, V., Hensel, A., Brand, E., and Lubitz. W. 2000. Improved protection against lung colonization by *Actinobacillus pleuropneumoniae* ghosts: characterization of a genetically inactivated vaccine. J. Biotechnol. 83: 161-172.

Jechlinger, W., Szostak, M.P., and Lubitz, W. 1998. Cold sensitive E-lysis systems. Gene 218: 1-7.

Jechlinger, W., Szostak, M.P., Witte, A., and Lubitz, W. 1999. Altered temperature induction sensitivity of the lambda PR/ cI857 system for controlled *gene E*-expression in *Escherichia coli*. FEMS Microbiol. Lett. 173: 347-352.

Katinger, A., Lubitz, W., Szostak, M.P., Stadler, M., Klein, R., Indra, A., Huter, V., and Hensel, A. 1999. Pigs aerogenously immunized with genetically inactivated (ghosts) or irradiated *Actinobacillus pleuropneumoniae* are protected against a homologous aerosol challenge despite differing in pulmonary cellular and antibody responses. J. Biotech. 73: 251-260.

Kloos, D.U., Stratz, M., Guttler, A., Steffan R.J., and Timmis K.N. 1994. Inducible cell lysis system for the study of natural transformation and environmental fate of DNA released by cell death. J. Bacteriol. 176: 7352-7361.

Kuen, B., Koch, A., Asenbauer, W., Sara, M., and Lubitz, W. 1994. Sequence analysis of the *sbsA* gene encoding the 130-kDa surface-layer protein of *Bacillus stearothermophilus* PV72. Gene 145: 115-120.

Kuen, B., Sara, M., and Lubitz, W. 1995. Heterologous expression and self-assembly of the S-layer protein *SbsA* of Bacillus stearothermophilus in *Escherichia coli*. Mol. Microbiol. 19: 495-503.

Kuen, B., Koch, A., Asenbauer, W., Sara, M., and Lubitz, W. 1997. Molecular characterization of the *Bacillus stearothermophilus* PV72 S-layer gene *sbsB* induced by oxidative stress. J. Bacteriol. 179: 1664-1670.

Lubitz, W., and Pugsley, A.P. 1985. Changes in host cell phospholipid composition of PhiX174 gene *E* product. FEMS Microbiol. Lett. 30: 171-175.

Mader, H.J., Szostak, M.P., Hensel, A., Lubitz, W., and Haslberger, A.G. 1997. Endotoxicity does not limit the use of bacterial ghosts as candidate vaccine. Vaccine 15: 195-202.

Paterson, M., Jennings, Z.A., Van Dui, M., and Aitken, R.J. 2000. Immunocontraception with zona pellucida proteins. Cells Tissues Organs 166: 228-232.

Resch, S., Gruber, K., Wanner, G., Slater, S., Dennis, D., and Lubitz, W. 1998. Aqueous release and purification of poly -β-hydroxybutyrate from *Escherichia coli*. J. Biotechnol. 65: 173-182.

Ronchel, M.C., Molina, L., Lubitz, W., Molin, S., Ramos, J.L., and Ramos, C. 1998. Characterization of cell lysis in *Pseudomonas putida* induced upon expression of heterologous killing genes. Appl. Environment. Microbiol. 64: 4904-4911.

Schätzlein, A.G., and Uchegbu, I.F. 2001. Non-viral vectors in gene delivery. Drug Deliv. Systems & Sci. 1: 17-23.

Schön, P., Schrot, G., Wanner, G., Lubitz, W., and Witte, A. 1995. Two-stage model for integration of the lysis protein E of PhiX174 into the cell envelope of *Escherichia coli*. FEMS Microbiol. Rev. 17: 207-212.

Schüller, A., Harkness, R.E., Rüther, U., and Lubitz, W. 1985. Deletion of C-terminal amino acid codons of PhiX174 gene *E*, Effects of its lysis inducing properties. Nucleic Acids Res. 13: 4143-4153.

Szostak, M.P., and Lubitz, W. 1991. Recombinant bacterial ghosts as multivaccine vehicles. In: Modern Approaches to New Vaccines Including Prevention of AIDS. Vaccines 91. R.M. Chanock *et al.*, eds. Cold Spring Harbor Laboratory Press, New York.p. 409-414.

Szostak, M.P., Hensel, A., Eko, F.O., Klein, R., Auer, T., Mader, H., Haslberger, A., Bunka, S., Wanner, G., and Lubitz, W. 1996. Bacterial ghosts, non-living candidate vaccines. J. Biotechnol. 44: 161-170.

Truppe, M., Howorka, S., Schroll, G., Lechleitner, S., Kuen, B., Resch, S., and Lubitz, W. 1997. Biotechnological applications of recombinant S-layer proteins rSbsA and rSbsB from *Bacillus stearothermophilus* PV72. FEMS Microbiol. Rev. 20: 47-98.

Witte, A., Wanner, G., Bläsi, U., Halfmann, G., Szostak, M., and Lubitz, W. 1990a. Endogenous transmembrane tunnel formation mediated by PhiX174 lysis protein E. J. Bacteriol. 172: 4109-4114.

Witte, A., Bläsi, U., Halfmann, G., Szostak, M., Wanner, G., and Lubitz, W. 1990b. PhiX174 protein E mediated lysis of *Escherichia coli*. Biochimie 72: 191-200.

Witte, A., Wanner, G., Sulzner, M., and Lubitz, W. 1992. Dynamics of PhiX174 protein E-mediated lysis of *Escherichia coli*. Arch. Microbiol. 157: 381-388.

Witte, A., Brand, E., Schrot, G., and Lubitz, W. 1993. Pathway of PhiX174 Protein E Mediated Lysis of *Escherichia coli*. In: Bacterial Growth and Lysis. M.A. dePedro, J.-V. Höltje, and W. Löffelhardt, eds. Plenum Press, New York. p. 277-283.

Witte, A., Schrot, G., Schön, P., and Lubitz, W. 1997. Proline 21, a residue within the alpha-helical domain of PhiX174 lysis protein E, is required for its lysis function in *Escherichia coli*. Mol. Microbiol. 26: 337-346.

Witte, A., Brand, E., Mayrhofer, P., Narendja, F., and Lubitz, W. 1998a. Dependence of PhiX174 protein E-mediated lysis on cell division activities of *Escherichia coli*. Arch. Microbiol. 170: 259-268.

Witte, A., Wanner, G., Lubitz, W., and Höltje, J.-V. 1998b. Effect of PhiX174 E-mediated lysis on murein composition of *Escherichia coli*. FEMS Microbiol. Lett. 164: 149-157.

From: *Vaccine Delivery Strategies*
Edited by: Guido Dietrich and Werner Goebel

Chapter 8

Attenuated *Salmonella* and *Shigella* Live Vectors

Myron M. Levine, James E. Galen, Eileen Barry, Marcela F. Pasetti, Carol O. Tacket, and Marcelo B. Sztein

ABSTRACT

Attenuated strains of *Salmonella enterica* serovar Typhi (*S. typhi*) or Typhimurium (*S. typhimurium*) and *Shigella* can serve as mucosally administered live vectors that express foreign protein or polysaccharide antigens and deliver them to the immune system, eliciting protective immune responses. Multiple factors influence the immunogenicity of these bacterial vectors, including the robustness of the vector strain itself, the nature of the foreign antigen, the promoter controlling expression, gene copy number, whether the foreign antigen gene is stabilized, the site of foreign antigen accumulation and the type of immune response that is desired. Extensive studies in animal models and limited human clinical trials emphasize the importance of optimizing these parameters in order to enhance the immunogenicity of the vector construct. Attenuated strains of *Salmonella* and *Shigella* can also carry plasmids with foreign genes under control of eukaryotic expression systems (DNA vaccines) and, following mucosal administration, can deliver those plasmids to antigen presenting cells. The immune response to foreign antigens stimulated by live vectors carrying either prokaryotic or eukaryotic expression systems can be modulated by having the bacteria concomitantly carry genes encoding relevant cytokines. The extraordinary versatility of *Salmonella* and *Shigella* live vectors makes them a promising live antigen delivery system.

INTRODUCTION

A vaccinology strategy that offers unusual flexibility as a "platform technology" is based on the use of bacterial live vectors. Attenuated strains of *Salmonella* and *Shigella* are particularly versatile because they can deliver to the mammalian immune system either foreign antigens produced by the vectors themselves by means of prokaryotic expression systems or eukaryotic expression plasmids (i.e., DNA vaccines) that allow mammalian antigen presenting cells (APCs) to produce the antigens. Potential advantages of these live vector vaccines include their administration by mucosal (oral or intranasal) rather than parenteral routes (which increases compliance and avoids problems of injection safety in developing countries) and their relatively economical manufacture compared to tissue culture-based, conjugate and purified subunit vaccines. This review will focus on attenuated *Salmonella* (mainly *S. typhi*) and *Shigella* live vectors as human vaccines.

PATHOGENESIS OF WILD TYPE INFECTION

A fundamental feature of the pathogenesis of both *S. typhi* and *Shigella* infection in humans that contributes to their success as live vectors is their ability to invade the intestinal mucosa. The invasion process begins with their uptake by microfold (M) cells and is followed by their passage to the underlying gut-associated lymphoid tissue (GALT) where they are ingested by professional phagocytes (including macrophages and dendritic cells) that function as APCs. *S. typhi*, an enteropathogen restricted to human hosts, is transmitted by the ingestion of contaminated food or water. Upon reaching the small intestine, *S. typhi* enters M cells and then passes to the GALT. However, *S. typhi* can also be pinocytosed by enterocytes that subsequently extrude the bacteria into the lamina propria where they elicit an influx of macrophages that ingest the typhoid bacilli. *S. typhi* is endowed with virulence attributes that allow survival within the phagocytic vacuoles of APCs (Miller and Mekalanos, 1990; Miller *et al.*, 1990). The typhoid bacilli are transported successively to draining lymph nodes, the lymph circulation and the bloodstream (via the thoracic duct). During this primary bacteremia they are filtered by fixed macrophages in the reticuloendothelial system (spleen, liver, bone marrow, etc.); typhoid bacilli also reach the gall bladder at this time. The clinically silent primary bacteremia is believed to ensue within 24 hours of having ingested the typhoid bacilli. After an incubation of ~8-14 days, clinical illness begins characterized by fever, headache, malaise, abdominal discomfort and secondary bacteremia.

Shigella is restricted to humans and higher primate hosts. Typically, 18-24 hours of watery diarrhea and fever precede the onset of dysentery (scanty stools of blood and mucus). Two enterotoxins mediate the watery diarrhea: *Shigella* enterotoxin 1 (ShET1) (Fasano *et al.*, 1995 and 1997), expressed mainly by the *S. flexneri* 2a serotype (Noriega *et al.*, 1995), is encoded by a gene located on a chromosomal pathogenicity island; *Shigella* enterotoxin 2 (ShET2) is encoded by a gene found on the large invasiveness plasmid carried by all pathogenic *Shigella* strains (Nataro *et al.*, 1995).

Shigella invades M cells and intestinal epithelial cells by a macropinocytotic process, leading to intense mucosal inflammation (Perdomo *et al.*, 1994; Sansonetti, 1992; Sansonetti and Phalipon, 1999). Invasion plasmid antigens (Ipas) secreted by the bacteria upon contact with M cells or epithelial cells cause cytoskeletal reorganization and internalization of the bacterium. The bacterium lyses the phagocytotic vacuole in which it resides and initiates intracytoplasmic movement, resulting from the polar assembly of actin filaments caused by the bacterial surface protein, VirG (also called IcsA). Bacteria pass to the underlying GALT of the terminal ileum and colon where they are ingested by macrophages. Within the macrophage, *Shigella* escapes from the phagolysosome by the action of IpaB and enters the cytoplasm. IpaB expressed by *Shigella* causes apoptosis of the macrophages in the follicular dome, resulting in the release of mature IL-1β and IL-1α precursors which induce a strong polymorphonuclear leukocyte inflammatory reaction, release of pro-inflammatory cytokines and an undermining of the integrity of the epithelial layer (Perdomo *et al.*, 1994).

Attractive attenuated *S. typhi* and *Shigella* live vector strains complete the early steps in pathogenesis and gain access to APCs in the GALT (and perhaps other lymphoid tissue) but do not cause adverse clinical responses (e.g., fever, diarrhea, malaise) or detectable bacteremia.

THE ARRAY OF IMMUNE RESPONSES ELICITED BY *SALMONELLA* AND *SHIGELLA*

Infection with wild type organisms or mucosal immunization with attenuated *Salmonella* and *Shigella* stimulate every arm of the immune system. This fact engenders optimism that relevant immune responses against foreign antigens can be generated when these bacterial live vectors carry prokaryotic expression systems encoding foreign antigens. Specific serum IgG (Hohmann *et al.*, 1996; Tacket *et al.*, 1992a, 1992b, 1997a, and 1997b), intestinal secretory IgA (SIgA) (Forrest *et al.*, 1990 and 1991; Viret *et al.*, 1999), lymphocyte proliferation and interferon-γ secretion (Sztein *et al.*, 1994), specific MHC I-restricted CD8$^+$ cytotoxic lymphocytes (CTL) (Sztein *et al.*, 1995) and specific antibody-dependent mononuclear cell killing responses (Tagliabue *et al.*, 1985 and 1986) have all been described in humans and in animal models. Thus, depending on the type of immune response that must be stimulated to prevent infection by the pathogen of interest, *Salmonella* and *Shigella* live vectors expressing protective foreign antigens can usually elicit the relevant humoral or cell-mediated immune response (Anderson *et al.*, 2000; Barry *et al.*, 1996; Chatfield *et al.*, 1992a; Galen *et al.*, 1997; Gomez-Duarte *et al.*, 2001; Gonzalez *et al.*, 1994 and 1998; Hess *et al.*, 1996; Noriega *et al.*, 1996a).

STUDIES IN ANIMAL MODELS WITH *SALMONELLA* AND *SHIGELLA* LIVE VECTORS EXPRESSING FOREIGN ANTIGENS ENCODED BY PROKARYOTIC EXPRESSION SYSTEMS

Salmonella

Attenuated *S. typhimurium* strains have been extensively studied as live vector vaccines in mice as a model to predict the responses that would occur when humans are fed homologous strains of *S. typhi*. *S. typhimurium* strains commonly used as live vectors harbor mutations in: 1) *cya* (encoding adenylate cyclase) and *crp* (encoding the cyclic AMP receptor protein), that together comprise a global regulatory system affecting multiple virulence and housekeeping genes (Curtiss and Kelly, 1987). 2) *aroA*, *aroC* or *aroD*, encoding enzymes in the biosynthesis of aromatic metabolites, including folate, enterochelin, and aromatic amino acids (Dougan *et al.*, 1988). Aro⁻

mutants require substrates (para-aminobenzoic acid and 2, 3 dihydroxybenzoate) that are not available in sufficient concentration once the bacteria have become intracellular. 3) *phoP, phoQ*, a regulatory system controlling genes that allow *Salmonella* to survive within phagolysosomes in macrophages (Miller *et al.*, 1989). 4) *htrA*, encoding a stress response protein that functions as a serine protease (Chatfield *et al.*, 1992b).

Studies in the mouse model with *S. typhimurium* expressing foreign antigens encoded by plasmids or by genes integrated into the chromosome have demonstrated the feasibility and versatility of this vaccinology strategy. Proteins and polysaccharide antigens from various genera of bacteria, viruses and parasites have been expressed in *Salmonella*. Following mucosal (usually oral, sometimes nasal) immunization with the live vectors, specific serum IgG antibodies, SIgA mucosal antibody or cell-mediated immune responses are stimulated that confer protection against challenge with wild type organisms or toxins (Aggarwal *et al.*, 1990; Ascon *et al.*, 1998; Chatfield *et al.*, 1992a; Clements *et al.*, 1986; Gomez-Duarte *et al.*, 1998; Huang *et al.*, 2001; Karem *et al.*, 1997; Nayak *et al.*, 1998; Sadoff *et al.*, 1988; Toebe *et al.*, 1997; Xu *et al.*, 1997; Zhang *et al.*, 1996).

A mouse model of intranasal immunization with attenuated *S. typhi* live vectors has been developed that overcomes the host restriction in mice of oral immunization with *S. typhi* and allows pre-clinical immunogenicity studies to be performed (Galen *et al.*, 1997; Pasetti *et al.*, 2000; Pickett *et al.*, 2000). In this murine model, *S. typhi* live vectors expressing various bacterial and protozoal antigens elicit relevant immune responses (Barry *et al.*, 1996; Galen *et al.*, 1997; Gomez-Duarte *et al.*, 2001; Pasetti *et al.*, 1999; Wu *et al.*, 2000); some studies have included challenges that document vaccine efficacy (Galen *et al.*, 1997).

Shigella

Attenuated *Shigella* also functions admirably as a live vector for carrying prokaryotic systems to express foreign antigens. Most work has been performed with *S. flexneri* 2a live vectors harboring mutations in *aroA*, *guaBA* and *virG* in a guinea pig model involving mucosal (intranasal) immunization (Altboum *et al.*, 2001; Anderson *et al.*, 2000; Koprowski *et al.*, 2000; Noriega *et al.*, 1996a and 1996b). The foreign antigens expressed have included cytoplasmic fragment C of tetanus toxin (Anderson *et al.*, 2000), periplasmic heat labile enterotoxin (LT) of enterotoxigenic *Escherichia coli* (ETEC) (Koprowski *et al.*, 2000) and ETEC fimbrial antigens (Altboum *et al.*, 2001;

Table1. Phase I and II human clinical trials evaluating the safety, immunogenicity and efficacy of attenuated *Salmonella enterica* serovar *typhi* and *typhimurium* constructs expressing foreign protein or polysaccharide antigens under the control of prokaryotic expression systems

S. typhi live vector, attenuating mutations	Contruct designation	Foreign antigen expressed	Site of foreign gene	Accumu-lation of antigen	Clinical response	No. of doses, route	Immune response to vector antigens	Immune response to foreign antigen	Protection
Ty21a[*], *rpoS, galE,* Vi-	5076-1C	*Shigella sonnei* O polysaccharide	plasmid	surface	well tolerated	3, oral	weak	9/9[+], 9/16[$]	variable efficacy against *S. sonnei* in several challenge studies
(Black *et al.*, 1987; Herrington *et al.*, 1990)									
Ty21a[*], *rpoS, galE,* Vi-	EX 645	*Vibrio cholerae* O1 Inaba LPS	plasmid	surface	well tolerated	3, oral	moderate	5/14[&]	25% efficacy against El Tor Inaba cholera challenge
(Tacket *et al.*, 1990)									
Ty21a[*], *rpoS, galE,* Vi-	Ty21a(pDB1)	*H. pylori* urease A & B	plasmid	cytoplasm	well tolerated	3, oral	modest	3/9[!]	NA
(Bumann *et al.*, 2001)									

CVD 908, *aroC, aroD*	CVD 908 Ω (*aroC*1019::_{tac}P-r*csp*)	*Plasmodium falciparum* CSP	chromo-some	cytoplasm	well tolerated	2, oral	strong	3/10^	NA

(Gonzalez *et al.*, 1994)

CVD 908-*htrA*, *aroC, aroD*, *htrA*	CVD 908-*htrA*(pTET1*pp*)	fragment C of tetanus toxin	plasmid	cytoplasm	well tolerated	1, oral	strong	low dose, 0/2# ; high dose, 1/1#	NA

(Tacket *et al.*, 2000)

X4073, *cya, crp, cdt*	X4632 (pYQ3167)	HBV core pre-S	stabilized plasmid	cytoplasm	well tolerated	1, oral	moderate	0/10	NA

(Tacket *et al.*, 1997a)

X4073, *cya, crp, cdt*	X4632 (pYQ3167)	HBV core pre-S	stabilized plasmid	cytoplasm	well tolerated	1, oral (N=7) 1, rectal (N=6)	strong after oral; weak after rectal	0/7 oral; 1/6 rectal**	NA

(Nardelli-Haefliger *et al.*, 1996)

Table 1, continued

| Ty800, *phoP, phoQ, purB* | Ty1033 | *H. pylori* urease A & B | stabilized plasmid | cytoplasm | well tolerated | 1, oral | strong | 0/8 | NA |

(DiPetrillo *et al.*, 1999)

S. typhimurium

| ATCC 14028 *phoP, phoQ, purB* | LH1160 | *H. pylori* urease A & B | stabilized plasmid | cytoplasm | moderately reactogenic | 1, oral | strong | 3/6[++] | NA |

(Angelakopoulos and Hohmann, 2000)

* Ty21a was developed using chemical mutagenesis and therefore has many other mutations besides the three listed
+ IgA antibody secreting cell response
$ Serum IgA antibody response
& Serum virbriocidal antibody
! Cell-mediated immune responses
^ Two subjects manifested serum antibody responses (ELISA against purified protein or indirect immunofluorescent assay against whole sporozoites. One subject mounted a specific MHC I-restricted, CD8+ cytotoxic lymphocyte response.
# Results in subjects lacking tetanus antitoxin at baseline
** Serum antibody
++ Detection of antibody secreting cells making anti-urease antibody

Noriega *et al.*, 1996a) as bacterial surface structures. These *Shigella* live vectors have stimulated serum IgG tetanus antitoxin and serum IgG and secretory IgA mucosal antibodies to LT and ETEC fimbriae. Strain SC 602 has been used as a live vector expressing a hybrid IpaC protein that incorporates the C3 neutralizing epitope of poliovirus VP1 protein (Barzu *et al.*, 1998).

Experience In Human Clinical Trials With Attenuated *S. typhi* And *S. typhimurium* And *Shigella* Expressing Foreign Antigens

Although studies in murine, guinea pig and other animal models with attenuated *Salmonella* live vectors expressing foreign antigens have clearly demonstrated the feasibility of this vaccinology strategy, heretofore, only a small number of Phase I and II clinical trials have been carried out in humans. Clinical trials with *Shigella* live vectors have not yet been initiated but are imminent. Salient results of these trials are summarized in Table 1.

Early studies with Ty21a expressing *Shigella sonnei* O polysaccharide or *Vibrio cholerae* O1 Inaba lipopolysaccharide established that *S. typhi* live vectors bearing foreign surface antigens could stimulate relevant immune responses (*S. sonnei* O antibody and Inaba vibriocidal antibody) and could confer protection against experimental shigellosis and cholera, respectively. However, the efficacy of the Ty21a construct expressing *S. sonnei* was inconsistent (Black *et al.*, 1987; Herrington *et al.*, 1990) and the level of protection (25% efficacy) of the Ty21a construct expressing Inaba LPS was low (Tacket *et al.*, 1990), impeding further development of those vaccines. Oral immunization of young adults with two doses of *S. typhi* live vector CVD 908 expressing the circumsporozoite of *Plasmodium falciparum* set two milestones (Gonzalez *et al.*, 1994). First, this construct documented that *S. typhi* live vectors could elicit antibody responses to a heterologous protein antigen in humans. Second, this *S. typhi* live vector stimulated CD8$^+$ MHC I-restricted cytotoxic lymphocytes that recognized targets bearing CSP, demonstrating that *typhi* live vectors could elicit relevant cell-mediated effector responses in humans (Gonzalez *et al.*, 1994).

Immunization of adults with a single oral dose of CVD 908-*htrA* carrying a plasmid encoding fragment C of tetanus toxin stimulated protective levels of tetanus antitoxin in a seronegative subject (Tacket *et al.*, 2000). The importance of this observation is to demonstrate that a single oral dose of a

S. typhi live vector can elicit a type of protective immune response that is generally thought to require parenteral immunization. A Phase I clinical trial of an attenuated *S. typhimurium* live vector expressing *H. pylori* urease A and B (Angelakopoulos and Hohmann, 2000) stimulated anti-urease antibodies in 3 of 6 subjects but this live vector was not well tolerated clinically.

Clinical trials with other live vector constructs have given generally modest results (Black *et al.*, 1987; Bumann *et al.*, 2001; DiPetrillo *et al.*, 1999; Herrington *et al.*, 1990; Nardelli-Haefliger *et al.*, 1996; Tacket *et al.*, 1997a; Tramont *et al.*, 1984). In some of these clinical trials, the *S. typhi* live vectors failed to elicit a detectable immune response to the foreign antigen, despite immunogenicity of the identical (or homologous *S. typhimurium*) constructs when tested in pre-clinical animal models. Regrettably, none of the human clinical trials with *Salmonella* live vectors, heretofore, have utilized constructs that would be considered optimal. The section below discusses the factors that influence the ability of *S. typhi* constructs to function successfully as oral live vector vaccines.

PARAMETERS THAT AFFECT THE IMMUNOGENICITY OF FOREIGN ANTIGENS EXPRESSED BY ATTENUATED *SALMONELLA* AND *SHIGELLA*

Choice of *S. typhi* or *Shigella* Strain

The choice of which attenuated *Salmonella* or *Shigella* strain to use as the live vector is critical. Attenuated strains that function admirably as live oral typhoid or *Shigella* vaccines may not necessarily work well as live vectors. The usual reason is that they are too attenuated *a priori* and become hyper-attenuated because of metabolic stress when they carry prokaryotic expression plasmids. Generally, the strength of the immune response to the vector and the heterologous antigen go in parallel. For example, Ty21a, the well-tolerated and protective licensed live oral typhoid vaccine strain, is only modestly immunogenic and thus has been disappointing as a live vector. Depending on the attenuating mutations, strains may differ in their capacity to elicit antibody or cell-mediated immune responses. For example, *Salmonella* that harbor mutations in the *phoPQ* operon, which limits survival within the phagolysosomes of macrophages, appear to elicit antibody responses preferentially (Benyacoub *et al.*, 1999). Strains harboring mutations in *aro* genes and *htrA* stimulate both Th1 and Th2 type responses.

Attenuated *S. typhi* strains that have been used as live vectors in clinical trials include: licensed strain Ty21a (Black *et al.*, 1987; Bumann *et al.*, 2001; Tacket *et al.*, 1990; Tramont *et al.*, 1984); CVD 908 (mutations in *aroC* and *aroD*) (Gonzalez *et al.*, 1994), CVD 908-*htrA* (mutations in *aroC*, *aroD* and *htrA*) (Tacket *et al.*, 2000), derivatives of Ty800 (mutations in *phoP, Q*) (DiPetrillo *et al.*, 1999), and derivatives of X4073 (Nardelli-Haefliger *et al.*, 1996; Tacket *et al.*, 1997a).

The most likely attenuated *Shigella* strains that may enter clinical trials as live vectors include CVD 1204 (Anderson *et al.*, 2000), CVD 1207 (Kotloff *et al.*, 2000), CVD 1208 (Koprowski *et al.*, 2000) and SC 602 (Barzu *et al.*, 1998).

Choice of Protective Foreign Antigens

Although the *Salmonella* system is versatile, it has limitations. For example, *Salmonella* cannot glycosylate proteins. Thus, if protective epitopes reside within a viral protein and post-translational modifications such as glycosylation are required to achieve correct folding of the antigen in order to stimulate specific antibodies against the conformational epitopes, *Salmonella* would not be the preferred vector system. On the other hand, if the critical immune response against a glycosylated viral protein target is cell-mediated (and therefore based on linear epitopes), *Salmonella* may function admirably.

Because of the broad immune response that *Salmonella* elicits, there is much interest in utilizing *Salmonella* to deliver to the immune system antigens from human parasites (Levine *et al.*, 1997). However, it is challenging to express these eukaryotic proteins and IT often requires protein engineering to delete highly hydrophobic regions usually found on the N-terminus or C-terminus. When such regions are removed, these eukaryotic proteins can usually be expressed (Gomez-Duarte *et al.*, 2001; Gonzalez *et al.*, 1994).

Optimization of Codon Usage

The level of expression of foreign proteins can be influenced by codon usage. For example, expression of certain eukaryotic proteins in bacteria such as *Salmonella* and *Escherichia coli,* and even expression of proteins from Gram positive genera such as *Clostridium tetani* in *Salmonella* and *Shigella,* may be notably improved by optimizing codon usage of the foreign gene for *Salmonella* or *Shigella* preferences.

Selection of a Promoter

Selection of the promoter used to control expression of a foreign gene in *Salmonella* or *Shigella* has proven to be critical in affecting the immunogenicity of the construct. For some antigens that are well tolerated by *Salmonella*, powerful constitutive promoters that achieve high level continuous expression of the antigen are advantageous (Galen *et al.*, 1997). However, the expression of certain other antigens has a deleterious effect on the live vector, taking a metabolic toll that alters its growth curve *in vitro* and its colonizing propensity *in vivo* (Coulson *et al.*, 1994). For such antigens, delaying the onset of full expression until the live vector has successfully reached a protected immunologically relevant site, such as within APCs, can be beneficial. The "*in vivo*-activated" promoters used in attempts to regulate expression include *nirB*, *nir*15 and *dmsA* (activated by low redox potential) (Chatfield *et al.*, 1992a; Gomez-Duarte *et al.*, 1995; Huang *et al.*, 2001; McSorley *et al.*, 1997; Orr *et al.*, 2001), *ompC* and *osmC* (activated by iso-osmolar conditions) (Galen *et al.*, 1999; McSorley *et al.*, 1997), *pagC* (activated by conditions in the phagolysosome) (Dunstan *et al.*, 1999) and *htrA* (activated by various environmental stresses) (Everest *et al.*, 1995). Irrespective of results obtained *in vitro*, studies in animal models and human clinical trials are required to judge whether the promoter has the desired effect *in vivo*.

Stabilization of Foreign Genes

Foreign genes encoding antigens of interest may be stabilized either by chromosomal integration or by a plasmid stabilization system. Integration into the chromosome assures stability but provides only a single gene copy and in some instances is technically difficult to accomplish (Gonzalez *et al.*, 1994; Hone *et al.*, 1988). In contrast, plasmid stabilization provides the potential benefits of multi-copy plasmids. A "balanced lethal system" assures that bacteria carrying the plasmid survive, whereas those that lose it die (post-segregational killing) (Nakayama *et al.*, 1988). One well known balanced lethal system is based on deleting *asd*, a gene that encodes an enzyme necessary for the synthesis of diaminopimelic acid (DAP), a substrate that Gram negative bacteria must have in order to synthesize their cell walls (Nakayama *et al.,* 1988). Inactivation of *asd* is lethal unless DAP, which is not present in mammalian tissues, is provided. A plasmid that carries *asd* plus the gene encoding the foreign antigen is introduced into a *Salmonella* harboring a chromosomal deletion in *asd*. This plasmid complements the Δ*asd* mutation *in trans* and the plasmid becomes stabilized because the bacterium would die if the plasmid was lost. One deficiency of such a balanced lethal system alone is that whereas it assures maintenance of the plasmid in an individual bacterium, it does not account for equitable distribution of the plasmid to daughter cells when replication occurs. This problem was solved by Galen *et al.* (1999) who constructed expression plasmids containing a post-segregational killing system as well as partitioning loci that enhance the probability that upon replication both daughter cells will inherit the plasmid.

Site of Expression

The site of accumulation of the expressed foreign antigen within *Salmonella* or *Shigella* can affect immunogenicity markedly. Some antigens, such as fragment C of tetanus toxin, are immunogenic when accumulated as cytoplasmic antigens (Chatfield *et al.,* 1992a; Galen *et al.,* 1997) in *Salmonella* and *Shigella*. Other antigens are more immunogenic when amassed in the periplasmic space (where conditions may foster correct folding to achieve conformational epitopes), when accumulated on the surface of the bacterium or when secreted out of the bacterial vector. This is true not only for stimulating antibodies (Lee *et al.,* 2000; Schorr *et al.,* 1991) but also for eliciting cell-mediated immune responses. Hess *et al.* (Hess *et al.,* 1996) have shown that the outright secretion of foreign antigens by *Salmonella* using the Hemolysin A secretion system results in significantly enhanced cytotoxic lymphocyte responses. Other secretion systems to export antigens or epitopes out of *Salmonella* include a modified type III secretion system (Russmann *et al.,* 1998) and the *clyA* system (Galen and Levine, 2001).

Metabolic Burden

The efficiency of a bacterial live vector vaccine correlates with its ability to present to the human immune system sufficient foreign antigen so that the desired protective immune response can be elicited. As reviewed by Galen and Levine (2001), often overlooked in live vector engineering is the effect on the fitness of the live vector that derives from high copy number expression plasmids and the heterologous antigens they encode. Expression of foreign antigens often leads to deleterious effects on the overall fitness of the live vector because of the increased metabolic load. Galen and Levine (2001) have described a novel highly stabilized plasmid-based prokaryotic expression system that incorporates a ClyA hemolysin secretion system to export foreign antigens out of the *S. typhi* live vector.

Co-expression of Adjuvants and Cytokines

It has been shown in animal models that the immune response can be enhanced or modulated towards a preferred Th1 or Th2 bias by co-expressing cytokines or biological adjuvants in the live vector (Carrier *et al.,* 1993; Chen *et al.,* 1998; Denich *et al.,* 1993; Dunstan *et al.,* 1996; Whittle *et al.,* 1997). For example, IL-4 and IL-5 expressed by attenuated *Salmonella* increase the serum and mucosal antibody responses (Denich *et al.,* 1993; Whittle *et al.,* 1997).

Cholera toxin (CT) and the related heat-labile enterotoxin (LT) of enterotoxigenic *E. coli* (ETEC) are powerful adjuvants that augment the serum and mucosal antibody responses to co-administered antigens. Mutant CT and LT molecules have been engineered that retain the adjuvanticity property but are virtually devoid of the ability to elicit intestinal secretion (Rappuoli *et al.,* 1999; Yamamoto *et al.,* 1997). Some investigators have reported that secretion of mutant LT by attenuated *Salmonella* can enhance immune responses to the bacteria (Covone *et al.,* 1998). In contrast, co-expression of mutant LT by attenuated *Shigella* did not enhance the immune response to co-expressed ETEC fimbrial antigens (Koprowski *et al.,* 2000).

ATTENUATED *SHIGELLA* AND *SALMONELLA* AS LIVE VECTORS DELIVERING DNA VACCINES

A startling observation made in the 1990s is that immune responses and protection can be elicited in animal models by inoculating with "naked DNA". Prototype DNA vaccines consist of a plasmid with the gene of interest placed under the control of a eukaryotic promoter (such as the cytomegalovirus immediate early promoter) to drive transcription in mammalian cells, a polyadenylation signal at the 3' end of the insert to stabilize mRNA and ensure translation, and an origin of replication (e.g., from SV40 or Epstein-barr virus) that allows some rounds of plasmid replication within eukaryotic cells. When such plasmids enter APCs, the eukaryotic cell machinery actually produces the foreign protein. An advantage is that, for viral proteins in particular, the protein receives all the appropriate post-translational modifications.

Initially, DNA vaccines were inoculated intramuscularly or adsorbed to gold particles and inoculated intradermally via a gene gun. Most investigations of DNA vaccines still utilize parenteral routes of administration. However, it has been demonstrated that mucosal immunization with attenuated *Shigella* and *Salmonella* can successfully deliver DNA vaccine plasmids directly to APCs in which eukaryotic expression of the foreign protein ensues, resulting in immune responses (Anderson *et al.*, 2000; Darji *et al.*, 1997; Fennelly *et al.*, 1999; Flo *et al.*, 2001; Pasetti *et al.*, 1999; Shata *et al.*, 2001a and 2001b; Sizemore *et al.*, 1995; Woo *et al.*, 2001). Many attenuated *Shigella* strains retain a functional IpaB that allows the bacteria to break out of the phagolysosome and enter the cytosol. Upon death and disruption of the attenuated bacteria, the DNA vaccine plasmid is released and can enter the nucleus of the eukaryotic cell. Thus, it is readily apparent why *Shigella* live vectors work well for delivering DNA vaccine plasmids. Nevertheless, attenuated *S. typhi* and *S. typhimurium* also function well, even though these bacteria are believed to remain within phagosomes within the APC and do not enter the cytoplasm. Gentschev *et al.* (2001) devised a way to improve *Salmonella* as a delivery system for DNA vaccines by equipping the bacteria with the ability to express Listeriolysin, which disrupts the phagosomal membrane and releases the *Salmonella* into the cytosol.

Shigella and *Salmonella* vectors can be modified to carry genes encoding cytokines in conjunction with the DNA vaccine encoding antigens of interest, in order to modify the immune response, as desired. Human clinical trials with DNA vaccines delivered by attenuated *Shigella* or *Salmonella* have not yet been undertaken. However, given the enthusiasm that live vector constructs carrying DNA vaccines are generating based on results in pre-clinical models, it is expected that clinical trials with constructs carrying *P. falciparum*, HIV and measles DNA vaccines will be initiated soon.

EFFECT OF PRIOR ANTI-VECTOR IMMUNITY ON THE IMMUNE RESPONSE TO FOREIGN ANTIGENS

It is appropriate to ponder what effect background immunity against *S. typhi* and *Shigella* can have on the ability of the live vectors to prime and boost immune responses in humans. This is relevant not only for immunizing populations in developing areas of the world where *Shigella* and *S. typhi* infections are endemic but also for subsequent re-immunization of subjects with the same vector carrying either the identical or different foreign antigens. There have been four reports in animal models assessing the effect of anti-*Salmonella* immunity upon the immune response to a foreign antigen when the same *Salmonella* is used as a mucosal live vector carrying the foreign antigen under control of a prokaryotic expression system. Two reports suggest that prior anti-vector immunity down modulates the response to the foreign antigen (Attridge *et al.*, 1997; Roberts *et al.*, 1999); one report describes an enhancing effect on the immune response to the foreign antigen (Bao *et al.*, 1991) and one report relates neither an enhancing nor a notable depressing effect of prior anti-vector immunity on the serologic response to the foreign antigen studied (Kohler *et al.*, 2000). In the recent human clinical trial of a *S. typhi* Ty21a construct expressing *H. pylori* urease A and B peptides, it was noted that the two subjects who had strong cell-mediated immune responses to the urease antigen had a history of prior antigenic contact with *S. typhi* (Bumann *et al.*, 2001).

There have been no reports on whether prior anti-*Shigella* immunity modifies the immune response to foreign antigens expressed by that live vector. There have also been no reports of the influence of anti-*Salmonella* or anti-*Shigella* immunity on the ability of these bacteria to function as live vectors that deliver DNA vaccines.

SUMMARY

Attenuated *Salmonella* and *Shigella* constitute highly versatile live vectors for delivering to the immune system either antigens expressed by the bacteria or DNA vaccines. During the past decade, the parameters that influence expression and immunogenicity have been elucidated and are now being applied to prepare more immunogenic constructs for use in clinical trials in humans. Even more promising is the use of these bacterial vectors to deliver DNA vaccines. It is anticipated that clinical trials with *Salmonella* and *Shigella* live vectors carrying DNA vaccines will be undertaken shortly.

REFERENCES

Aggarwal, A., Kumar, S., Jaffe, R., Hone, D., Gross, M., and Sadoff, J. 1990. Oral *Salmonella* - Malaria circumsporozoite recombinants induce specific CD8+ cytotoxic T-Cells. J. Exp. Med. 172: 1083-1090.

Altboum, Z., Barry, E.M., Losonsky, G., Galen, J.E., and Levine, M.M. 2001. Attenuated *Shigella flexneri* 2a Δ*guaBA* strain CVD 1204 expressing enterotoxigenic *Escherichia coli* (ETEC) CS2 and CS3 fimbriae as a live mucosal vaccine against *Shigella* and ETEC infection. Infect. Immun. 69: 3150-3158.

Anderson, R., Pasetti, M.F., Sztein, M.B., and Levine, M.M. 2000. Δ*guaBA* attenuated *Shigella flexneri* 2a strain CVD 1204 as a *Shigella* vaccine and as a live mucosal delivery system for fragment C of tetanus toxin. Vaccine 18: 2193-2202.

Angelakopoulos, H., and Hohmann, E.L. 2000. Pilot study of *phoP/phoQ*-deleted *Salmonella enterica* serovar Typhimurium expressing *Helicobacter pylori* urease in adult volunteers. Infect. Immun. 68: 2135-2141.

Ascon, M.A., Hone, D.M., Walters, N., and Pascual, D.W. 1998. Oral immunization with a *Salmonella typhimurium* vaccine vector expressing recombinant enterotoxigenic *Escherichia coli* K99 fimbriae elicits elevated antibody titers for protective immunity. Infect. Immun. 66: 5470-5476.

Attridge, S.R., Davies, R., and LaBrooy, J.T. 1997. Oral delivery of foreign antigens by attenuated *Salmonella*: consequences of prior exposure to the vector strain. Vaccine 15: 155-162.

Bao, J.X. and Clements, J.D. 1991. Prior immunologic experience potentiates the subsequent antibody response when *Salmonella* strains are used as vaccine carriers. Infect. Immun. 59: 3841-3845.

Barry, E.M., Gomez-Duarte, O., Chatfield, S., Pizza, M., Rappuoli, R., Losonsky, G.A., Galen, J.E., and Levine, M.M. 1996. Expression and immunogenicity of pertussis toxin S1 subunit-tetanus toxin fragment C fusions in *Salmonella typhi* vaccine strain CVD 908. Infect. Immun. 64: 4172-4181.

Barzu, S., Arondel, J., Guillot, S., Sansonetti, P.J., and Phalipon, A. 1998. Immunogenicity of IpaC-hybrid proteins expressed in the *Shigella flexneri* 2a vaccine candidate SC602. Infect. Immun. 66: 77-82.

Benyacoub, J., Hopkins, S., Potts, A., Kelly, S., Kraehenbuhl, J.P., Curtiss, R., III, De Grandi, P., and Nardelli-Haefliger, D. 1999. The nature of the attenuation of *Salmonella typhimurium* strains expressing human papillomavirus type 16 virus-like particles determines the systemic and mucosal antibody responses in nasally immunized mice. Infect. Immun. 67: 3674-3679.

Black, R.E., Levine, M.M., Clements, M.L., Losonsky, G., Herrington, D., Berman, S., and Formal, S.B. 1987. Prevention of shigellosis by a *Salmonella typhi-Shigella sonnei* bivalent vaccine. J. Infect. Dis. 155: 1260-1265.

Bumann, D., Metzger, W.G., Mansouri, E., Palme, O., Wendland, M., Hurwitz, R., Haas, G., Aebischer, T., von Specht, B., and Meyer, T.F. 2001. Safety and immunogenicity of live recombinant *Salmonella enterica* serovar Typhi Ty21a expressing urease A and B from *Helicobacter pylori* in human volunteers. Vaccine 20: 845-852.

Carrier, M.J., Chatfield, S.N., Dougan, G., Nowicka, U.T.A., O'Callaghan, D., Beesley, J.E., Milano, S., Cillari, E., and Liew, F.Y. 1993. Expression of Human IL-1β in *Salmonella typhimurium*: a model system for the delivery of recombinant therapeutic proteins *in vivo*. Infect. Immun. 61: 4818-4827.

Chatfield, S., Charles, I., Makoff, A., Oxer, M., Dougan, G., Pickard, D., Slater, D., and Fairweather, N. 1992a. Use of the *nirB* promoter to direct the stable expression of heterologous antigens in *Salmonella* oral vaccine strains: development of a single-dose oral tetanus vaccine. Biotechnology 10: 888-892.

Chatfield, S.N., Strahan, K., Pickard, D., Charles, I.G., Hormaeche, C.E., and Dougan, G. 1992b. Evaluation of *Salmonella typhimurium* strains harbouring defined mutations in *htrA* and *aroA* in the murine salmonellosis model. Microb. Pathog. 12: 145-151.

Chen, I., Pizza, M., Rappuoli, R., and Newton, S.M. 1998. Effects of the insertion of a nonapeptide from murine IL-1beta on the immunogenicity of carrier proteins delivered by live attenuated *Salmonella*. Arch. Microbiol. 169: 113-119.

Clements, J.D., Lyon, F.L., Lowe, K.L., Farrand, A.L., and El-Morshidy, S. 1986. Oral immunization of mice with attenuated *Salmonella enteritidis* containing a recombinant plasmid which encodes for production of the B subunit of heat-labile *Escherichia coli* enterotoxin. Infect. Immun. 53: 685-692.

Coulson, N.M., Fulop, M., and Titball, R.W. 1994. *Bacillus anthracis* protective antigen, expressed in *Salmonella typhimurium* SL 3261, affords protection against anthrax spore challenge. Vaccine 12: 1395-1401.

Covone, M.G., Brocchi, M., Palla, E., Dias, d.S., Rappuoli, R., and Galeotti, C.L. 1998. Levels of expression and immunogenicity of attenuated *Salmonella enterica* serovar typhimurium strains expressing *Escherichia coli* mutant heat-labile enterotoxin. Infect. Immun. 66: 224-231.

Curtiss, R., III, and Kelly, S.M. 1987. *Salmonella typhimurium* deletion mutants lacking adenylate cyclase and cyclic AMP receptor protein are avirulent and immunogenic. Infect. Immun. 55: 3035-3043.

Darji, A., Guzman, C.A., Gerstel, B., Wachholz, P., Timmis, K.N., Wehland, J., Chakraborty, T., and Weiss, S. 1997. Oral somatic transgene vaccination using attenuated *S. typhimurium*. Cell 91: 765-775.

Denich, K., Börlin, P., O'Hanley, P.D., Howard, M., and Heath, A.W. 1993. Expression of the murine interleukin-4 gene in an attenuated *aroA* strain of *Salmonella typhimurium*: Persistence and immune response in BALB/c mice and susceptibility to macrophage killing. Infect. Immun. 61: 4818-4827.

DiPetrillo, M.D., Tibbetts, T., Kleanthous, H., Killeen, K.P., and Hohmann, E.L. 1999. Safety and immunogenicity of *phoP/phoQ*-deleted *Salmonella typhi* expressing *Helicobacter pylori* urease in adult volunteers. Vaccine 18: 449-459.

Dougan, G., Chatfield, S., Pickard, D., Bester, J., O'Callaghan, D., and Maskell, D. 1988. Construction and characterization of vaccine strains of *Salmonella* harbouring mutations in two different *aro* genes. J. Infect. Dis. 158: 1329-1335.

Dunstan, S.J., Ramsay, A.J., and Strugnell, R.A. 1996. Studies of immunity and bacterial invasiveness in mice given a recombinant *Salmonella* vector encoding murine interleukin-6. Infect. Immun. 64: 2730-2736.

Dunstan, S.J., Simmons, C.P., and Strugnell, R.A. 1999. Use of *in vivo*-regulated promoters to deliver antigens from attenuated *Salmonella enterica* var. *typhimurium*. Infect. Immun. 67: 5133-5141.

Everest, P., Frankel, G., Li, J., Lund, P., Chatfield, S., and Dougan, G. 1995. Expression of LacZ from the *htrA*, *nirB*, and *groE* promoters in a *Salmonella* vaccine strain: influence of growth in mammalian cells. FEMS Microbiol. Lett. 126: 97-102.

Fasano, A., Noriega, F.R., Liao, F.M., Wang, W., and Levine, M.M. 1997. Effect of *Shigella* enterotoxin 1 (ShET1) on rabbit intestine *in vitro* and *in vivo*. Gut 40: 505-511.

Fasano, A., Noriega, F.R., Maneval, D.R., Jr., Chanasongcram, S., Russell, R., Guandalini, S., and Levine, M.M. 1995. *Shigella* enterotoxin 1: an enterotoxin of *Shigella flexneri* 2a active in rabbit small intestine *in vivo* and *in vitro*. J. Clin. Invest. 95: 2853-2861.

Fennelly, G.J., Khan, S.A., Abadi, M.A., Wild, T.F., and Bloom, B.R. 1999. Mucosal DNA vaccine immunization against measles with a highly attenuated *Shigella flexneri* vector. J. Immunol. 162: 1603-1610.

Flo, J., Tisminetzky, S., and Baralle, F. 2001. Oral transgene vaccination mediated by attenuated *Salmonellae* is an effective method to prevent *Herpes simplex* virus-2 induced disease in mice. Vaccine 19: 1772-1782.

Forrest, B.D., LaBrooy, J.T., Dearlove, C.E., and Shearman, D.J.C. 1991. The human humoral immune response to *Salmonella typhi* Ty21a. J. Infect. Dis. 163: 336-345.

Forrest, B.D., Shearman, D.J.C., and LaBrooy, J.T. 1990. Specific immune response in humans following rectal delivery of live typhoid vaccine. Vaccine 8: 209-211.

Galen, J.E., Gomez-Duarte, O.G., Losonsky, G.A., Halpern, J.L., Lauderbaugh, C.S., Kaintuck, S., Reymann, M.K., and Levine, M.M. 1997. A murine model of intranasal immunization to assess the immunogenicity of attenuated *Salmonella typhi* live vector vaccines in stimulating serum antibody responses to expressed foreign antigens. Vaccine 15: 700-708.

Galen, J.E., and Levine, M.M. 2001. Can a 'flawless' live vector vaccine strain be engineered? Trends Microbiol. 9: 372-376.

Galen, J.E., Nair, J., Wang, J.Y., Wasserman, S.S., Tanner, M.K., Sztein, M.B., and Levine, M.M. 1999. Optimization of plasmid maintenance in the attenuated live vector vaccine strain *Salmonella typhi* CVD 908-*htrA*. Infect. Immun. 67: 6424-6433.

Gentschev, I., Dietrich, G., Spreng, S., Kolb-Maurer, A., Brinkmann, V., Grode, L., Hess, J., Kaufmann, S.H., and Goebel, W. 2001. Recombinant attenuated bacteria for the delivery of subunit vaccines. Vaccine 19: 2621-2628.

Gomez-Duarte, O., Galen, J., Chatfield, S.N., Rappuoli, R., Eidels, L., and Levine, M.M. 1995. Expression of fragment C of tetanus toxin fused to a carboxyl-terminal fragment of diphtheria toxin in *Salmonella typhi* CVD 908 vaccine strain. Vaccine 13: 1596-1602.

Gomez-Duarte, O.G., Lucas, B., Yan, Z.X., Panthel, K., Haas, R., and Meyer, T.F. 1998. Protection of mice against gastric colonization by *Helicobacter pylori* by single oral dose immunization with attenuated *Salmonella typhimurium* producing urease subunits A and B. Vaccine 16: 460-471.

Gomez-Duarte, O.G., Pasetti, M.F., Santiago, A., Sztein, M.B., Hoffman, S.L., and Levine, M.M. 2001. Expression, extracellular secretion and immunogenicity of the *Plasmodium falciparum* sprozoite surface protein-2 in *Salmonella* vaccine strains. Infect. Immun. 69: 1192-1198.

Gonzalez, C., Hone, D., Noriega, F., Tacket, C.O., Davis, J.R., Losonsky, G., Nataro, J.P., Hoffman, S., Malik, A., Nardin, E., Sztein, M.B., Heppner, D.G., Fouts, T.R., Isibasi, A., and Levine, M.M. 1994. *Salmonella typhi* vaccine strain CVD 908 expressing the circumsporozoite protein of *Plasmodium falciparum*: Strain construction and safety and immunogenicity in humans. J. Infect. Dis. 169: 927-931.

Gonzalez, C.R., Noriega, F.R., Huerta, S., Santiago, A., Vega, M., Paniagua, J., Ortiz-Navarrete, V., Isibasi, A., and Levine, M.M. 1998.

Immunogenicity of a *Salmonella typhi* CVD 908 candidate vaccine strain expressing the major surface protein gp63 of *Leishmania mexicana*. Vaccine 16: 1043-1052.

Herrington, D.A., Van de Verg, L., Formal, S.B., Hale, T.L., Tall, B.D., Cryz, S.J., Tramont, E.C., and Levine, M.M. 1990. Studies in volunteers to evaluate candidate *Shigella* vaccines: further experience with a bivalent *Salmonella typhi- Shigella sonnei* vaccine and protection conferred by previous *Shigella sonnei* disease. Vaccine 8: 353-357.

Hess, J., Gentschev, I., Miko, D., Welzel, M., Ladel, C., Goebel, W., and Kaufmann, S.H.E. 1996. Superior efficacy of secreted over somatic antigen display in recombinant *Salmonella* vaccine induced protection against listeriosis. Proc. Natl. Acad. Sci. USA. 93: 1458-1463.

Hohmann, E.L., Oletta, C.A., Killeen, K.P., and Miller, S.I. 1996. *phoP/ phoQ*-deleted *Salmonella typhi* (Ty800) is a safe and immunogenic single-dose typhoid fever vaccine in volunteers. J. Infect. Dis. 173: 1408-1414.

Hone, D., Attridge, S., van den Bosch, L., and Hackett, J. 1988. A chromosomal integration system for stabilization of heterologous genes in *Salmonella* based vaccine strains. Microb. Pathog. 5: 407-418.

Huang, Y., Hajishengallis, G., and Michalek, S.M. 2001. Induction of protective immunity against *Streptococcus mutans* colonization after mucosal immunization with attenuated *Salmonella enterica* serovar Typhimurium expressing an *S. mutans* adhesin under the control of *in vivo*-inducible *nirB* promoter. Infect. Immun. 69: 2154-2161.

Karem, K.L., Bowen, J., Kuklin, N., and Rouse, B.T. 1997. Protective immunity against herpes simplex virus (HSV) type 1 following oral administration of recombinant *Salmonella typhimurium* vaccine strains expressing HSV antigens. J. Gen. Virol. 78 (Pt 2): 427-434.

Kohler, J.J., Pathangey, L.B., Gillespie, S.R., and Brown, T.A. 2000. Effect of preexisting immunity to *Salmonella* on the immune response to recombinant *Salmonella enterica* serovar *typhimurium* expressing a *Porphyromonas gingivalis* hemagglutinin. Infect. Immun. 68: 3116-3120.

Koprowski, H., Levine, M.M., Anderson, R.J., Losonsky, G., Pizza, M., and Barry, E.M. 2000. Attenuated *Shigella flexneri* 2a vaccine strain CVD 1204 expressing colonization factor antigen I and mutant heat-labile enterotoxin of enterotoxigenic *Escherichia coli*. Infect. Immun. 68: 4884-4892.

Kotloff, K.L., Noriega, F.R., Samandari, T., Sztein, M.B., Losonsky, G.A., Nataro, J.P., Picking, W.D., Barry, E.M., and Levine, M.M. 2000. *Shigella flexneri* 2a Strain CVD 1207, with specific deletions in *virG, sen, set*, and *guaBA*, is highly attenuated in humans. Infect. Immun. 68: 1034-1039.

Lee, J.S., Shin, K.S., Pan, J.G., and Kim, C.J. 2000. Surface-displayed viral antigens on *Salmonella* carrier vaccine. Nat. Biotechnol. 18: 645-648.

Levine, M.M., Galen, J.E., Sztein, M.B., Beier, M., and Noriega, F. 1997. *Salmonella* expressing protozoal antigens. In: New Generation Vaccines. M.M.Levine *et al.*, eds. Marcel Dekker, New York. p. 351-361.

McSorley, S.J., Xu, D., and Liew, F.Y. 1997. Vaccine efficacy of *Salmonella* strains expressing glycoprotein 63 with different promoters. Infect. Immun. 65: 171-178.

Miller, S.I., Kukral, A.M., and Mekalanos, J.J. 1989. A two-component regulatory system (*phoP phoQ*) controls *Salmonella typhimurium* virulence. Proc. Natl. Acad. Sci. USA. 86: 5054-5058.

Miller, S.I., and Mekalanos, J.J. 1990. Constitutive expression of the *phoP* regulon attenuates *Salmonella* virulence and survival within macrophages. J. Bacteriol. 172: 2485-2490.

Miller, S.I., Pulkkinen, W.S., Selsted, M.E., and Mekalanos, J.J. 1990. Characterization of defensin resistance phenotypes associated with mutations in the *phoP*-virulence regulon of *Salmonella typhimurium*. Infect. Immun. 58: 3706-3710.

Nakayama, K., Kelly, S., and Curtiss, R. 1988. Construction of an ASD+ expression-cloning vector: stable maintenance and high level expression of cloned genes in a *Salmonella* vaccine strain. Biotechnology 6: 693-697.

Nardelli-Haefliger, D., Kraehenbuhl, J.P., Curtiss, R., III, Schodel, F., Potts, A., Kelly, S., and De Grandi, P. 1996. Oral and rectal immunization of adult female volunteers with a recombinant attenuated *Salmonella typhi* vaccine strain. Infect. Immun 64: 5219-5224.

Nataro, J.P., Seriwatana, J., Fasano, A., Maneval, D.R., Guers, L.D., Noriega, F., Dubovsky, F., Levine, M.M., and Morris, J.G., Jr. 1995. Identification and cloning of a novel plasmid-encoded enterotoxin of enteroinvasive *Escherichia coli* and *Shigella strains*. Infect. Immun. 63: 4721-4728.

Nayak, A.R., Tinge, S.A., Tart, R.C., McDaniel, L.S., Briles, D.E., and Curtiss, R., III 1998. A live recombinant avirulent oral *Salmonella* vaccine expressing pneumococcal surface protein A induces protective responses against *Streptococcus pneumoniae*. Infect. Immun. 66: 3744-3751.

Noriega, F.R., Liao, F.M., Formal, S.B., Fasano, A., and Levine, M.M. 1995. Prevalence of *Shigella* enterotoxin 1 among *Shigella* clinical isolates of diverse serotypes. J. Infect. Dis. 172: 1408-1410.

Noriega, F.R., Losonsky, G., Lauderbaugh, C., Liao, F.M., Wang, M.S., and Levine, M.M. 1996b. Engineered Δ*guaB-A*, Δ*virG Shigella flexneri* 2a strain CVD 1205: construction, safety, immunogenicity and potential efficacy as a mucosal vaccine. Infect. Immun. 64: 3055-3061.

Noriega, F.R., Losonsky, G., Wang, J.Y., Formal, S.B., and Levine, M.M. 1996a. Further characterization of Δ*aroA, ΔvirG Shigella flexneri* 2a strain CVD 1203 as a mucosal *Shigella* vaccine and as a live vector vaccine for delivering antigens of enterotoxigenic *Escherichia coli*. Infect. Immun. 64: 23-27.

Orr, N., Galen, J.E., and Levine, M.M. 2001. Novel use of anaerobically induced promoter, *dmsA*, for controlled expression of Fragment C of tetanus toxin in live attenuated *Salmonella enterica* serovar *typhi* strain CVD 908-*htrA*. Vaccine 19: 1694-1700.

Pasetti, M.F., Anderson, R.J., Noriega, F.R., Levine, M.M., and Sztein, M.B. 1999. Attenuated Δ*guaBA Salmonella typhi* vaccine strain CVD 915 as a live vector utilizing prokaryotic or eukaryotic expression systems to deliver foreign antigens and elicit immune responses. Clin. Immunol. 92: 76-89.

Pasetti, M.F., Pickett, T.E., Levine, M.M., and Sztein, M.B. 2000. A comparison of immunogenicity and *in vivo* distribution of *Salmonella enterica* serovar *typhi* and *typhimurium* live vector vaccines delivered by mucosal routes in the murine model. Vaccine 18: 3208-3213.

Perdomo, O.J., Cavaillon, J.M., Huerre, M., Ohayon, H., Gounon, P., and Sansonetti, P.J. 1994. Acute inflammation causes epithelial invasion and mucosal destruction in experimental shigellosis. J. Exp. Med. 180: 1307-1319.

Pickett, T.E., Pasetti, M.F., Galen, J.E., Sztein, M.B., and Levine, M.M. 2000. *In vivo* characterization of the murine intranasal model for assessing the immunogenicity of attenuated *Salmonella enterica* serovar *typhi* strains as live mucosal vaccines and as live vectors. Infect. Immun. 68: 205-213.

Rappuoli, R., Pizza, M., Douce, G., and Dougan, G. 1999. Structure and mucosal adjuvanticity of cholera and *Escherichia coli* heat-labile enterotoxins. Immunol. Today 20: 493-500.

Roberts, M., Bacon, A., Li, J., and Chatfield, S. 1999. Prior immunity to homologous and heterologous *Salmonella* serotypes suppresses local and systemic anti-fragment C antibody responses and protection from tetanus toxin in mice immunized with *Salmonella* strains expressing fragment C. Infect. Immun. 67: 3810-3815.

Russmann, H., Shams, H., Poblete, F., Fu, Y., Galan, J.E., and Donis, R.O. 1998. Delivery of epitopes by the *Salmonella* type III secretion system for vaccine development. Science 281: 565-568.

Sadoff, J., Ballou, W.R., Baron, L., Majarian, W., Hockmeyer, W., Young, J., Cryz, S., Ou, J., Lowell, G., and Chulay, J. 1988. Oral *Salmonella typhimurium* vaccine expressing circumsporozoite protein protects against malaria. Science 240: 336-338.

Sansonetti, P.J. 1992. Molecular and cellular biology of *Shigella flexneri* invasiveness: From cell assay systems to shigellosis. Curr. Top. Microbiol. Immunol. 180: 1-19.

Sansonetti, P.J., and Phalipon, A. 1999. M cells as ports of entry for enteroinvasive pathogens: mechanisms of interaction, consequences for the disease process. Semin. Immunol. 11: 193-203.

Schorr, J., Knapp, B., Hundt, E., Küpper, H.A., and Amann, E. 1991. Surface expression of malarial antigens in *Salmonella typhimurium:* induction of serum antibody response upon oral vaccination of mice. Vaccine 5: 675-681.

Shata, M.T., and Hone, D.M. 2001a. Vaccination with a *Shigella* DNA vaccine vector induces antigen-specific CD8(+) T cells and antiviral protective immunity. J. Virol. 75: 9665-9670.

Shata, M.T., Reitz, M.S., Jr., DeVico, A.L., Lewis, G.K., and Hone, D.M. 2001b. Mucosal and systemic HIV-1 Env-specific CD8(+) T-cells develop after intragastric vaccination with a *Salmonella* Env DNA vaccine vector. Vaccine 20: 623-629.

Sizemore, D.R., Branstrom, A.A., and Sadoff, J.C. 1995. Attenuated *Shigella* as a DNA delivery vehicle for DNA-mediated immunization. Science 270: 299-302.

Sztein, M.B., Tanner, M.K., Polotsky, Y., Orenstein, J.M., and Levine, M.M. 1995. Cytotoxic T lymphocytes after oral immunization with attenuated vaccine strains of *Salmonella typhi* in humans. J. Immunol. 155: 3987-3993.

Sztein, M.B., Wasserman, S.S., Tacket, C.O., Edelman, R., Hone, D., Lindberg, A.A., and Levine, M.M. 1994. Cytokine production patterns and lymphoproliferative responses in volunteers orally immunized with attenuated vaccine strains of *Salmonella typhi*. J. Infect. Dis. 170: 1508-1517.

Tacket, C.O., Forrest, B., Morona, R., Attridge, S.R., LaBrooy, J., Tall, B.D., Reymann, M., Rowley, D., and Levine, M.M. 1990. Safety, immunogenicity, and efficacy against cholera challenge in humans of a typhoid-cholera hybrid vaccine derived from *Salmonella typhi* Ty21a. Infect. Immun. 58: 1620-1627.

Tacket, C.O., Galen, J., Sztein, M.B., Losonsky, G., Wyant, T.L., Nataro, J., Wasserman, S.S., Edelman, R., Chatfield, S., Dougan, G., and Levine, M.M. 2000. Safety and immune responses to attenuated *Salmonella enterica* serovar typhi oral live vector vaccines expressing tetanus toxin fragment C. Clin. Immunol. 97: 146-153.

Tacket, C.O., Hone, D.M., Curtiss, R.I., Kelly, S.M., Losonsky, G., Guers, L., Harris, A.M., Edelman, R., and Levine, M.M. 1992b. Comparison of the safety and immunogenicity of *aroC, aroD* and *cya, crp Salmonella typhi* strains in adult volunteers. Infect Immun 60: 536-541.

Tacket, C.O., Hone, D.M., Losonsky, G.A., Guers, L., Edelman, R., and Levine, M.M. 1992a. Clinical acceptability and immunogenicity of CVD 908 *Salmonella typhi* vaccine strain. Vaccine 10: 443-446.

Tacket, C.O., Kelly, S.M., Schodel, F., Losonsky, G., Nataro, J.P., Edelman, R., Levine, M.M., and Curtiss, R., III 1997a. Safety and immunogenicity in humans of an attenuated *Salmonella typhi* vaccine vector strain expressing plasmid-encoded hepatitis B antigens stabilized by the ASD balanced lethal system. Infect. Immun. 65: 3381-3385.

Tacket, C.O., Sztein, M.B., Losonsky, G.A., Wasserman, S.S., Nataro, J.P., Edelman, R., Pickard, D., Dougan, G., Chatfield, S.N., and Levine, M.M. 1997b. Safety of live oral *Salmonella typhi* vaccine strains with deletions in *htrA* and *aroC aroD* and immune response in humans. Infect. Immun. 65: 452-456.

Tagliabue, A., Nencioni, L., Cafferena, A., Villa, L., Boraschi, D., Cazzola, G., and Cavalieri, S. 1985. Cellular immunity against *Salmonella typhi* after live oral vaccines. Clin. Exp. Immunol. 52: 242-247.

Tagliabue, A., Villa, L., De Magistiris, M.T., Romano, M., Silvestri, S., Boraschji, D., and Nencioni, L. 1986. IgA-driven T-Cell-mediated antibacterial immunity in man after live oral Ty21a vaccine. J. Immunol. 137: 1504-1510.

Toebe, C.S., Clements, J.D., Cardenas, L., Jennings, G.J., and Wiser, M.F. 1997. Evaluation of immunogenicity of an oral *Salmonella* vaccine expressing recombinant *Plasmodium berghei* merozoite surface protein-1. Am. J. Trop. Med. Hyg. 56: 192-199.

Tramont, E.C., Chung, R., Berman, S., Keren, D., Kapfer, C., and Formal, S.B. 1984. Safety and antigenicity of typhoid-*Shigella sonnei* vaccine (strain 5076-1C). J. Infect. Dis. 149: 133-136.

Viret, J.F., Favre, D., Wegmuller, B., Herzog, C., Que, J.U., Cryz, S.J., Jr., and Lang, A.B. 1999. Mucosal and systemic immune responses in humans after primary and booster immunizations with orally administered invasive and noninvasive live attenuated bacteria. Infect. Immun. 67: 3680-3685.

Whittle, B.L., Smith, R.M., Matthaei, K.I., Young, I.G., and Verma, N.K. 1997. Enhancement of the specific mucosal IgA response *in vivo* by interleukin- 5 expressed by an attenuated strain of *Salmonella serotype* Dublin. J. Med. Microbiol. 46: 1029-1038.

Woo, P.C., Wong, L.P., Zheng, B.J., and Yuen, K.Y. 2001. Unique immunogenicity of hepatitis B virus DNA vaccine presented by live-attenuated *Salmonella typhimurium*. Vaccine 19: 2945-2954.

Wu, S., Beier, M., Sztein, M.B., Galen, J.E., Pickett, T., Holder, A.A., Gómez-Duarte, O.G., and Levine, M.M. 2000. Construction and immunogenicity in mice of attenuated *Salmonella typhi* expressing *Plasmodium falciparum* merozoite surface protein 1 (MSP-1) fused to tetanus toxin fragment C. J. Biotechnol. 83: 125-135.

Xu, D., McSorley, S.J., Chatfield, S.J., Dougan, G., and Liew, F.Y. 1997. Protection against *Leishmania major* infection in genetically susceptible BALB/c mice by gp63 delivered orally in attenuated *Salmonella typhimurium* (*AroA- AroD-*). Immunology 85: 1-7.

Yamamoto, S., Kiyono, H., Yamamoto, M., Imaoka, K., Fujihashi, K., Van Ginkel, F.W., Noda, M., Takeda, Y., and McGhee, J.R. 1997. A nontoxic mutant of cholera toxin elicits Th2-type responses for enhanced mucosal immunity. Proc. Natl. Acad. Sci.USA. 94: 5267-5272.

Zhang, T. and Stanley, S.L., Jr. 1996. Oral Immunization with an attenuated vaccine strain of *Salmonella typhimurium* expressing the serine-rich *Entamoeba histolytica* protein induces an antiamebic immune response and protects gerbils from amebic liver abscess. Infect.Immun. 64: 1526-1531.

From: *Vaccine Delivery Strategies*
Edited by: Guido Dietrich and Werner Goebel

Chapter 9

Use of the α-Hemolysin Secretion System (Type I) of *Escherichia coli* in Vaccine Development

Ivaylo Gentschev, Guido Dietrich,
Juergen Hess and Werner Goebel

ABSTRACT

Many gram-negative bacteria use a type I secretion machinery for the translocation of proteins across the two membranes into the extracellular surroundings (e. g. pore-forming toxins, proteases, lipases and S-layer proteins). This work is a review on the application of the α-hemolysin secretion system (type I) of *Escherichia coli* for development of live vaccines on the basis of attenuated bacteria.

INTRODUCTION

Vaccination is the most important preventive measure against widespread infectious diseases. Conventional vaccines directed against infectious microorganisms are mainly based on non-viable microorganisms which are inactivated through chemical or physical processes, or on isolated protective antigens or parts thereof. These vaccines were successful in some cases, but of limited or no value in many others. This limitation is mainly due to the fact that such vaccines, although often very efficient in triggering humoral responses, are rather restricted in the induction of Th1 and especially cytotoxic T cell (CTL) responses. T-cell immunity is, however, crucial for the elimination of pathogenic intracellular microorganisms, such as most viruses, intracellular bacteria and parasites. The causative agents of many of the severe infectious diseases for which efficient vaccines do not exist belong to this category of microorganisms.

Among the various delivery systems, orally given live virulence-attenuated viruses and bacteria are promising candidates to circumvent this problem. Vaccines administered by a mucosal route mimic the immune response elicited by natural infection and can lead to long-lasting protective mucosal and systemic responses (McGhee *et al.*, 1992; Shata *et al.*, 2000). Moreover vaccination via a mucosal route is also associated with less side effects and in many cases lower delivery costs.

The most successful live vaccines existing today are based on whole polio and vaccinia virus. Among the bacterial live vaccines applied to humans are *Salmonella typhi* Ty21 (against typhoid fever) and the *Mycobacterium bovis* strain Calmette-Guerin (BCG) (active against certain forms of human tuberculosis). The vaccination of virtually billions of people with these bacterial live vaccine strains was successful and the application of these live bacterial vaccines proved to be rather harmless for the vaccinees (Hormaeche and Khan, 1996; Lindberg, 1998).

In more recent years, strategies were developed to produce foreign antigens by such virulence attenuated bacteria. Especially auxotrophic mutants of *Salmonella* serotypes (Cardenas and Clement, 1992; Chatfield and Dougan, 1997), but also of *Shigella flexneri* (Noriega *et al.*, 1997; Lindberg *et al.*, 1998), *Listeria monocytogenes* (Jensen *et al.*, 1997; Weiskirch and Paterson, 1997), and *Mycobacterium bovis* BCG (Matsumoto *et al.*, 1998; Edelman *et al.*, 1999) were used as carriers for suitable antigens to provide protective immunity against the pathogen from which the antigen is derived. These bacterial carriers belong to the group of intracellular bacteria which are able to survive and replicate inside phagocytic, antigen-presenting cells (dendritic cells and macrophages). While *Salmonella* and *Mycobacterium tuberculosis* (and *bovis*) reside in specialized vacuoles within the host cell, *Shigella spp.* and *L. monocytogenes* escape into the cytosol, replicate in this compartment and are able to spread from one infected cell into a neighboring one. Advantages of these bacterial carriers are their immunogenicity, ease of genetic manipulation, and established methods to grow and process the organisms.

The best-characterized attenuated bacteria are salmonellae harboring mutations in the aromatic amino acids pathway e.g. *aroA*, *aroC* and *aroD* (Hoiseth and Stocker 1981; Hone *et al.*, 1991). Aro mutants cause an obligate requirement for all aromatic amino acids including *p*-aminobenzoic acid (PABA) which is absent in mammalian tissues relevant to infection. The result is a block in protein biosynthesis due to a lack of fMet-tRNA^{fMet} (Stocker, 1990). Hovewer, the *Salmonella aro* vaccines were shown to trigger efficient humoral and/or cell-mediated immune responses to a large number of heterologous antigens from a wide range of pathogens (Roberts *et al.*, 1994; Hormaeche and Khan, 1996).

ANTIGEN DELIVERY VIA A TYPE I SECRETION SYSTEM

Heterologous Antigen Presentation in Virulence-Attenuated Gram-Negative Bacteria by the Use of the *Escherichia coli* α-Hemolysin (HlyA) Secretion System (Type I)

The expression level of heterologous antigens can strongly influence the immune responce that is induced by live recombinant bacterial vaccines. In order to achieve stable expression of heterologous antigens, several different strategies were developed (Tijhaar *et al.*, 1994, Gentschev *et al.*, 1996b; Rüssmann *et al.*, 1998; Xu *et al.*, 1998; Roberts *et al.*, 1998). One of the most efficient approaches is the use of the *Escherichia coli* α-hemolysin (HlyA) secretion system for delivery of heterologous antigens in virulence-attenuated gram-negative bacteria. The HlyA export machinery is the best-studied type I secretion system and consists of the three components HlyB, HlyD and TolC (Wagner *et al.*, 1983; Wandersman and Delepelaire, 1990). Whereas the inner membrane proteins HlyB and HlyD are specific components of the transport apparatus of α-hemolysin, the third component, TolC, is a multifunctional protein located in the outer membrane of *E. coli*.

HlyB is an inner membrane (IM) protein with ATPase activity (Koronakis *et al.*, 1993). It belongs to the ABC (ATP-binding cassette) superfamily of eukaryotic and prokaryotic protein exporters and couples ATP hydrolysis to the protein export (Holland *et al.*, 1990; Young and Holland, 1999). The second component (HlyD) is an IM-anchored protein that spans the periplasm; such proteins are termed membrane fusion proteins (MFP) (Dinh *et al.*, 1994). The third component (TolC) is a general outer membrane protein (OMF; Paulsen *et al.*, 1997), which is a part of at least four different export systems (Zgurskaya and Nikaido, 2000). HlyA carries at its C-terminus a secretion signal of about 50-60 amino acids in length (termed in the following HlyAs), which is recognized by the HlyB/HlyD/TolC-translocator, promoting direct secretion of the entire protein into the extracellular medium without the formation of periplasmic intermediates. This secretion signal (HlyAs) differs completely from the N-terminal signal sequences. Until now the precise nature of HlyAs is basically unknown. HlyAs seems to be necessary and sufficient for secretion of HlyA, since a peptide consisting of the C-terminal 60 amino acids of HlyA is secreted in the presence of HlyB/HlyD/TolC with the same efficiency as HlyA itself (Jarchau *et al.*, 1994). In addition, a large number of hybrid proteins (more than 400) have been generated by gene fusion with the 3′ end of *hlyA* which encodes HlyAs. For this purpose, several different systems have been developed (e.g. plasmid vectors, chromosomal integration vectors and a transposon encoding HlyAs), allowing the generation of such hybrid proteins and their secretion (Hess *et al.*, 1990, 1996 and 1997; Blight and Holland 1994; Blight *et al.*, 1994a; Gentschev *et al*, 1994, 1996a,1996b, 1997, and 2000; Mollenkopf *et al.*, 1996; Tzschaschel *et al.*, 1996a and 1996b).

From studies concerned with the expression and secretion of HlyAs fusion proteins (e. g. Blight and Holland, 1994; Gentschev *et al.*, 1994, 1996a and 1996b; Mollenkopf *et al.*, 1996), the following rather general rules can be deduced:

- Most hemolysin fusion proteins can be secreted via the hemolysin secretion system.
- Efficient secretion can be achieved for heterologous proteins ranging from 20 amino acids to 1000 amino acids.
- Some of the HlyAs fusion proteins are still enzymatically active (Nakano *et al.*, 1992; Gentschev *et al.*, 1995; Hess *et al.*, 1995; Chervaux *et al.*, 1995; Kern and Ceglowski, 1995; Hahn *et al.*1998).

As recently shown, the Hly plasmid system stably replicates in many other gram-negative bacteria, including different *Salmonella* serotypes, *Shigella spp.* and *Vibrio cholerae* (Gentschev *et al.*, 1996b; Spreng *et al.*, 1999) and the encoded HlyAs-fused antigen is likewise secreted by these bacterial carriers. These gram-negative bacteria contain TolC or TolC-analogous proteins in the outer membrane, the genes encoding HlyB and HlyD are generally provided by the plasmid which we use for the expression of HlyAs-fusion proteins (Spreng *et al.*, 1999; Gentschev *et al.*, 2000 and 2001). Since the latter bacteria colonize different compartments of the infected host cell, *i.e.* cell surface (*V. cholerae*), specialized phagosome of APCs (*Salmonella*) and cytosol (*Shigella*), the same antigen can be introduced into different compartments of APCs and hence will trigger different immune responses against the same antigen (see Figure 1).

Normally HlyA or the generated HlyAs-fusion proteins are completely secreted into the extracellular surroundings and only a small pool remains inside the producing bacterial cells (Gentschev *et al.*, 1996a; Spreng *et al.*, 1999). However, specifically engineered plasmid variants allow the complete retainment of the protein antigen in the cytoplasm or its accumulation on the surface of the producing bacterial cell without proteolytic degradation of the antigen *in vitro* (Figure 1; Hess *et al.* 1996). Thus, the HlyA system offers the possibility to trigger different immune responses against a given protein antigen by using bacterial carriers which will deliver the same antigen to different compartments of APCs (extracellular, phagosomal, cytosolic).

Live Bacterial Vaccines on the Basis of the Hemolysin Secretion System

On the basis of attenuated *Salmonella* spp., *V. cholerae* and *S. flexneri* carriers, several live vaccines were developed using the hemolysin secretion system. The first reports on successful delivery of heterologous antigens by this system were published simultaneously by two groups in 1992 (Gentschev *et al.*,1992; Su *et al.*, 1992). Su and co-workers demostrated that Shiga toxin B-subunit fused to the 23 kDa C-terminus of *E. coli* hemolysin was exported from recombinant *S. typhimurium aroA* (SL3261) via the hemolysin secretion pathway and immunisation of BALB/c mice resulted in significant B-subunit specific mucosal and serum antibody responses.

The first live vaccine on the basis of hemolysin secretion system was published by Gentschev *et al.* (1992). Using a recombinant *S. typhimurium aroA* (SL7207) strain secreting the p60 protein, a major B- and T-cell antigen of the intracellular bacterium *Listeria monocytogenes* as HlyAs fusion

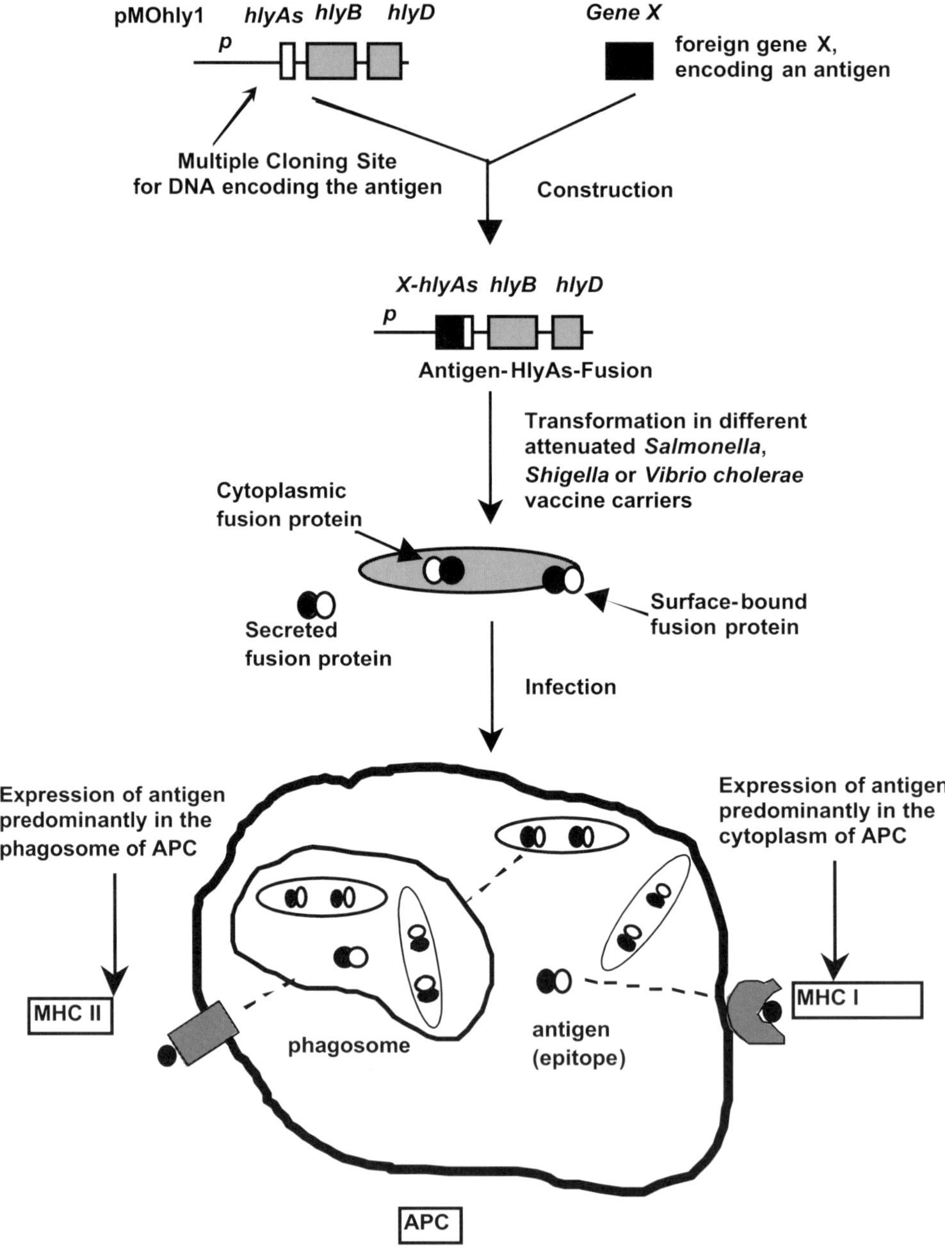

Figure 1. Variation of antigen presentation in APC by different attenuated gram-negative vaccine carriers via the hemolysin secretion machinery.

protein. These authors demonstrated that BALB/c mice infected intraperitoneally (i.p.) with this recombinant strain were protected partially against a *Listeria* infection.

However, these studies showed that the two-plasmid-systems employed (one plasmid provided effective HlyA-specific secretion functions HlyB and HlyD and a second one carryed *hlyAs* for the in frame insertion of heterologous proteins) are rather unstable in *Salmonella* strains under *in vivo* conditions. This fact rendered these constructs unsuitable for vaccination purposes. In order to resolve this problem, Tzschaschel and coworkers combined all the genes necessary for expression and export of the StxB-HlyAs fusion in one *Not*I cassette, which was then integrated into the chromosome of attenuated *S. flexneri aroA* or *S. typhimurium aroA* vaccine strains via a mini-transposon (Tzschaschel *et al.*, 1996a and 1996b). This new system led to a higher stability of the gene fusion under *in vivo* conditions (Tzschaschel *et al.*, 1996a). However, this techniques reduces gene copy number to one per bacterial cell and the expression level of the heterologous antigen is normally quite low (Hormaeche and Khan, 1996).

An alternative strategy was developed by the construction of a single plasmid system for heterologous protein expression and secretion via the hemolysin pathway (Gentschev *et al.*, 1994 and 1996). This plasmid system (prototype pMOhly1) contains a cassette allowing the insertion of any gene or gene fragment encoding antigens in-frame with HlyAs. All genes (including the *hlyAs*-fused gene for the respective antigen) are transcribed from the original *cis*-acting expression sites in front of *hlyC* (Vogel *et al.*, 1988); synthesis of the fusion antigen protein and the translocator proteins, HlyB and HlyD, and hence secretion of the fusion protein are thereby optimally balanced. This system was very stable under *in vitro* conditions with the loss of plasmid being less than 1% in 20 generations (I. Gentschev, unpublished results). Under *in vivo* conditions (mouse infection) about 80% of all attenuated *Salmonella* still carried the plasmid 3 weeks after infection (J. Hess, unpublished results).

Using pMOhly1, Hess *et al.* (1996 and 1997) tested the impact of antigen display via the hemolysin secretion system for vaccine development. In these experiments, various virulence-attenuated *S. typhimurium aroA* (SL7207) strains have been engineered to express either listeriolysin, the p60 protein or superoxide dismutase (SOD) of *Listeria monocytogenes*. While the first two proteins are extracellular virulence proteins (Portnoy *et al.*, 1992) and immunologically well characterized (Vijh and Pamer, 1997), SOD (Brehm *et al.*, 1992) is a cytoplasmic protein and immunologically

Table 1. Antigen expression by and host-cell localization of the r-*S. typhimurium aroA* strains used for vaccination against *L. monocytogenes*

Recombinant *S. typhimurium* (SL7207)	Antigen and antigen display by the vaccine strain	Preferred host-cell localization of r-constructs	Protection[A] against *L. monocytogenes*
Secreted antigen vaccines			
SL7207 Hlys	active listeriolysin Secreted/somatic	Endosomal/cytosolic	+++
SL7207 Hly492	inactive listeriolysin Secreted/somatic	Endosomal	+
SL7207 p60s	p60-protein Secreted/somatic	Endosomal	++
SL7207 SODs	SOD Secreted/somatic	Endosomal	+
Somatic antigen vaccines			
SL7207Hlyc	active listeriolysin Somatic	Endosomal	-
SL7207 p60c	p60-protein Somatic	Endosomal	-
SL7207 SODc	SOD Somatic	Endosomal	-
SL7207 control	-	Endosomal	-

[A] Analyzed by survival rates of r-*S. typhimurium* SL7207 vaccinated mice after *lethal L. monocytogenes* EGD infection or by *L. monocytogenes* CFU in livers and spleens of infected mice. +++ = strong, ++ = intermediate, + = weak protection.

uncharacterized. C57BL/6 mice were infected with different recombinant *S. typhimurium* strains displaying listeriolysin-, p60- or SOD-HlyAs fusion protein in secreted or somatic form (Table 1; Hess *et al.*, 1996 and 1997).

The vaccinated mice were challenged with a high, normally lethal dose of *L. monocytogenes*. All mice vaccinated with *S. typhimurium aroA* secreting a HlyAs fusion protein survived subsequent a *L. monocytogenes* infection, whereas all mice vaccinated with the *Salmonella* control strain died (Table 1). Interestingly, this anti-listerial protection was not observed when attenuated *Salmonella* strains were used as live vaccines which stably retained similar amounts of these hybrid proteins in the bacterial cytosol. *In vitro*, both secreted and nonsecreted antigens delivered by *Salmonella* carriers were presented by major histocompatibility complex (MHC) class I molecules but followed different kinetics (Catic *et al.*, 1999). Secreted antigens were recognized by CD8+ T cells more rapidly than their nonsecreted derivatives. Taken together, the faster availability of antigens secreted by *S. typhimurium* strains apparently augments CD8+ T cell-mediated immune responses *in vivo* which in turn lead to the beneficial outcome in listeriosis. Moreover, even SOD-HlyAs-secreting *Salmonella* microorganisms induced protective immunity, although SOD represents a naturally nonsecreted protein of the target-pathogen becoming only accessible for MHC class I presentation after killing of *L. monocytogenes* within antigen presenting cells (Hess *et al.*, 1997). The phagosomal escape of *S. typhimurium* secreting cytolytically active listeriolysin-HlyAs hybrid protein additionally enhanced antigen availability for the classical MHC class I presentation pathway via endoplasmic reticulum and Golgi network, thus inducing the most potent anti-listerial protection after oral *Salmonella* administration (Gentschev *et al.*, 1995; Hess *et al.*, 1996, 2000a and 2000c). It should be noted that *S. typhimurium* microbes secreting a nonhemolytic version of listeriolysin remain in the phagosome of macrophages only allowing CD8+ T cell priming via non-classical MHC class I presentation pathways (Hess *et al.*, 2000a and 2000c; Gentschev *et al.*, 2001). The data thus far show that three listerial fusion proteins - when secreted by the attenuated *S. typhimurium* strain - provide protective cell-mediated immunity against subsequent infection with the intracellular pathogen, *L. monocytogenes* (Table 1).

Clostridium difficile causes pseudomembranous colitis through the action of Rho-modifying proteins, toxins A and B (Kelly *et al.*, 1994) Antibodies directed against toxin A limit or prevent the disease in humans; however no effective *C. difficile* vaccine has yet been developed. An attenuated *V. cholerae* strain, O395-NT was used successfully for antigen presentation and secretion of a nontoxic, immunogenic portion of *C. difficile* toxin A fused to HlyAs (Ryan *et al.*, 1997). Vaccination with this recombinant strain produced significant systemic anti-*C. difficile* toxin A immunoglobulin G and anti-*V. cholerae* vibriocidal antibody responses (Ryan *et al.*, 1997). These results suggest that the hemolysin system can be used successfully in *V. cholerae* carrier strains to obtain secretion of large heterologous antigens and to induce protective systemic and mucosal immunity against a given antigen.

An attenuated *Salmonella typhi* CVD 908-*htrA* strain has also been employed for the delivery of antigens by utilizing the hemolysin A secretion system

(Orr *et al.*, 1999). In this study a mutant diphtheria toxin molecule CRM(197) and fragments thereof were expressed and secreted by the hemolysin secretion system, and the constructs were tested for their ability to induce serum antitoxin. Hovewer, mice immunized intranasally with CVD 908-*htrA* secreting CRM(197) failed to manifest serologic responses against DT (Orr *et al.*, 1999). In this case, it is likely that the low level of expression of the fusion protein precluded elicitation of an immune response by the live carrier.

The p30-protein (antigen 85B or 30-kDa antigen) of *M. bovis* strain BCG was fused in frame to the HlyA secretion signal and secreted via the HlyB/HlyD/TolC export machinery (Hess *et al.*, 2000b). For analyzing the potective efficacy of recombinant *S. typhimurium* p30, C57BL/6 mice were vaccinated p.o. and then challenged i.v. with *M. tuberculosis* H37Rv 120 days later. After *in vitro* restimulation with *M. tuberculosis* H37a lysate, splenocytes of recombinant *S. typhimurium* p30-immunized mice showed an enhanced anti-TB immune response [significantly increased production of interferon-gamma (IFN-γ) and tumor necrosis factor-alpha (TNF-α)] compared with that in BCG or r-*Salmonella* control immunized mice. In addition, the r-*S. typhimurium* p30 strain induced partial protection against *M. tuberculosis* infections in the murine model (Hess *et al.*, 2000b).

The first demonstration that complete antigens of eukaryotic origin can be fused to the C-terminal portion of *E. coli* hemolysin and secreted by attenuated *Salmonella* strains and that such secreted antigens can protect in an animal model against subsequent parasite challenge, was published by Gentschev *et al.* (1998). In this report, the p67 sporozoite antigen of *Theileria parva*, a tick-borne protozoan parasite, has been fused to the C-terminal secretion signal of *E. coli* hemolysin and expressed in secreted form by attenuated *S. dublin aroA* strain SL5631. Immunization of cattle with the recombinant SL5631 strain provoked specific antibody responses to p67, and a proportion of the immunized animals were protected against challenge with *T. parva* sporozoites (Gentschev *et al.*, 1998).

In an initial approach, the HlyA secretion system was used to achieve stable expression of the sporozoite surface protein (SSP-2) of *Plasmodium falciparum* (Gomez-Duarte *et al.*, 2001). *S. typhimurium* SL3261 and *S. typhi* CVD 908-*htrA* constructs secreting SSP-2 stimulated greater IFN-γ splenocyte responses in mice than did nonsecreting constructs.

In order to enhance the expression of heterologous antigens, Spreng *et al.* (2000) tested a new cloning strategy which comprised the multiplication and adaptation of the sequence encoding the antigen to the codon usage of bacterial carriers. For this purpose, a live vaccine against *Measles virus* (MV) infection on the basis of attenuated *S. typhimurium aroA* secreting MV antigens via the *E. coli* α-hemolysin secretion system was constructed. The sequences encoding two well characterized measles virus epitopes, a B-cell epitope of the MV fusion protein and a T-cell epitope of the MV nucleocapsid protein were first adapted to the codon usage of *Salmonella*. Oral immunization of MV-susceptible C3H mice with *S. typhimurium aroA* secreting the triple B-cell epitope resulted in the induction of a humoral immune response, manifested by the presence of MV-specific antibodies in the sera of the vaccinated mice (Spreng *et al.*, 2000). Mice immunized with *S. typhimurium aroA* secreting the double T-cell epitope developed a MV-specific CD4+ T-cell response. Based on the immune responses elicited by vaccination with the B-cell and the T-cell epitopes, C3H mice were immunized with a combination of both recombinant *Salmonella* strains and subsequently challenged. This resulted in a slower mortality rate and complete protection of 30% of the animals after intracerebral challenge with a rodent-adapted, neurotropic MV strain.

These data demonstrated for the first time that the *E. coli* hemolysin secretion system is also suitable for the delivery of viral antigens.

CONCLUSIONS

On the basis of the hemolysin secretion system, several live vaccines against the bacterial pathogens *Listeria monocytogenes* (Hess *et al.*, 1996 and 1997), *Mycobacterium tuberculosis* (Hess *et al.*, 2000b) and *Clostridium difficile* (Ryan *et al.*, 1997), against the parasites *Theileria parva* (Gentschev *et al.*, 1998) and *Plasmodium falciparum* (Gomez-Duarte *et al.*, 2001) and against the *Measles virus* (Spreng *et al.*, 2000) were developed. Interestingly, protection was observed after vaccination with recombinant vaccine carriers secreting the heterologous antigens (Hess *et al.*, 1996 and 1997; Gentschev *et al.*, 1998; Hess *et al.*, 2000; Gomez-Duarte *et al.*, 2001). In contrast, protection was either low or absent when the corresponding antigens remained intracellularly in the vaccine strain, possibly due to the inefficient induction of T cell responses. These findings suggest that antigen localization plays a role and that antigen display is crucial for vaccine development on the basis of attenuated bacteria.

The HlyA antigen-delivery system offers possibilities to modulate the immune response against a given protein antigen, by either changing the localization of the antigen within the producing bacterial carrier (secreted versus cell-surface-bound, cytoplasmic) or by changing the bacterial carrier to one which will deliver the same antigen to different compartments of APCs (extracellular, phagosomal, cytosolic).

Last but not least, the HlyA system can find application not only in the classical field of anti-infective vaccines, but also in the immunoprophylaxis of tumors, as delivery system for immunocontraceptive vaccines and as a system for the co-expression and co-delivery of bioactive proteins such as cytokines or enzymes.

ACKNOWLEDGEMENTS

We thank Z. Sokolovic for stimulating discussions and M. Dietrich for crititical reading of the manuscript.

REFERENCES

Blight, M.A., Chervaux, C., and Holland I.B. 1994. Protein secretion pathway in *Escherichia coli*. Curr. Opin. Biotechnol. 5: 468-474.

Blight M.A., and Holland I.B. 1994. Heterologous protein secretion and the versatile *Escherichia coli* haemolysin translocator. Trends Biotechnol. 12: 450-455.

Brehm, K., Haas, A., Goebel, W., and Kreft, J. 1992. A gene encoding a superoxide dismutase of the facultative intracellular bacterium *Listeria monocytogenes*. Gene 118: 121-125

Cardenas, L., and Clements, J.D. 1992. Oral immunization using live attenuated *Salmonella* spp. as carriers of foreign antigens. Clin. Microbiol. Rev. 5: 328-342.

Catic, A., Dietrich, G., Gentschev, I., Goebel, W., Kaufmann. S.H.E., and Hess, J. 1999. Introduction of protein or DNA delivered via recombinant *Salmonella typhimurium* into the major histocompatibility complex class I presentation pathway of macrophages. Microbes and Infection 2: 111-121.

Chatfield, S.N., and Dougan, G. 1997. Attenuated *Salmonella* as a live vector for expression of foreign antigens In: New Generation Vaccines, 2nd edn. Levine, M.M., *et al.*, eds. Marcel Dekker, New York. p. 331-341.

Chervaux, C., Sauvonnet, N., Le Clainche, A., Kenny, B., Hung, A.L., Broome-Smith, J.K., and Holland, I.B. 1995. Secretion of active beta-lactamase to the medium mediated by the *Escherichia coli* haemolysin transport pathway. Mol. Gen. Genet. 249: 237-245.

Dinh, T., Paulsen, I.T., and Saier, Jr. M.H. 1994. A family of extracytoplasmic proteins that allow transport of large molecules across the outer membranes of Gram-negative Bacteria. J. Bacteriol. 176: 3825-3831.

Edelman, R., Palmer, K., Russ, K.G., Secrest, H.P., Becker, J.A., Bodison, S.A., Perry, J.G., Sills, A.R., Barbour, A.G., Luke, C.J., Hanson, M.S., Stover, C.K., Burlein, J.E., Bansal, G.P., Connor, E.M., and Koenig, S. 1999. Safety and immunogenicity of recombinant *Bacille Calmette-Guerin* (rBCG) expressing *Borrelia burgdorferi* outer surface protein A (OspA) lipoprotein in adult volunteers: a candidate Lyme disease vaccine. Vaccine 17: 904-914.

Gentschev, I., Sokolovic, Z., Köhler, S., Krohne, G.F., Hof, H., Wagner, J., and Goebel, W. 1992. Identification of p60 antibodies in human sera and presentation of this listerial antigen on the surface of attenuated salmonellae by the HlyB-HlyD secretion system. Infect. Immun. 60: 5091-5098.

Gentschev, I., Mollenkopf, H.-J., Sokolovic, Z., Ludwig, A., Tengel, C., Gross, R., Hess, J., Demuth, A., and Goebel, W. 1994. Synthesis and secretion of bacterial antigens by attenuated *Salmonela* via the *Escherichia coli* hemolysin system. Behring Inst. Mitt. 95: 57-66.

Gentschev, I., Sokolovic, Z., Mollenkopf, H.-J., Hess, J., Kaufmann, S.H.E., Kuhn, M., Krohne, G.F., and Goebel, W. 1995. *Salmonella* secreting active listeriolysin changes its intracellular localization. Infect. Immun. 63: 4202-4205.

Gentschev, I., Maier, G., Kranig, A., Goebel, W. 1996a. Mini-Tn*hlyA*s: a new tool for the construction of secreted fusion proteins. Mol. Gen. Genet. 252: 266-274.

Gentschev, I., Mollenkopf H., Sokolovic Z., Hess J., Kaufmann, S.H.E., and Goebel, W. 1996b. Development of antigen-delivery systems, based on the *Escherichia coli* hemolysin secretion pathway. Gene 179: 133-140.

Gentschev, I., Dietrich, G., Mollenkopf, H.-J., Sokolovic, Z., Hess, J., Kaufmann, S.H.E., and Goebel, W. 1997. The *Escherichia coli* hemolysin secretion apparatus - a versatile anti-gen delivery system in attenuated *Salmonella*. Behring Inst. Mitt. 98: 103-113.

Gentschev, I, Glaser, I., Goebel, W., McKeever, D.J., and Heussler V. 1998. Delivery of the p67 sporozoite antigen of *Theileria parva* using recombinant *Salmonella*: secretion of the product enhances specific antibody responses in cattle. Infect. Immun. 66: 2060-2064.

Gentschev, I., Dietrich, G., Spreng, S., Kolb-Maurer, A., Daniels, J., Hess, J., Kaufmann S.H.E., and Goebel, W. 2000. Delivery of protein antigens and DNA by virulence-attenuated strains of *Salmonella typhimurium* and *Listeria monocytogenes*. J. Biotechnol. 83: 19-26.

Gentschev, I., Dietrich, G., Spreng, S., Kolb-Mäurer, A., Brinkmann, J., Grode, V., Hess, J., Kaufmann, S.H.E., and Goebel, W. 2001. Recombinant attenuated bacteria for the delivery of subunit vaccines. Vaccine. 19: 2621-2628.

Gomez-Duarte, O.G., Pasetti, M.F., Santiago, A., Sztein, M.B., Hoffman, S.L., and Levine M.M. 2001. Expression, extracellular secretion, and immunogenicity of the *Plasmodium falciparum* sporozoite surface protein 2 in *Salmonella* vaccine strains. *Infect. Immun.* 69: 1192-1198.

Hahn, H.P., Hess, C., Gabelsberger, J., Domdey, H., von Specht, B.U.A. 1998. *Salmonella typhimurium* strain genetically engineered to secrete effectively a bioactive human interleukin (hIL)-6 via the *Escherichia coli* hemolysin secretion apparatus. *FEMS Immunol. Med. Microbiol.* 20: 111-119.

Hess, J., Gentschev, I., Goebel, W., and Jarchau, T. 1990. Analysis of the haemolysin secretion system by PhoA-HlyA fusion proteins. Mol. Gen. Genet. 224: 201-208.

Hess, J., Gentschev, I., Szalay, G., Ladel, C., Bubert, A., Goebel, W., and Kaufmann, S.H.E. 1995. *Listeria monocytogenes* p60 supports host cell invasion by and *in vivo* survival of attenuated *Salmonella typhimurium*. *Infect. Immun.* 63: 2047-2053.

Hess, J., Gentschev, I., Miko, D., Welzel, M., Ladel, Ch., Goebel, W., and Kaufmann, S.H.E. 1996. Superior efficacy of secreted over somatic antigen display in recombinant *Salmonella* vaccine induced protection against listeriosis. Proc. Natl. Acad. Sci. USA. 93: 1458-1463.

Hess, J., Dietrich, G., Gentschev, I., Miko, D., Goebel, W., and Kaufmann, S.H.E. 1997. Protection against murine Listeriosis by an attenuated recombinant *Salmonella typhimurium* vaccine strain that secretes the naturally somatic antigen superoxide dismutase. Infect. Immun. 65: 1286-1292.

Hess, J., Grode, L., Gentschev, I., Fensterle, J., Dietrich, G., Goebel, W., and Kaufmann, S.H.E. 2000a. Secretion of different listeriolysin cognates by recombinant attenuated *Salmonella typhimurium*: superior efficacy of haemolytic over non-haemolytic constructs after oral vaccination. Microbes Infect. 2: 1799-1806.

Hess, J., Grode, L., Hellwig, J., Gentschev, I., Goebel, W., Ladel, C., and Kaufmann, S.H.E. 2000b. Protection against murine tuberculosis by an attenuated recombinant *Salmonella typhimurium* vaccine strain that secreted the 30 kDa-antigen of *Mycobacterium bovis* BCG. FEMS Immunol. Med. Microbiol. 27: 283-289.

Hess, J., Schaible, U., Raupach, B., and Kaufmann, S.H.E. 2000c. Exploiting the immune system: toward new vaccines against intracellular bacteria. Adv. Immunol. 75: 1-88.

Hoiseth, S.K., and Stocker, B.A.D. 1981. Aromatic-dependent *Salmonella typhimurium* are non-virulent and effective as live vaccines. Nature 291: 238-239.

Holland, I.B., Blight, M.A., and Kenny, B. 1990. The mechanism of secretion of hemolysin and other polypeptides from gram-negative bacteria. J. Bioenerg. Biomembr. 22: 473-491.

Hone, D.M., Harris, A.M., Chatfield, S., Dougan, G., and Levine, M.M. 1991. Construction of genetically defined double *aro* mutants of *Salmonella typhi*. Vaccine 9: 810-816.

Hormaeche, C., and Khan, C. 1996. Recombinant bacteria as vaccine carriers of heterologous antigens. In: Concept in Vaccine Development. S.H.E. Kaufmann, ed. Walter de Gruyter, Berlin and New York. p. 327-349.

Jarchau, T., Chakraborty, T., Garcia, F., and Goebel W. 1994. Selection for transport competence of C-terminal polypeptides from *Escherichia coli* hemolysin: the shortest peptide capable of autonomous HlyB/HlyD-dependent secretion comprises the 62 C-terminal amino acids of HlyA. Mol. Gen. Genet. 245: 53-60.

Jensen, E.R., Shen, H., Wettstein, F.O., Ahmed, R., and Miller, J.F. 1997. Recombinant *Listeria monocytogenes* as a live vaccine vehicle and a probe for studying cell-mediated immunity. *Immunol. Rev.* 158: 147-157.

Kelly, C.P., Pothoulakis, C., and LaMont, J.T. 1994. *Clostridium difficile* colitis. N. Engl. J. Med. 330: 257-262.

Kern, I., and Ceglowski, P. 1995. Secretion of streptokinase fusion proteins from *Escherichia coli* cells through the hemolysin transporter. Gene 163: 53-57.

Koronakis, V., Hughes, C., and Koronakis, E. 1993. ATPase activity and ATP/ADP-induced conformational change in the soluble domain of the bacterial protein translocator HlyB. Mol. Microbiol. 8: 1163-1175.

Lindberg. A.A. 1998. Vaccination against enteric pathogens: from science to vaccine trials. Curr. Opin. Microbiol. 1: 116-124.

Lindberg, A.A., Karnell, A., Stocker, B.A.D., Katakura, S., Sweiha, H., and Reinholt, F.P. 1988. Development of an auxotrophic oral live *Shigella flexneri* vaccine. Vaccine 6: 146-150.

Matsumoto, S., Yukitake, H., Kanbara, H., and Yamada, T. 1998. Recombinant *Mycobacterium bovis bacillus* Calmette-Guerin secreting merozoite surface protein 1 (MSP1) induces protection against rodent malaria parasite infection depending on MSP1-stimulated interferon gamma and parasite-specific antibodies. J. Exp. Med. 188: 845-854.

McGhee, J.R., Mestecky, J., Dertzbaugh, M.T., Eldridge, J.H., Hirasawa, M., and Kiyono, H. 1992. The mucosal immune system: from fundamental concepts to vaccine development. Vaccine 10: 75-88.

Mollenkopf, H.-J., Gentschev, I., and Goebel, W. 1996. Conversion of bacterial gene products to secretion-competent fusion proteins. Biotechniques 21: 854-860.

Nakano, H., Kawakami, Y., and Nishimura, H. 1992. Secretion of genetically-engineered dihydrofolate reductase from *Escherichia coli* using an *E. coli* alpha-hemolysin membrane translocation system. *Appl.* Microbiol. Biotechnol. 37: 765-771.

Noriega, F., Formal, S.B., Kotloff, K.L., and Lindberg, A.A. 1997. Vaccines agaist *Shigella* infections Part II: engineered attenuated mutants of *Shigella* as oral vaccines. In New Generation Vaccines, 2nd edn. Levine, M.M., *et al.*, eds. Marcel Dekker, New York. p. 853.

Orr, N., Galen, J.E., and Levine, M.M. 1999. Expression and immunogenicity of a mutant diphtheria toxin molecule, CRM(197), and its fragments in *Salmonella typhi* vaccine strain CVD 908-htrA. Infect. Immun. 67: 4290-4294.

Paulsen, I.T., Park, J.H., Choi, P.S., and Saier Jr M.H.. 1997. A family of gram-negative bacterial outer membrane factors that function in the export of proteins, carbohydrates, drugs and heavy metals from gram-negative bacteria. FEMS Microbiol. Lett. 156: 1-8.

Portnoy, D.A., Chakraborty, T., Goebel, W., and Cossart, P. 1992. Molecular determinants of *Listeria monocytogenes* pathogenesis. Infect. Immun. 60: 1263-1267.

Roberts, M., Chatfield, S.N., and Dougan, G. 1994. *Salmonella* as carries of heterogous antigens. In: Novel Delivery Systems for Oral Vaccines. D.T.O'Hagan, ed. CRC Press, London. p. 27-58.

Roberts, M., Li, J., Bacon, A., and Chatfield, S. 1998. Oral vaccination against tetanus: comparison of the immunogenicities of *Salmonella* strains expressing fragment C from the *nirB* and *htrA* promoters. Infect. Immun. 66: 3080-3087.

Rüssmann, H., Shams, H., Poblete, F., Fu, Y., Galan, J.E., and Donis, R.O. 1998. Delivery of epitopes by the *Salmonella* type III secretion system for vaccine development. Science 281: 565-568.

Ryan, E.T., Butterton, J.R., Smith, R.N., Carroll, P.A., Crean, T.I., and Calderwood, S.B. 1997. Protective immunity against *Clostridium difficile* toxin A induced by oral immunization with a live, attenuated *Vibrio cholerae* vector strain. Infect. Immun. 65: 2941-2949.

Shata, M.T., Stevceva, L., Agwale, S., Lewis, G.K., and Hone, D.M. 2000. Recent advances with recombinant bacterial vaccine vectors. Mol. Med. Today 6: 66-71.

Spreng, S., Dietrich, G., Goebel, W., and Gentschev, I. 1999. The *Escherichia coli* haemolysin secretion apparatus: a potential universal antigen delivery system in gram-negative bacterial vaccine carriers. Mol. Microbiol. 31: 1596-1598.

Spreng, S., Gentschev, I., Goebel, W., Weidinger, G., ter Meulen, V., and Niewiesk S. 2000. *Salmonella* vaccines secreting measles virus epitopes induce protective immune responses against *measles virus* encephalitis. Microbes Infect. 2: 1687-1689.

Stocker, B.A.D. 1990. Aromatic-dependent *Salmonella* as live vaccine presenters of foreign epitopes as inserts in flagellin. Res.Microbiol. 141: 787-796.

Su, G.F., Brahmbhatt, H.N., de Lorenzo, V., Wehland, J., and Timmis, K.N. 1992. Extracellular export of Shiga toxin B-subunit/haemolysin A (C-terminus) fusion protein expressed in *Salmonella typhimurium aroA*-mutant and stimulation of B-subunit specific antibody responses in mice. Microb. Pathog. 13: 465-476.

Tijhaar, E.J., Zheng-Xin, Y., Karlas, J.A., Meyer, T.F., Stukart, M.J., Osterhaus, A.D., and Mooi, F.R. 1994. Construction and evaluation of an expression vector allowing the stable expression of foreign antigens in a *Salmonella typhimurium* vaccine strain. Vaccine 12: 1004-1011.

Tzschaschel, B.D., Guzman, C.A., Timmis K.N., and de Lorenzo, V. 1996a. An *Escherichia coli* hemolysin transport system-based vector for the export of polypeptides: export of Shiga-like toxin IIeB subunit by *Salmonella typhimurium aroA*. Nat. Biotechnol. 14: 765-769.

Tzschaschel, B.D., Klee, S.R., de Lorenzo, V., Timmis, K.N., and Guzman, C.A. 1996b. Towards a vaccine candidate against *Shigella dysenteriae* 1: expression of the Shiga toxin B-subunit in an attenuated *Shigella flexneri aroD* carrier strain. Microb. Pathog. 21: 277-288.

Vijh, S., and Pamer, E.G. 1997. Immunodominant and subdominant CTL responses to *Listeria monocytogenes* infection. J. Immunol. 158: 3366-3371.

Vogel, M., Hess, J., Then, I., Juarez, A., and Goebel, W. 1988. Characterization of a sequence (*hlyR*) which enhances synthesis and secretion of hemolysin in *Escherichia coli*. Mol. Gen. Genet. 212: 76-84.

Wagner, W., Vogel, M., and Goebel, W. 1983. Transport of hemolysin across the outer membrane of *Escherichia coli* requires two functions. J. Bacteriol. 154: 200-210.

Wandersman, C., and Delepelaire, P. 1990. TolC, an *Escherichia coli* outer membrane protein required for hemolysin secretion. Proc. Natl. Acad. Sci. USA. 87: 4776-4780.

Weiskirch, L.M., and Paterson, Y. 1997. *Listeria monocytogenes*: a potent vaccine vector for neoplastic and infectious disease. Immunol. Rev. 158:159.

Xu, D., McSorley, S.J., Tetley, L., Chatfield, S., Dougan, G., Chan, W.L., Satoskar, A., David, J.R., and Liew, F.Y. 1998. Protective effect on *Leishmania major* infection of migration inhibitory factor, TNF-alpha, and IFN-gamma administered orally via attenuated *Salmonella typhimurium*. J. Immunol. 160: 1285-1289.

Young J., and Holland I.B. 1999. ABC transporters: bacterial exporters-revisited five years on. Biochim. Biophys. Acta. 1461: 177-200.

Zgurskaya, H.L., and Nikaido, H. 2000. Multidrug resistance mechanisms: drug efflux across two membranes. Mol. Microbiol. 37: 219-225.

From: *Vaccine Delivery Strategies*
Edited by: Guido Dietrich and Werner Goebel

Chapter 10

Use of Type III Secretion Systems to Induce MHC Class I-Restricted Immune Responses

Holger Rüssmann

ABSTRACT

The chapter will focus on the use of the type III secretion system of *Salmonella* and *Yersinia* to target heterologous antigens directly to the cytosol of eukaryotic cells. Type III secretion systems are currently discovered in an increasing number of taxonomically diverse Gram-negative animal and plant pathogens. These systems are specialized for the export of bacterial virulence factors delivered directly into the cytosol of target cells to modulate host cellular functions. Certain *Salmonella* and *Yersinia* type III effector proteins with defined secretion and translocation domains can be used for delivery of large protein fragments derived from immunodominant viral and bacterial heterologous antigens into the MHC class I-restricted antigen processing pathway. In orally immunized mice, this novel vaccination strategy results in the induction of pronounced peptide-specific cytotoxic CD8 T cell responses.

INTRODUCTION

Research on the molecular and genetic bases of microbial pathogenicity has revealed that many Gram-negative bacteria exploit a common strategy to become successful pathogens (Finlay and Falkow, 1989). Virulence genes of bacterial microorganisms are often clustered in functionally related groups and, surprisingly, these clusters are probably acquired by horizontal gene transfer, as the base content of their DNA sequence differs significantly from the rest of the genome. These observations resulted in the concept of "pathogenicity islands" - defined segments of DNA that encode virulence factors (Knapp *et al.*, 1986; Hacker *et al.*, 1990, Hacker and Kaper, 2000).

In the past ten years, highly conserved, multicomponent secretion systems encoded by pathogenicity islands have been identified in many Gram-negative bacterial plant and human pathogens (Hueck, 1998). These secretion systems, termed type III, are used by bacteria to establish a remarkable relationship to eukaryotic cells. Composed of up to 40 proteins, type III secretion systems are among the most complex protein secretion systems known. Essential part of such complexity and probably the most fascinating aspect of type III secretion is the fact that proteins are not only secreted from the bacterial cytoplasm but also delivered directly to the inside of the eukaryotic host cell, therefore effectively working as a "molecular syringe" (Kubori *et al.*, 1998; Galán, 1998). First step of this sophisticated type III export mechanism is the secretion process: effector proteins cross the inner and outer membrane of Gram-negative bacteria without making an intermediate stop in the periplasm, thereby completely bypassing the general secretory pathway (Pugsley, 1993). This secretion process is reminiscent of the mechanism used by type I secretion systems (Fath and Kolter, 1993). Careful analysis of a number of type III proteins revealed that they span both the inner and outer membrane of the bacterial envelope (Kubori *et al.*, 1998). These components assemble into an organelle, termed the "needle complex" (Kubori *et al.*, 1998). The architecture of the neddle complex resembles that of the flagellar hook-basal body (Aizawa, 1996) and this molecular structure provides some understanding how type III secretion works. However, this model cannot elucidate the second step of the type III export mechanism by which the system mediates the translocation of secreted proteins into the host cell. To explain translocation, it has been proposed that some type III proteins form a pore or channel through which effector proteins cross the eukaryotic cell membrane (Hakansson *et al.*, 1996; Neyt and Cornelis, 1999).

USE OF TYPE III SECRETION SYSTEMS AS ANTIGEN DELIVERY TOOLS IN ATTENUATED BACTERIAL LIVE CARRIER VACCINES

Yersinia and *Salmonella* Exploit Type III Secretion Systems to Establish Their Ecological Niche

Probably two of the best studied bacterial microorganisms that use type III secretion systems are *Yersinia* and *Salmonella* species (Hueck, 1998). The life cycles of these enteropathogens differ significantly from each other: *Yersinia* species employ type III effector proteins to destroy key functions of immune cells (Cornelis *et al.*, 1998). When these bacteria bind to the surface of macrophages, at least six effector proteins (*Yersinia* outer proteins, Yops) are translocated in a type III-dependent fashion into the cytosol of the eukaryotic host cell (Lee, 1997) mediating the ability to resist phagocytosis (Rosqvist *et al.*, 1988; Black and Bliska, 1997) to trigger apoptosis (Ruckdeschel *et al.*, 1997), and to suppress TNF-α and IFN-γ release (Autenrieth and Heesemann, 1992). Thus, the consequence of the translocation process is that pathogenic *Yersinia* survive and proliferate extracellulary in the infected host (Simonet *et al.*, 1990). In contrast to this survival strategy of *Yersinia*, *Salmonella* uses type III effector proteins encoded in the *Salmonella* Pathogenicity Island 1 (SPI1) at centisome 63 of its chromosome to invade eukaryotic cells (Galán, 1996). After gaining access to the host cell, *Salmonella* species persist in membrane-bound vacuoles (macropinosomes) during their entire intracellular life cycle (Alpuche-Aranda *et al.,* 1994). From this endosomal compartment, *Salmonella* continues to translocate type III effector proteins into the eukaryotic cell cytosol (Galán, 1998).

Attenuated *Yersinia* and *Salmonella* Strains as Live Carrier Vaccines

Attenuated *Yersinia* and *Salmonella* strains are attractive candidates as live carrier vaccines because they induce complex mucosal and systemic immune responses in the vaccinated host after oral administration (Schödel *et al.*, 1995; Levine *et al.*, 1996, Igwe *et al.*, 1999). A fascinating aspect of utilizing recombinant *Yersinia* and *Salmonella* strains is that both have the potential to be used as delivery sytems for expressing foreign proteins from pathogens of viral, bacterial, and parasitic origin. Immunization with these genetically manipulated carrier vaccines can result in the induction of both humoral and cell-mediated immune responses to the heterologous antigen being expressed and, in some cases, protection against the pathogen and the host bacterium.

Virtually all viruses and many bacterial pathogens invade mammalian host cells, thereby potentially escaping complement- and antibody-mediated defense mechanisms. Once inside the infected cell, viruses and some bacteria - such as *Shigella, Rickettsia*, and *Listeria monocytogenes* - enter the host cell cytosol whereas other intracellular bacteria (e. g. *Mycobacterium tuberculosis* and *Salmonella*) remain confined in membrane-bound vacuoles. These different subcellular localizations of the pathogens have important implications for their detection and elimination by host T lymphocytes (Harding *et al.*, 1995; Jondal *et al.*, 1996; Harty and Bevan, 1999; Kerksiek and Pamer, 1999). Before the infected cell can be recognized by T cells, microbial proteins must be degraded into peptides within the host cell. These peptides bind to major histocompatibility complex (MHC) proteins, and the peptide-MHC complex is displayed on the host cell surface, where it can interact specifically with corresponding T cell receptors. CD4 T cells recognize peptide antigens in the context of MHC class II molecules, which are loaded with antigen within acidic intracellular vacuoles and vesicles of antigen presentining cells (APC). It is a well investigated concept in immunobiology that peptides presented by MHC class II molecules may derive from exogenous proteins or from pathogens residing within membrane-bound compartments. In contrast, CD8 T cells detect peptides bound to MHC class I molecules. Most peptides presented by MHC class I molecules derive from endogenous proteins degraded by proteasomes in the cytosol of the host cell. The resulting peptides are transported by TAP (transporter associated with antigen processing) molecules into the endoplasmic reticulum, where they are loaded onto newly synthesized MHC class I molecules. Thus, CD4 T cells have been implicated in defense against microbial pathogens residing in vacuolar compartments, whereas CD8 T cells defend against cytosolic microorganisms. In many settings, the successful defense against intracellular pathogens is achieved by cooperative work of CD4 and CD8 T cells.

To elicit suitable CD8 T cell responses, a live vaccine vector must be capable of delivering pathogen-derived antigenic peptides in the vaccinated individual in a way that they are made available for binding to MHC class I molecules of appropriate APC (Germain, 1994; Germain, 1995). Taking into account the knowledge about antigen presentation and T cell stimulation, it is clear that extracellular *Yersinia* and endosomal-bound *Salmonella* are not ideal vectors to deliver heterologous proteins to the cytosol of host cells. In fact, secretion of foreign proteins into the extracellular environment by attenuated *Yersinia* results in a strong antigen-specific antibody response (Igwe *et al.*, 1999) whereas secretion of heterologous antigens into the macropinosome by *Salmonella* induces peptide-specific CD4 T cell priming (Wick *et al.*, 1994). The question arises, how could one genetically manipulate attenuated *Yersinia* and *Salmonella* strains in a way that they become efficient inducers of MHC class I-restricted immune responses? The fact that both bacterial species employ a type III secretion system to inject effector proteins directly into the cytosol of the host cell, makes it conceivable to use these translocated molecules as carrier proteins for heterologous antigen delivery into the MHC class I processing pathway of APC.

THE PROOF OF PRINCIPLE: VIRAL EPITOPE DELIVERY BY *SALMONELLA*'S TYPE III SECRETION SYSTEM

In an effort to improve the ability of *Salmonella* to elicit MHC class I-restricted immune responses, the potential of its type III secretion system was investigated by our laboratory to deliver heterologous viral epitopes into the host cell cytosol (Rüssmann *et al.*, 1998). CD8 nonamer peptides from the influenza virus nucleoprotein ($IVNP_{366-374}$) or from the murine lymphocytic choriomeningitis virus nucleoprotein ($LCMVNP_{118-126}$) were inserted in frame between two functional domains of the *Salmonella* protein tyrosine phosphatase (SptP), a type III effector molecule delivered into the host cell (Kaniga *et al.*, 1996; Fu and Galán, 1998). Biochemical analysis of tissue culture cells infected with *Salmonella* expressing chimeric SptP revealed that hybrid $SptP-IVNP_{366-374}$ or $SptP-LCMVNP_{118-126}$ were translocated into the cytosol of eukaryotic cells at concentrations indistinguishable from those of wild-type SptP. RMA thymoma cells used as APC were infected with *Salmonella* expressing $SptP-IVNP_{366-374}$ and subsequently recognized by the epitope-specific T cell hybridoma. This antigen presentation was strictly dependent on the cytosolic delivery of the epitope by *Salmonella*'s type III secretion system, as RMA cells infected with a *Salmonella* mutant strain which can secrete $SptP-IVNP_{366-374,}$ but is unable to translocate it into the cell cytosol, did not stimulate the T cell hybridoma. To assess the ability of the type III-mediated antigen delivery system to induce a protective CD8 T cell response, mice were orally immunized with a single dose of an attenuated *Salmonella typhimurium* mutant strain expressing translocated SptP-LCMVNP$_{118-126}$. Vaccinated animals were completely protected against a lethal intracerebral challenge with a virulent strain of LCMV. This induction of protective immunity in mice by *Salmonella* vaccination was correlated with the presence of LCMV-specific splenic CD8 T cells. Thus, for the first time, it was demonstrated that delivery of epitopes by the *Salmonella* type III secretion system results in efficient stimulation of MHC class I-restricted protective antiviral immune responses.

STATE-OF-THE-ART: IDENTIFICATION OF A TYPE III EFFECTOR PROTEIN TO BE USED IN *YERSINIA* AND *SALMONELLA* FOR ANTIGEN DELIVERY OF LARGE PROTEIN FRAGMENTS

The use of SptP as a carrier protein for heterologous antigens was limited to deliver small protein fragments of 45-55 amino acids inserted between two independent domains of this molecule (Rüssmann *et al.*, 1998). Because a versatile antigen delivery system should be capable of targeting large protein fragments derived from diverse pathogens, our laboratory was interested in identifying a type III effector protein that could be used in both *Yersinia* and *Salmonella* for this purpose.

Among different bacterial species, many components of type III secretion systems reveal functional conservation probably due to the fact that shared type III genes were recruited by horizontal transfer during evolution (Hueck, 1998). One of the best studied type III effector proteins is the 25-kDa *Yersinia* outer protein E (YopE). During the interaction of *Yersinia* species with professional phagocytes, YopE translocation mediates the ability of the bacteria to resist phagocytosis and to survive at extracellular sites (Rosqvist *et al.*, 1991, and 1994). Cytosolic delivery of YopE into host cells was first observed using immunofluorescence microscopy (Rosqvist *et al.*, 1991, and 1994). Alternative techniques to demonstrate YopE translocation were based on reporter enzymes such as a calmodulin-dependent adenylate cyclase, a neomycin phosphotransferase, and the green fluorescent protein fused to various residues of YopE (Sory and Cornelis, 1994; Sory *et al.*, 1995; Schesser *et al.*, 1996; Jacobi *et al.*, 1998; Lee *et al.*, 1998). These studies led to the characterization of N-terminal signals required for type III-dependent secretion and translocation of YopE. The minimal sequence shown to be

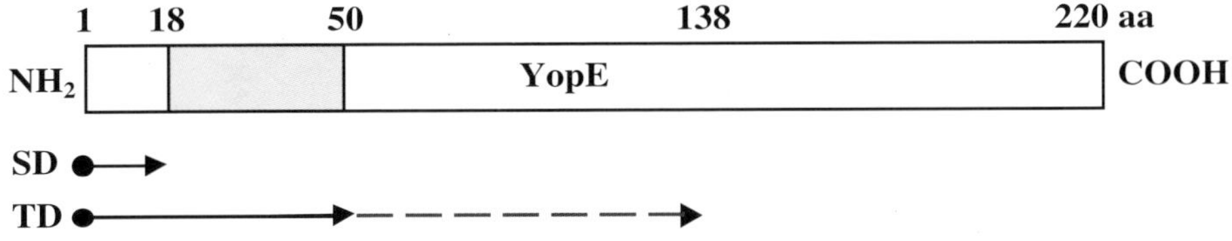

Figure 1. Defined amino-terminal secretion (SD) and translocation domains (TD) of the *Yersinia* type III effector molecule YopE. It has been shown that foreign proteins fused to the N-terminal 138 amino acids (aa) of YopE are more efficiently translocated into the cytosol of infected cells than heterologous antigens fused to the minimal YopE translocation domain comprised of 50 residues (Jacobi *et al.*, 1998; Rüssmann *et al.*, 2000).

sufficient for secretion of YopE was found to comprise 11-15 amino acids, whereas the minimal domain required for translocation of YopE across the eukaryotic cell membrane was reduced to 50 residues (Figure 1). The YopE-specific chaperone SycE, which is required for YopE translocation, binds to amino acids 15-50 of this domain (Lee *et al.*, 1998).

The waste information about YopE prompted us to use *Yersinia enterocolitica* for the injection of a heterologous antigen into the cytosol of infected host cells and to deliver foreign antigenic peptides to the MHC class I-restricted antigen presentation pathway (Rüssmann *et al.*, 2000). The p60 protein of *Listeria monocytogenes*, an intracellular bacterium, was used as a model antigen to construct various hybrid YopE proteins (Bubert *et al.*, 1992). In the cytosol of infected cells, *L. monocytogenes* constitutively secretes the murein hydrolase p60 that enters the MHC class I processing pathway. Two immunodominant p60 nonamer peptides (p60$_{217-225}$ and p60$_{449-457}$) are presented to CD8 T cells by MHC class I molecules and it has been shown that CD8 T cells specific for p60$_{217-225}$ can transfer immunity against *L. monocytogenes* to naive mice (Pamer, 1994; Harty and Pamer, 1995; Sijts *et al.*, 1996; Vijh and Pamer, 1997; Harty and Bevan, 1999). To assess the ability of YopE to secrete and translocate large foreign protein fragments, the C-terminal 354 amino acids of p60 were fused to various N-terminal parts of YopE (Rüssmann *et al.*, 2000). Immunoblot analysis of *Yersinia*-infected epithelial or macrophage-like tissue culture cells revealed that hybrid YopE$_{1-18}$-p60$_{130-484}$ lacking the YopE translocation domain was secreted into the culture supernatant, but was not translocated into the host cell cytosol. In contrast, chimeric YopE$_{1-138}$-p60$_{130-484}$ containing both the secretion and translocation domain of YopE was translocated into the cytosol of infected cells in a type III-dependent fashion. These results were confirmed by immunofluorescence staining of *Yersinia*-infected APC (H. Rüssmann,

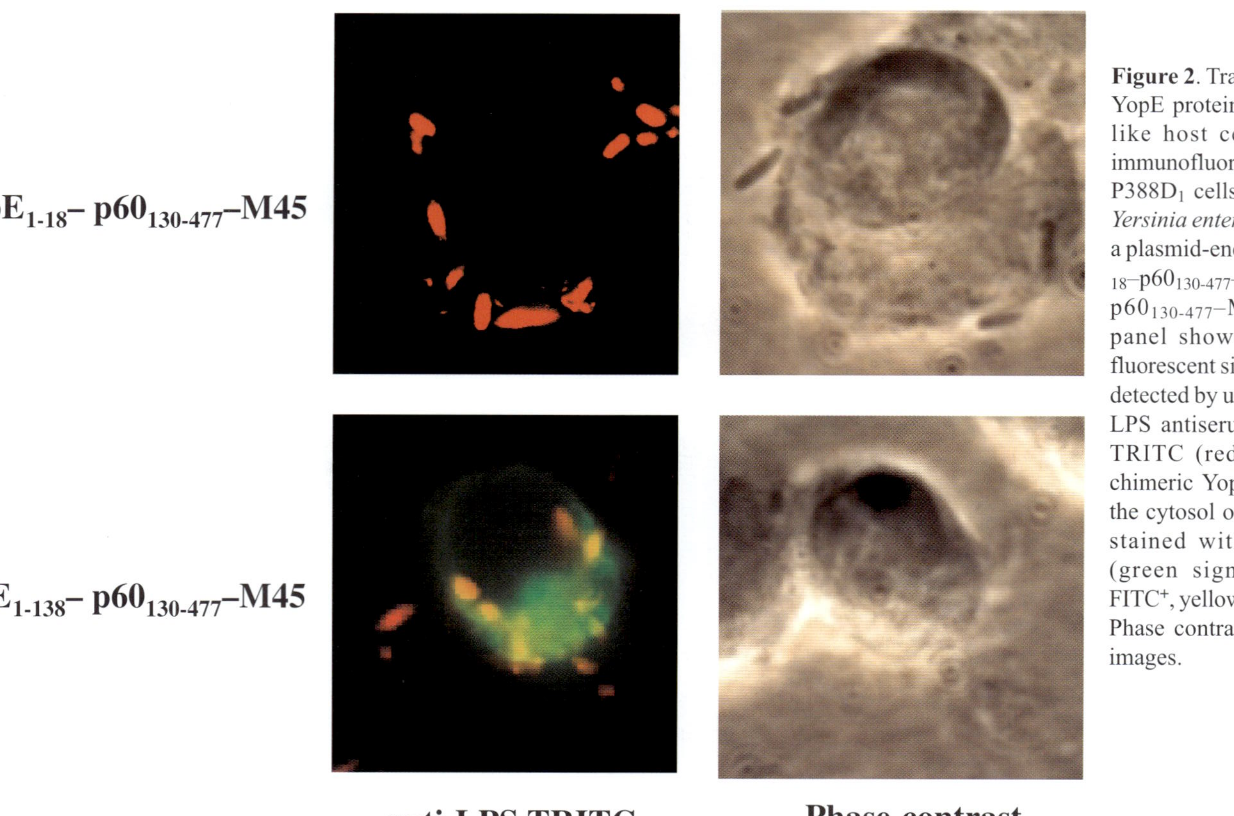

Figure 2. Translocation of hybrid YopE proteins into macrophage-like host cells visualized by immunofluorescence microscopy. P388D$_1$ cells were infected with *Yersinia enterocolitica* expressing a plasmid-encoded hybrid YopE$_{1\text{-}18}$–p60$_{130\text{-}477}$–M45 or YopE$_{1\text{-}138}$–p60$_{130\text{-}477}$–M45 protein. Left panel showing an overlay of fluorescent signals: Bacteria were detected by using an anti-*Yersinia* LPS antiserum conjugated with TRITC (red signal), whereas chimeric YopE translocated into the cytosol of the target cell was stained with anti-M45 FITC (green signal). TRITC[+] and FITC[+], yellow signal. Right panel: Phase contrast of corresponding images.

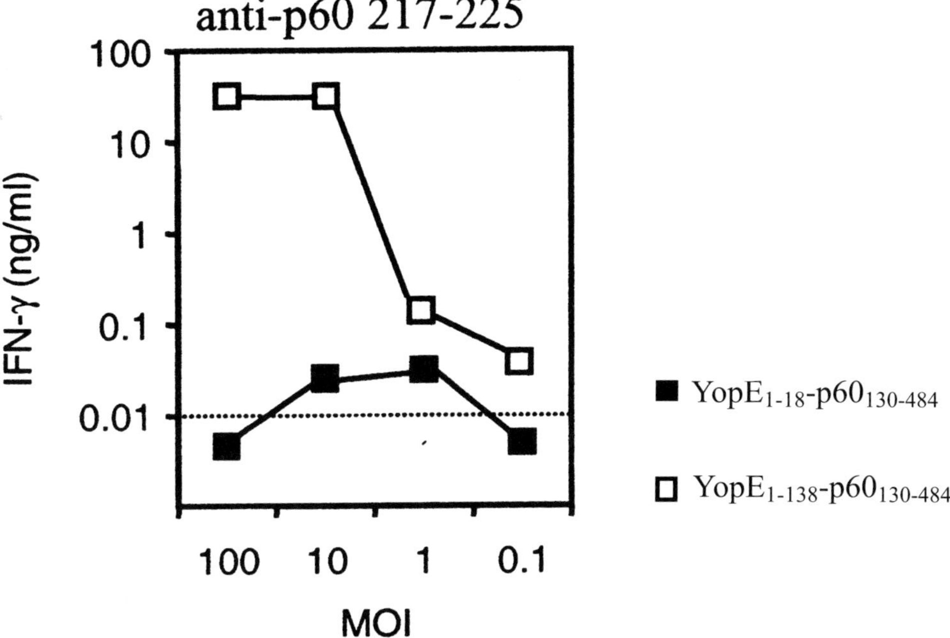

Figure 3. Antigen presentation of p60 nonamer peptide 217-225 by murine P388D$_1$ cells. APC were infected with the attenuated *Yersinia enterocolitica* WA-314 *sodA* strain (Igwe *et al.*, 1999) expressing secreted or translocated hybrid YopE-p60 protein. Cells were infected at various multiplicities of infection (MOI). Activation of anti-p60 217-225 T cells was determined by measurement of the IFN-γ concentration in culture supernatants using a IFN-γ-specific sandwich ELISA kit. The dotted line at 0.01 ng/ml indicates the detection limit of the ELISA. This figure was kindly provided by Dr. Gernot Geginat, Institut für Medizinische Mikrobiologie und Hygiene, Klinikum Mannheim, Germany.

unpublished). For this purpose, both hybrid YopE$_{1\text{-}18}$-p60$_{130\text{-}477}$ and YopE$_{1\text{-}138}$-p60$_{130\text{-}477}$ proteins were tagged at their C-terminus with an 18 amino acid M45 epitope derived from an adenovirus protein. Translocated chimeric YopE proteins were detected by an anti-M45 FITC-conjugated monoclonal antibody (Figure 2).

In further experiments, the ability of *Yersinia enterocolitica* to deliver the C-terminal amino acids 130-484 containing the antigenic nonamer peptides 217-225 and 449-457 of the p60 molecule to the MHC class I-restricted antigen presenting pathway was studied (Rüssmann *et al.*, 2000). APC infected with *Yersinia* expressing and translocating YopE$_{1\text{-}138}$-p60$_{130\text{-}484}$ stimulated specifically both p60$_{217\text{-}225}$- and p60$_{449\text{-}457}$-specific T cells. CD8 T cell stimulation was strictly dependent on the cytosolic delivery of the C-terminal portion of p60 by the *Yersinia* type III apparatus, as APC infected with an attenuated *Yersinia enterocolitica* strain secreting but not translocating YopE$_{1-18}$-p60$_{130-484}$ did not stimulate p60-specific T cells (Figure 3). Efficient translocation and subsequent MHC class I-restricted antigen presentation of chimeric YopE-p60 required co-localized expression of recombinant *sycE* in direct vicinity to the plasmid-borne hybrid *yopE* gene fusion. Thus, the chaperone SycE not only fulfills an important role concerning the stability and conformation of wild-type YopE, but also of YopE$_{1-138}$ fused to heterologous antigens.

In a previous study, it has been shown that full-length wild-type YopE can be secreted and translocated by *Salmonella typhimurium* in a type III-dependent manner (Rosqvist *et al.*, 1995). This observation, combined with our promising experiences with YopE as a carrier molecule in *Yersinia*, prompted our laboratory to investigate the possible employment of YopE for the delivery of heterologous antigens by attenuated *Salmonella*. The immunodominant T cell antigens listeriolysin O (LLO) and p60 of *L. monocytogenes* (Pamer *et al.*, 1991) were fused to the above mentioned defined secretion and translocation domains of YopE (Rüssmann *et al.*, 2000). *In vitro* experiments showed that *S. typhimurium* allows secretion and translocation of large hybrid YopE proteins in a type III-dependent fashion. Translocation and cytosoloc delivery of these chimeric proteins into host cells, but not secretion into endosomal macropinosomes, led to efficient MHC class I-restricted antigen presentation of listerial nonamer peptides. As determined by ELISPOT assay, mice orally vaccinated with a single dose of attenuated *S. typhimurium* expressing translocated hybrid YopE proteins revealed high numbers of IFN-γ-producing cells reactive with LLO$_{91-99}$ or p60$_{217-225}$, respectively. This CD8 T cell response protected mice against a challenge with *L. monocytogenes* (Rüssmann *et al.*, 2001) In conclusion, by engaging well-defined type III secretion and translocation signals of YopE, cytosolic delivery of large foreign proteins by attenuated *Yersinia* and *Salmonella* strains can be achieved resulting in an excellent MHC class I-restricted antigen presentation of nonamer peptides.

FUTURE PERSPECTIVES

Use of type III secretion systems will expand the efficiency of *Salmonella*- and *Yersinia*-based live vaccines to induce MHC class I-restricted immune and antigen-specific CD8 T cell responses (Figure 4). In the case of *Yersinia*, efficient MHC class I-restricted antigen presentation of heterologous proteins has been demonstrated using *in vitro* assays (Rüssmann *et al.*, 2000).

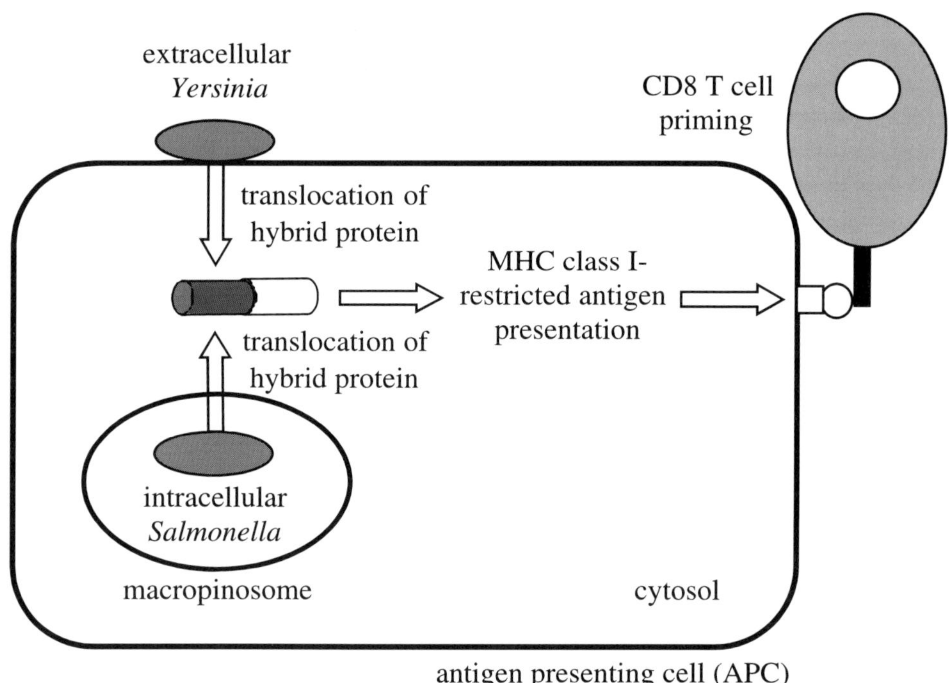

Figure 4. Scheme of type III secretion system-mediated translocation of heterologous antigens by *Yersinia* and *Salmonella*. Cytosolic delivery of hybrid proteins from different cellular compartments results in MHC class I-restricted antigen presentation and antigen-specific cytotoxic CD8 T cell priming.

However, in mice orally vaccinated with attenuated *Yersinia enterocolitica* expressing translocated foreign antigens, no such immune response could be detected (H. Rüssmann, unpublished). One of the major problems associated with expression of heterologous antigens is the stability of DNA within *Yersinia* during infection of mice. Expression vectors carrying foreign genes tend to get lost by segregation following growth of the attenuated bacterial strain in the animal. An alternative approach is to integrate the gene for the foreign antigen into the 70 kb virulence plasmid pYVO8 of *Y. enterocolitica*. This plasmid carries the genetic information for the entire virulence-associated *Yersinia* type III secretion system and is therefore mandatory for the survival of the bacterium in the host resulting in its stable maintenance. Our laboratory currently tries to identify non-coding regions of pYVO8 that can be chosen for stable integration of gene fusions. Future experiments will demonstrate whether this expression strategy leads to efficient CD8 T cell priming *in vivo* by attenuated *Yersinia* vaccine carriers.

REFERENCES

Aizawa, S.I. 1996. Flagellar assembly in *Salmonella typhimurium*. Mol. Microbiol. 19: 1-5.

Alpuche-Aranda, C.M., Racoosin, E.L., Swanson, J.A., and Miller, S.I. 1994. *Salmonella* stimulate macrophage macropinocytosis and persist within spacious phagosomes. J. Exp. Med. 179: 601-608.

Autenrieth, I.B. and Heesemann, J. 1992. *In vivo* neutralization of tumor necrosis factor-alpha and interferon-gamma abrogates resistance to *Yersinia enterocolitica* infection in mice. Med. Microbiol. Immunol. Berl. 181: 333-338.

Black, D.S. and Bliska, J.B. 1997. Identification of p130Cas as a substrate of *Yersinia* YopH (Yop51), a bacterial protein tyrosine phosphatase that translocates into mammalian cells and targets focal adhesions. EMBO J. 16: 2730-2744.

Bubert, A., Kuhn, M., Goebel, W., and Köhler, S. 1992. Structural and functional properties of the p60 protein from different *Listeria* species. J. Bacteriol. 174: 8166-8171.

Cornelis, G.R., Boland, A., Boyd, A.P., Geuijen, C., Iriarte, M., Neyt, C., Sory, M.-P., and Stanier, I. 1998. The virulence plasmid of *Yersinia*, an antihost genome. Microbiol. Mol. Rev. 62: 1315-1352.

Fath, M.J., and Kolter, R. 1993. ABC transporters: bacterial exporters. Microbiol. Rev. 57: 997-1017.

Finlay, B.B., and Falkow, S. 1989. Common themes in microbial pathogenicity. Microbiol. Rev. 53: 210-230.

Fu, Y., and Galán, J.E. 1998. The *Salmonella typhimurium* tyrosine phosphatase SptP is translocated into host cells and disrupts the actin cytoskeleton. Mol. Microbiol. 27: 359-368.

Galán, J.E. 1996. Molecular genetic bases of *Salmonella* entry into host cells. Mol. Microbiol. 20: 263-271.

Galán, J.E. 1998. Interactions of *Salmonella* with host cells: Encounters of the closest kind. Proc. Natl. Acad. Sci. USA. 95: 14006-14008.

Germain, R.N. 1994. MHC-dependent antigen processing and peptide presentation: providing ligands for T lymphocyte avtivation. Cell 76: 287-299.

Germain, R.N. 1995. The biochemistry and cell biology of antigen presentation by MHC class I and II molecules: implications for development of combination vaccines. Ann. NY Acad. Sci. 754: 114-125.

Hacker, J., Bender, L., Ott, M., Wingender, J., Lund, B., Marre, R., and Goebel, W. 1990. Deletions of chromosomal regions coding for fimbriae and hemolysins occur *in vitro* and *in vivo* in various extraintestinal *Escherichia coli* isolates. Microb. Pathog. 8: 213-225.

Hacker, J., and Kaper, J.B. 2000. Pathogenicity islands and the evolution of micobes. Annu. Rev. Microbiol. 54: 641-679.

Hakansson, S., Schesser, K., Persson, C., Galyov, E.E., Rosqvist, R., Homble, F., and Wolf-Watz, H. 1996. The YopB protein of *Yersinia pseudotuberculosis* is essential for the translocation of Yop effector proteins across the target cell membrane and displays a contact-dependent membrane disrupting activity. EMBO J. 15: 5812-5823.

Harding, C.V., Song, R., Griffin, J., France, J., Wick, M.J., Pfeifer, J.D., and Geuze, H.J. 1995. Processing of bacterial antigens for presentation to class I and II MHC-restricted T lymphocytes. Infect. Agents Dis. 4: 1-12.

Harty, J.T., and Pamer, E.G. 1995. CD8 T lymphocytes specific for the secreted p60 antigen protect against *Listeria monocytogenes* infection. J. Immunol. 154: 4642-4650.

Harty, J.T., and Bevan, M.J. 1999. Responses of CD8+ T cells to intracellular bacteria. Curr. Opin. Immunol. 11: 89-93.

Hueck, C.J. 1998. Type III protein secretion systems in bacterial pathogens of animals and plants. Microbiol. Mol. Biol. Rev. 62: 379-433.

Igwe, E.I., Rüssmann, H., Roggenkamp, A., Noll, A., Autenrieth, I.B. and Heesemann, J. 1999. Rational live oral carrier vaccine design by mutating virulence-associated genes of *Yersinia enterocolitica*. Infect. Immun. 67: 5500-5507.

Jacobi, C.A., Roggenkamp, A., Rakin, A., Zumbihl, R., Leitritz, L., and Heesemann, J. 1998. *In vitro* and *in vivo* expression studies of YopE from *Yersinia enterocolitica* using the *gfp* reporter gene. Mol. Microbiol. 30: 865-882.

Jondal, M., Schirmbeck, R., Reimann, J. 1996. MHC class I-restricetd CTL responses to exogenous antigens. Immunity 5: 295-302.

Kaniga, K., Uralil, J., Bliska, J.B., and Galán, J.E. 1996. A secreted protein tyrosin phosphatase with modular effector domains in the bacterial pathogen *Salmonella typhimurium*. Mol. Microbiol. 21: 633-641.

Kerksiek, K.M., and Pamer, E.G. 1999. T cell responses to bacterial infection. Curr. Opin. Immunol. 11: 400-405.

Knapp, S., Hacker, J., Jarchau, T., and Goebel, W. 1986. Large, unstable inserts in the chromosome affect virulence properties of uropathogenic *Escherichia coli* O6 strain 536. J. Bacteriol. 168: 22-30.

Kubori, T., Matsushima, Y., Nakamura, D., Uralil, J., Lara-Tejero, M., Sukhan, A., Galán, J.E., and Aizawa, S.I. 1998. Supramolecular structure of the *Salmonella typhimurium* type III protein secretion system. Science 280: 602-605.

Lee, C.A. 1997. Type III secretion systems: machines to deliver bacterial proteins into eukaryotic cells. Trends Microbiol. 5: 148-156.

Lee, V.T., Anderson, D.M. and Schneewind, O. 1998. Targeting of *Yersinia* Yop proteins into the cytosol of HeLa cells: one-step translocation of YopE across bacterial and eukaryotic membranes is dependent on SycE chaperone. Mol. Microbiol. 28: 593-601.

Levine, M.M., Galen, J., Barry, E., Noriega, F., Chatfield, S., Sztein, M., Dougan, G., and Tacket, C. 1996. Attenuated *Salmonella* as live oral vaccine against typhoid fever and as live vectors. J. Biotechnol. 44: 193-196.

Neyt, C., and Cornelis, G.R. 1999. Insertion of a Yop translocation pore into the macrophage plasma membrane by *Yersinia enterocolitica*: requirement for translocators YopB and YopD, but not LcrG. Mol. Microbiol. 33: 971-981.

Pamer, E.G., Harty, J.T., and Bevan, M.J. 1991. Precise prediction of a dominant class I-restricted epitope of *Listeria monocytogenes*. Nature 353: 852-855.

Pamer, E.G. 1994. Direct sequence identification and kinetic analysis of an MHC class I-restricted *Listeria monocytogenes* CTL epitope. J. Immunol. 152: 686-694.

Pugsley, A.P. 1993. The complete general secretory pathway. Microbiol. Rev. 57: 50-108.

Rosqvist, R., Bolin, I. and Wolf-Watz, H. 1988. Inhibition of phagocytosis in *Yersinia pseudotuberculosis*: a virulence plasmid-encoded ability involving the Yop2b protein. Infect. Immun. 56: 2139-2143.

Rosqvist, R., Forsberg, A., and Wolf-Watz, H. 1991. Intracellular targeting of the *Yersinia* YopE cytotoxin in mammalian cells induces actin microfilament disruption. Infect. Immun. 59: 4562-4569.

Rosqvist, R., Magnusson, K.E., and Wolf-Watz, H. 1994. Target cell contact triggers expression and polarized transfer of *Yersinia* YopE cytotoxin into mammalian cells. EMBO J. 13: 964-972.

Rosqvist, R., Hakansson, S., Forsberg, A., and Wolf-Watz, H. 1995. Functional conservation of the secretion and translocation machinery for virulence proteins of Yersiniae, Salmonellae and Shigellae. EMBO J. 14: 4187-4195.

Ruckdeschel, K., Roggenkamp, A., Lafont, V., Mangeat, P., Heesemann, J. and Rouot, B. 1997. Interaction of *Yersinia enterocolitica* with macrophages leads to macrophage cell death through apoptosis. Infect. Immun. 65: 4813-4821.

Rüssmann, H., Shams, H., Poblete, F., Fu, Y., Galán, J.E., and Donis, R.O. 1998. Delivery of epitopes by the *Salmonella* type III secretion system for vaccine development. Science 281: 565-568.

Rüssmann, H., Weissmüller, A., Geginat, G., Igwe, E.I., Roggenkamp, A., Bubert, A., Goebel, W., Hof, H., and Heesemann, J. 2000. *Yersinia enterocolitica*-mediated translocation of defined fusion proteins to the cytosol of mammalian cells results in MHC class I-restricted antigen presentation. Eur. J. Immunol. 30: 1375-1384.

Rüssmann, H., Igwe, E.I., Sauer, J., Hardt, W.-D., Bubert, A., and Geginat, G. 2001. Protection against murine listeriosis by oral vaccination with recombinant *Salmonella* expressing hybrid *Yersinia* type III proteins. J. Immunol. 167: 357-365.

Schesser, K., Frithz-Lindsten, E. and Wolf-Watz, H. 1996. Delineation and mutational analysis of the *Yersinia pseudotuberculosis* YopE domains which mediate translocation across bacterial and eukaryotic cellular membranes. J. Bacteriol. 178: 7227-7233.

Schödel, F., and Curtiss III, R. 1995. Salmonellae as oral vaccine carriers. Dev. Biol. Stand. 84: 245-253.

Sijts, A.J.A.M., Neisig, A., Neefjes, J., and Pamer, E.G. 1996. Two *Listeria monocytogenes* CTL epitopes are processed from the same antigen with different efficiencies. J. Immunol. 156: 683-692.

Simonet, M., Richard, S. and Berche, P. 1990. Electron microscopic evidence for *in vivo* extracellular localization of *Yersinia pseudotuberculosis* harboring the pYV plasmid. Infect. Immun. 58: 841-845.

Sory, M.-P. and Cornelis, G.R. 1994. Translocation of a hybrid YopE-adenylate cyclase from *Yersinia enterocolitica* into HeLa cells. Mol. Microbiol. 14: 583-594.

Sory, M.-P., Boland, A., Lambermont, I. and Cornelis, G.R. 1995. Identification of the YopE and YopH domains required for secretion and internalization into the cytosol of macrophages, using the *cyaA* gene fusion approach. Proc. Natl. Acad. Sci. USA. 92: 1998-2002.

Vijh, S., and Pamer, E.G. 1997. Immunodominant and subdominant CTL responses to *Listeria monocytogenes* infection. J. Immunol. 158: 3366-3371.

Wick, M.J., Harding, C.V., Normark, S.J., and Pfeifer, J.D. 1994. Parameters that influence the processing efficiency of antigenic epitopes expressed in *Salmonella typhimurium*. Infect. Immun. 62: 4542-4548.

From: *Vaccine Delivery Strategies*
Edited by: Guido Dietrich and Werner Goebel

Chapter 11

Live Mycobacterial Vaccine Candidates

Jürgen Hess

ABSTRACT

Vaccination provides the most potent measure against infectious diseases and recombinant (r)-live antigen carriers expressing defined pathogen-derived proteins represent promising candidates for future vaccination trials. Novel techniques in genome manipulation allow the construction of virulence-attenuated. *Mycobacterium tuberculosis* and r-*Mycobacterium* bovis Bacille Calmette-Guérin (BCG) strains that could be used as homologous vaccines or as heterologous antigen delivery systems, respectively, for priming pathogen-specific immunity against infectious diseases, including tuberculosis (TB). On the basis of recent achievements in complete genome analysis of various target-pathogens, combined with a better understanding of protective pathogen-specific immune responses, rational design of a novel mycobacterial vaccine generation against a multitude of infectious diseases has become possible.

INTRODUCTION

Viable bacterial carriers like *Mycobacterium bovis* Bacille Calmette-Guérin (BCG) elicit very potent Th1-mediated immune responses. In comparison to subunit vaccines, live bacterial vectors require no additional adjuvant component in their vaccine formulations to evoke protective immunity in several animal models of experimental infectious diseases. For attenuated microorganisms, usually a single inoculation at a modest dose is sufficient for a protective immune response, since these microbes will grow *in vivo* to a sufficiently large immunogenic dose and at the same time will produce a multitude of antigens usually expressed during the natural course of infection. Most importantly, recombinant (r)-antigens delivered by these carrier strains are not only targeted to appropriate pathways of major histocompatibility complex (MHC) antigen processing, but also stimulate the innate immune system to provide the adequate cytokine milieu and appropriate expression of costimulatory molecules for promoting the protective immune response. It should be noted that the presentation and processing events of antigenic components of bacterial origin additionally mimic a natural infection of pathogens, resulting in immune responses similar to the ones elicited in infected individuals. Therefore, attenuated r-bacterial strains expressing heterologous target antigens are effective devices for protecting against challenge with pathogenic bacterial, viral or parasitic microorganisms which are primarily controlled by Th1 cell responses.

BCG

BCG, the currently used vaccine against tuberculosis (TB), was developed in 1908 by 230 serial *in vitro* passages of a virulent *M. bovis* strain (Calmette *et al.*, 1927). During *in vitro* passage, the *M. bovis* microbes became attenuated due to the loss of numerous gene complexes that have recently been identified (Behr *et al.*, 1999). For comparative genome analysis between BCG, *M. bovis* and *Mycobacterium tuberculosis,* a DNA microarray platform was established which revealed virtually all genetic differences between *M. tuberculosis* H37Rv, *M. bovis* and some BCG substrains by DNA-DNA hybridisation (Cole *et al.*, 1998; Behr *et al.*, 1999). In summary, 129 *M. tuberculosis* H37Rv-specific open reading frames were absent in 16 regions of the genome of nearly all BCG substrains (Cole *et al.*, 1998; Behr *et al.*, 1999), underlining the virulence-attenuated state of BCG.

Although the anti-TB vaccine BCG is considered as very safe, it is also among the current vaccines with highest reactogenicity which in turn gradually depends on the respective BCG 'sub-strain' used for vaccination. BCG is currently recommended at birth, or at first contact with health services. Interestingly, World Health Organization (WHO) reported that in the years 1989-1996 the annual global vaccination coverage of infants with BCG by 12 months of age was beyond 80 % (Fine *et al.*, 1999). In general, successful BCG vaccination causes minor lesions, local self-limiting bacterial multiplication, and delayed-type hypersensitivity (DTH) to mycobacterial protein preparations such as purified protein derivative (PPD), which may persist for several years. In the absence of BCG vaccination, the DTH response to PPD is considered as a tentative indicator of *M. tuberculosis* infection, and hence BCG is not recommended for general TB control in countries with low TB incidences, such as the EU member states or the US. Interestingly, a leucine-auxotrophic BCG mutant strain was recently identified that protects guinea pigs against hematogenous spread of *M. tuberculosis* without sensitization to PPD, simultaneously conferring a similar vaccine efficacy as the parental BCG strain (Chambers *et al.*, 2000). In addition, there has been particular concern over the implications of HIV for the safety of BCG vaccination, after early case reports of systemic BCG infection in individuals with AIDS. Several studies available to date have supported the WHO policy of exempting only individuals with symptomatic HIV infection (AIDS) from routine BCG vaccination at birth.

TB AND BCG IN ANTI-TB CONTROL

Since the discovery of the causative agent of TB, *M. tuberculosis*, by Robert Koch in 1882, TB remains a major health problem even in our days. Whilst approximately 95 percent of TB cases occur in the developing world, several countries of Eastern Europe, including Russia, have been witnessing increasing incidences of TB. There were an estimated 8.4 million new tuberculosis cases in 1999, up from 8.0 million in 1997; the rise is due largely to a 20 % increase in incidence in African countries most affected by the epidemic of HIV/AIDS. If present trends continue, 10.2 million new cases are expected in 2005, and Africa will have more cases than any other WHO region (WHO Report, 2001). Global mortality ranges from 1.6 to 2.2 million lives per year, depending on whether the half million individuals suffering co-infection with HIV and *M. tuberculosis* are included in the toll of HIV/ AIDS or TB (WHO Report, 2001). The situation is further worsened by the increasing incidence of multidrug resistant *M. tuberculosis* strains, which is in part due to incomplete compliance with chemotherapy. In several countries, e.g. Estonia and the Dominican Republic, as many as 10-20 % of all mycobacterial isolates are of the multidrug resistant type. Each year, 55 million people become newly infected with the pathogen, resulting in as many as 2 billion infected people world-wide. Of these infected individuals, 8 million annually will develop disease. Thus, less than 10 % of infected people will develop TB during their lifetime, although they are all at risk of doing so. This low ratio of diseased over infected individuals indicates that the immune system can control *M. tuberculosis* efficiently, as long as it remains competent. In contrast, immunodeficiency will markedly increase the risk of active disease to about 10 % per year.

Although BCG represents the most widely used viable vaccine, its protective value as anti-TB vaccine is still questionable. General agreement exists that BCG can protect against, or at least ameliorate, severe forms of systemic TB in children, particularly meningitis (Huebner, 1996). However, it seems to be of low or no protective value in adults with TB. (Colditz *et al.*, 1994). Comparison by a meta-analysis of various controlled trials revealed that the average protective efficacy of BCG in adults reaches 50 % with an efficacy range from ineffective to 80 % protection (Colditz *et al.*, 1994). Therefore, the most prevalent form of TB, namely reactivation of latent pulmonary TB in adults, cannot be prevented by BCG in a satisfactory way (Parrish *et al.*, 1998). In pulmonary TB, the lung represents the port of *M.tuberculosis* entry and disease manifestation. In general, at the site of mycobacterial growth, granulomas are formed whereby the microbes are contained efficaciously in immunocompetent persons. However, weakening of the immune response results in reactivation of pathogens, transforming infection into an active disease stage. Infection of immunocompromised individuals, including newborns, results in microbial dissemination, directly leading to miliary TB.

Importantly, the BCG vaccine could be better at protecting against primary disease than against either reactivation- or reinfection-type disease. Recent data from South India indicate a complex interaction of age and time effects: BCG imparted consistent protection in children, but no protection for subjects older than 15 years, and may even have imparted negative protection among these older individuals. If true, these findings have important implications for efforts to develop a vaccine against adult pulmonary tuberculosis (Fine *et al.*, 2001). In conclusion, general agreement exists that a novel vaccine is required for satisfactory TB control mostly in developing countries, but in the light of the increasing incidence of multidrug resistant *M. tuberculosis* strains, this medical need for efficacious TB vaccines will not be limited to the developing world. Several reasons and experimental evidences may help to explain the failure of BCG in the control of TB:

- the genetic variability amongst, and different age of, the vaccinated individuals.
- the immunological cross-reactivity between BCG and environmental mycobacterial strains prevalent in different parts of the world.
- latent *M. tuberculosis* infection in vaccinees.
- lack of comparability between different vaccination studies due to the current use of 6 different BCG 'sub-strains' (Copenhagen-1131, Pasteur-1173P, Glaxo-1077, Tokyo-172, Russian, Moreau) (Fine *et al.*, 1999), variable doses, and different immunisation schedules (BCG only at birth, BCG once in childhood or repeated/booster BCG) (Fine *et al.*, 1999) and routes of administration (BCG was given to humans orally between 1921 and the late 1940s and administered mainly by percutaneous or intradermal routes since the late 1940s) (Fine *et al.*, 1999).
- genetic differences between BCG and *M. tuberculosis* provide several possible explanations for the failure of BCG as an anti-TB vaccine (Cole *et al.*, 1998; Behr *et al.*, 1999).

From an immunological point of view, one of BCG's major drawbacks is its failure to stimulate adequate anti-mycobacterial CD8 T cell responses required for *M. tuberculosis* control. It should be noted that the course of BCG infection in β2-microglobulin-deficient mice lacking CD8 T cells revealed that CD4 T cells are virtually sufficient for the control of BCG (Flynn *et al.*, 1992; Ladel *et al.*, 1995). Taken together, it is evident that the balanced combination of CD4 and CD8 T lymphocytes required for protection against TB cannot be induced by the current BCG vaccine. In general, one major aspect should be taken into consideration when interpreting the results obtained with screening anti-TB vaccines in animal models, as most of these models mimic the acute primary-type disease and not the reactivation-type of TB. Therefore future screening strategies should be developed identifying vaccine candidates that could be used for prevention and therapy of TB.

MODIFIED BCG OR ATTENUATED *M. TUBERCULOSIS* STRAINS AS ANTI-TB VACCINE CANDIDATES

The recent success in the generation of gene-deletion mutants of *M. tuberculosis* by allelic exchange and transposon mutagenesis is promising (Pelicic *et al.*, 1997; Berthet *et al.*, 1998). These mycobacterial mutant strains do not survive in the host, either because they are auxotrophic, e.g. due to *purC* deficiency (Pelicic *et al.*, 1997) or because they have lost their virulence for unknown reasons as is the case in *erp* or *acr* deletion mutants (Berthet *et al.*, 1998; Yuan *et al.*, 1998). Erp represents a secreted protein of *M. tuberculosis*, whilst the 14 kDa Acr protein of *M. tuberculosis* is related to the α-crystallin family of low-molecular-weight Hsp (Verbon *et al.*, 1992). Notably, Acr is primarily produced during the stationary growth phase *in vitro*, but undetectable during logarithmic growth of *M. tuberculosis*. By growing bacilli at defined oxygen concentrations, *acr* transcription was strongly induced at mildly hypoxic conditions and during *in vitro* infection of macrophages (Yuan *et al.*, 1998). The precise functional basis of the role of both Erp and Acr in virulence and persistence remains to be established. In addition, no data are yet available regarding the protective capacity of such attenuated *M. tuberculosis* strains. Transposon mutagenesis was also used to generate enhanced attenuated strains of BCG for their potential use to vaccinate HIV-infected individuals during the asymptomatic phase of disease (Guleria *et al.*, 1996; Berthet *et al.*, 1998). Severe combined immunodeficiency (SCID)-mice lacking virtually all T cells and B cells were infected with methionine- and leucine-auxotrophic BCG strains and were able to control these infections for at least 230 days. In contrast, all SCID mice succumbed to a conventional BCG vaccine within eight weeks (Guleria *et al.*, 1996).

An obvious alternative approach is to improve the immunogenicity of BCG by genetic engineering. Recombinant BCG strains were constructed which express cytokines such as IFN (interferon)-γ or IL (interleukin)-2 in an attempt to evoke more potent immune responses against *M. tuberculosis* (Murray *et al.*, 1996). In this line of r-BCG constructs with enhanced immunostimulatory properties, BCG was genetically engineered to secrete r-human IFN-α (rhIFNα) under control of the mycobacterial heat shock protein (Hsp) 60 promoter and the α-antigen signal sequence (Luo *et al.*, 2001). When compared with control BCG, rhIFNα BCG was substantially more active in inducing the production of IFNγ from human peripheral blood mononuclear cells. These effects were reversible upon antibody neutralization of rhIFNα. Among 10 patients tested, rhIFNα BCG enhanced IFNγ production in all patients compared to responses induced by parental BCG. The onset of IFNγ production induced by rhIFNα BCG was also more rapid, occurring within 4 h after stimulation versus more than 24 h with wild-type BCG. The observation that the maximum IFNγ induction depends on the simultaneous presence of both IFNα and BCG highlights the advantages of rhIFNα BCG. Taken together, the immunostimulatory properties of rhIFNα BCG suggest that it may be a superior agent for immunotherapeutic protocols involving live BCG in humans (Luo *et al.*, 2001).

In an effort to improve access to the MHC class I pathway of antigen processing, r-BCG strains were generated which secrete a hemolytic fusion protein containing listeriolysin (Hly) of *Listeria monocytogenes* (Hess *et al.*, 1998). Hly enables *L. monocytogenes* to escape from the phagosome of infected cells. However, Hly secretion did not allow escape of BCG from the phagosomal vacuole. Yet, it enhanced presentation of co-phagocytosed soluble ovalbumin to CD8 T cells, suggesting that the release of Hly into the phagosome improved the translocation of antigen into the MHC class I pathway (Hess *et al.*, 1998). Future experiments should be directed at clarifying whether these r-BCG strains possess increased vaccine efficacy against TB in experimental guinea pig and mouse models. Preliminary data from an *in vitro* system consisting of human macrophages or dendritic cells infected with BCG secreting Hly revealed improved cytotoxic T lymphocyte (CTL) responses (Conradt *et al.*, 1999).

Another research approach towards improved anti-TB vaccines focused on the dose of well-established and protective antigens like Ag85B stably overexpressed by a r-BCG strain (Horwitz *et al.*, 1995; Horwitz *et al.*, 2000). It should be noted that Ag85B of *M. tuberculosis* and BCG are nearly homologous proteins (only 2 amino acid alterations) and belong to a family of gene products with fibronectin-binding capacity and mycolyl transferase activity which is involved in the final stages of mycobacterial cell wall assembly (Wiker and Harboe, 1992; Belisle *et al.* 1997). Horwitz and colleagues tested the efficacy of two r-BCG strains (Connaught and Tice) overexpressing Ag 85B in the highly susceptible guinea pig model of pulmonary TB, a model noteworthy for its close resemblance to human TB. Animals immunized with the r-BCG vaccines and challenged by aerosol with a highly virulent strain of *M. tuberculosis* had 0.5 logs colony forming units (CFU) fewer microorganisms in their lungs and 1 log fewer bacilli in their spleens on average than animals immunized with their parental appropriate BCG vaccine strain. These r-BCG vaccines are the first anti-TB vaccine candidates more potent than the current commercially available BCG vaccine (Horwitz *et al.*, 2000). In contrast, overexpression of the 19-kDa antigen as a r-protein in two saprophytic mycobacteria - *Mycobacterium vaccae* and *Mycobacterium smegmatis* - resulted in abrogation of their ability to confer protection against *M. tuberculosis* in a murine challenge model, and in their ability to prime a DTH response to cross-reactive mycobacterial antigens. The 19-kDa antigen is a cell wall-associated lipoprotein present in *M. tuberculosis* and in BCG vaccine strains. Induction of an immune response to the 19-kDa antigen by an alternative approach of DNA vaccination had no effect on subsequent *M. tuberculosis* challenge. These results are consistent with a model in which the presence of the 19-kDa protein has a detrimental effect on the efficacy of vaccination with live mycobacteria (Yeremeev *et al.*, 2000a). Recently, Yeremeev and colleagues addressed the question whether expression of the 19-kDa antigen has an analogous detrimental effect on the efficacy of BCG vaccination. In contrast to the results in saprophytes, neither overexpression of the 19-kDa antigen, nor deletion of the endogenous gene encoding the 19-kDa lipoprotein altered the ability of BCG to protect against *M. tuberculosis* challenge in a mouse model (Yeremeev *et al.*, 2000b). Additionally, it should be noted that r-*M. tuberculosis* microbes were constructed which overexpress a Hsp70. Although this mycobacterial mutant strain was fully virulent in the initial stage of murine infection, it was significantly impaired in its ability to persist during the subsequent chronic phase (Stewart *et al.*, 2001). Therefore, induction of mycobacterial Hsp might provide a novel strategy to boost the individual immune response with latent *M. tuberculosis* infection. An additional strategy to improve the current BCG vaccine is based on the recent knowledge of the genes absent from BCG as compared to *M. tuberculosis* (Behr *et al.*, 1999; Cole, 1999). It is an obvious goal to endow BCG with *M. tuberculosis*-specific genes in order to enhance its immunogenicity and protective efficacy against TB. Obviously, genes encoding putative virulence factors of *M. tuberculosis* should not be introduced in active form into the genome of BCG in order to maintain its attenuated state.

BCG As Carrier For Heterologous Antigens Of Different Target Pathogens

BCG represent an effective vehicle for delivery of heterologous antigens due to their preferred intracellular replication in professional antigen presenting cells such as macrophages or dendritic cells (Inaba *et al.*, 1993; Kaufmann, 1998). The preferred intraphagosomal location of this vector strain determines the trafficking of bacterial antigens through different MHC processing pathways. BCG microorganisms target their antigens mainly to the MHC class II presentation pathway and, therefore, stimulate predominantly CD4 T cells. However, with respect to the induction of CD4 versus CD8 T cell responses, this impact of intracellular compartmentalization on antigen trafficking should not be taken as absolute. Various antigen delivery systems based on BCG (Aldovini and Young, 1999; Hess *et al.*, 1998) have been described which allow antigen-specific stimulation of CD8 T lymphocytes in addition to the prominent CD4 T cell induction. About 10 years ago, two groups reported the construction of *E. coli*-mycobacteria shuttle vectors capable of expressing foreign antigens (Aldovini and Young,

1991; Stover *et al.*, 1991). Since then, several studies have demonstrated that strong cellular and humoral immune responses can be induced against heterologous proteins delivered by r-BCG. With BCG being the currently used vaccine against TB, the question arises whether immunization with r-BCG strains would successfully induce immune responses to heterologous antigens in populations that were already BCG vaccinated. By using β-galactosidase as marker antigen for r-BCG, it was found that proliferative T cell responses were suppressed to approximately 50 % of those in naive animals, whereas antibody responses were enhanced (Gheorghiu *et al.*, 1994). These results may indicate that pre-exposure to BCG can reduce T cell responses but is not a limiting factor, especially when antibody and Th2-dominated immune responses are important for control of the target pathogen. In this respect, experiments in which mice were immunized with different numbers of BCG provided evidence that the mycobacterial dose defines the Th1/Th2 nature of the immune response independently of the route of administration (Bretscher, 1992; Power *et al.*, 1998). A high BCG dose apparently polarized the immune response towards Th2, whereas low BCG inocula induced Th1-like, IFNγ-mediated defense mechanisms (Bretscher, 1992; Power *et al.*, 1998). In the case of anti-bacterial vaccination, such a dose-dependent polarization of the immune response should also be considered important because Th1-biased immunity is central to the control of intracellular bacteria like *M. tuberculosis*.

Besides the vaccine dose antigen compartmentalization represents an important feature for modulating the immune response induced by r-BCG strains. A protective antigen, p60 of *L. monocytogenes*, was displayed in secreted, cytosolic or membrane-attached form by different r-BCG constructs for T cell recognition. Anti-listerial protection evoked by the membrane-linked p60 lipoprotein of r-BCG and that of the p60 derivative secreted by rBCG were nearly equal, whereas cytosolic p60 displayed by r-BCG failed to protect mice from *L. monocytogenes* infection (L. Grode, S.H.E. Kaufmann, and J. Hess; unpublished). Interestingly, *in vivo* depletion of CD4 or CD8 T cell subpopulations in mice immunized with r-BCG expressing the membrane-anchored p60 lipoprotein prior to listerial challenge revealed interactions of both T cell subsets in anti-listerial protection (L. Grode, S.H.E. Kaufmann, and J. Hess; unpublished). In animals vaccinated with r-BCG secreting a p60 cognate, CD4 T cells predominantly contributed to anti-listerial control as shown by the failure of anti-CD8 monoclonal antibody treatment to impair the outcome of infectious disease after *L. monocytogenes* challenge (L. Grode, S.H.E. Kaufmann, and J. Hess; unpublished). Hence, differential antigen display by r-BCG influences cell-mediated immunity, which in turn may impact vaccine efficacy due to the different requirements of CD4 or CD8 T cells for pathogen elimination. Importantly, this study provides new insights into the importance of targeting r-antigens, for instance those specifically expressed by *M. tuberculosis*, to highly immunostimulatory compartments of BCG. We could learn from this study that antigen compartmentalization by r-BCG can apparently influence distinct cellular branches of cell mediated immunity. For achieving protective cell-mediated immunity with emphasis on CD4 and CD8 T lymphocytes, antigen display by means of membrane-anchored lipoprotein signal peptides appears to be the appropriate immunodominant mode for antigen delivery by improved BCG vaccines. In the case of humoral immune responses induced by r-BCG strains, compartmentalized expression of a model antigen, MalE, is additionally central to antibody titres. As quantified by MalE-specific ELISA assays, a stronger and more rapid immune response was induced by r-BCG strains expressing the highest level of secreted MalE antigen in comparison to that of cytoplasmic- or membrane-directed MalE r-constructs of BCG (Himmelrich *et al.*, 2000).

Recombinant BCG vaccine candidates have already been developed against pneumonia and Lyme disease caused by *Streptococcus pneumoniae* or *Borrelia burgdorferi*, respectively (Stover *et al.*, 1993; Langermann *et al.*, 1994a, 1994b). These diseases are mainly controlled by antibodies. The pneumococcal surface protein A (PspA) of *S. pneumoniae* and the outer-surface protein (OspA) of *B. burgdorferi* were expressed by these r-BCG strains. More recently, r-BCG constructs expressing glutathione-S-transferase (GST) of *Schistosoma haematobium* or *Schistosoma mansoni* induced mixed neutralising anti-GST serum antibodies of different isotypes such as IgG1, IgG2a, IgG2b and IgA (Kremer *et al.*, 1996, and 1998). After intranasal (i.n.) administration, high levels of anti-GST IgA were found in the bronchoalveolar lavage fluid, demonstrating that r-BCG was capable of inducing long-lasting secretory and systemic immune responses to antigens expressed intracellularly (Kremer *et al.*, 1998). Interestingly, this i.n. route of immunisation has recently been of active interest in endeavours to improve the efficacy of vaccination against a number of respiratory infections including TB. I.n. application of the BCG Pasteur strain in mice was found to be highly protective against challenge infection with the pathogenic *M. tuberculosis* H37Rv strain given after a 4-week interval, reflected by the 100-fold reduction of CFU in both lungs and spleens. In conclusion, the strong protection demonstrated by BCG suggests that the i.n. route of vaccine delivery deserves further attention toward improving vaccination against tuberculosis (Falero-Diaz *et al.*, 2000).

Expression of foreign antigens with the signal sequence of the 19-kDa lipoprotein of *M. tuberculosis* improved induction of humoral immunity in mice consistent with a B cell activating capacity of these lipid residues (Stover *et al.*, 1993; Langermann *et al.*, 1994a). Recently, the potential immunostimulatory effects of the 19-kDa lipoprotein were also shown for the generation of T cell responses, as indicated by markedly increased interleukin-12 production by human macrophages (Brightbill *et al.*, 1999). The IL-12 induction in macrophages is mediated by Toll-like receptors (Brightbill *et al.*, 1999). Interestingly, the 19-kDa antigen was also found to traffic separately from live mycobacteria within infected macrophages by a pathway that was dependent on acylation of the protein. When expressed as a recombinant protein in rapid-growing mycobacteria, the 19-kDa lipoprotein was able to deliver peptides for recognition by MHC class I-restricted T cells (Neyrolles *et al.*, 2001).

However, it should be noted that a r-BCG strain expressing a fusion protein consisting of OspA of *Borrelia burgdorferi* and the 19-kDa lipoprotein failed to elicit primary antigen-specific antibody responses in humans (Edelman *et al.*, 1999). In this first phase-I-study with r-BCG microorganisms, the low immunization doses which had to be used for safety reasons induced a PPD-positive skin test in only half of the vaccinees. This relatively low seroconversion rate could also explain the ineffective induction of OspA-specific antibodies in r-BCG-vaccinated individuals (Edelman *et al.*, 1999).

The capacity of the r-BCG carrier strain to efficiently stimulate cell-mediated immunity against antigens originating from various infectious agents has been reported:

- Somatic expression of the leishmanial gp63 protein by r-BCG evoked potent protective immunity to *L. major* challenge in resistant and susceptible mice suggesting that CD4 T cells of Th1 type were induced (Connell *et al.*, 1993; Abdelhak *et al.*, 1995).
- Immunisation with r-BCG expressing the simian immunodeficiency virus (SIV$_{mac}$) Gag, Pol, Env, and Nef proteins elicited an antigen-specific CTL response in rhesus monkeys (Yasutomi *et al.*, 1993, and 1995; Leung *et al.*, 2000).
- Vaccination with r-BCG expressing the SIV$_{mac}$ Nef protein induced CTL responses against Nef synthetic peptides in mice (Winter *et al.*, 1995).
- Recombinant BCG producing the HIV-1 Env-V3-loop epitope evoked Env-specific CD8 CTL responses in mice (Kameoka *et al.*, 1994; Honda *et al.*, 1995).

- Recombinant BCG strains expressing the amino-terminal half of Env-antigen of SIV_{mac} induced neutralising antibodies and CTL responses in mice (Lim *et al.*, 1997).
- Recombinant BCG expressing pertussis toxin S1 subunit induced protection against an intracerebral challenge with live *Bordetella pertussis* in mice (Nascimento *et al.*, 2000).
- Induction of immune responses by r-BCG strains against human papillomavirus L1 and E7 proteins (Jabbar *et al.*, 2000).

CONCLUSIONS

Several approaches aimed at developing potent mycobacterial vaccines against TB and other infectious diseases are outlined in the present review. In the light of these successful preclinical attempts and past and ongoing field vaccination studies with parental and r-strains, BCG represents an ideal carrier for a multitude of antigens originating from different target pathogens. In the case of TB, the improvement of BCG remains the best choice for the rational design of a vaccine. Recently, this notion was supported by the successful vaccination of guinea pigs with r-BCG overexpressing a mycobacterial antigen against a pulmonary *M. tuberculosis* challenge (Horwitz *et al.*, 2000). It should be noted that this r-BCG construct was more efficacious in anti-TB protection than the parental BCG vaccine (Horwitz *et al.*, 2000). In the light of this success, the post-genomic era could lead to the identification of novel *M. tuberculosis*-specific antigens which are absent from the BCG proteome and could therefore be used for enhancing the immunogenicity of BCG even more effectively (Cole *et al.*, 1998; Behr *et al.*, 1999; Jungblut *et al.*, 1999; Young, 2001). In conclusion, if further attenuated while simultaneously improving its pathogen-specific immunogenicity, BCG may generally serve as a valuable vaccine carrier for heterologous antigens of numerous pathogenic microorganisms even in populations with uncertain HIV-status.

ACKNOWLEDGEMENTS

I thank Dr. Jürgen Walter for critically reading the manuscript.

REFERENCES

Abdelhak, S., Louzir, H., Timm, J., Blel, L., Benlasfar, Z., Lagranderie, M., Gheorghiu, M., Dellagi, K., and Gicquel, B. 1995. Recombinant BCG expressing the leishmania surface antigen Gp63 induces protective immunity against *Leishmania major* infection in BALB/c mice. Microbiology 141: 1585-1592.

Aldovini, A., and Young, R.A. 1991. Humoral and cell-mediated immune responses to live recombinant BCG-HIV vaccines. Nature 351: 479-482.

Aldovini, A., and Young, R.A. 1999. Recombinant BCG vaccines. In: Intracellular Bacterial Vaccine Vectors: Immunology, Cell Biology and Genetics. Y. Paterson, ed. John Wiley & Sons, New York, Chicester, Weinheim, Brisbane, Singapore, Toronto. p. 151-170.

Behr, M.A., Wilson, M.A., Gill, W.P., Salamon, H., Schoolnik, G.K., Rane, S., and Small, P.M. 1999. Comparative genomics of BCG vaccines by whole-genome DNA microarray. Science 284: 1520-1523.

Belisle, J.T., Vissa, V.D., Sievert, T., Takayama, K., Brennan, P.J., and Besra, G.S. 1997. Role of the major antigen of *Mycobacterium tuberculosis* in cell wall biogenesis. Science 276: 1420-1422.

Berthet, F.X., Lagranderie, M., Gounon, P., Laurent-Winter, C., Ensergueix, D., Chavarot, P., Thouron, F., Maranghi, E., Pelicic, V., Portnoi, D., Marchal, G., and Gicquel, B. 1998. Attenuation of virulence by disruption of the *Mycobacterium tuberculosis erp* gene. Science 282: 759-762.

Bretscher, P.A. 1992. A strategy to improve the efficacy of vaccination against tuberculosis and leprosy. Immunol. Today 13: 342-345.

Brightbill, H.D., Libraty, D.H., Krutzki, S.R., Yang, R.-B., Belisle, J.T., Bleharski, J.R., Maitland, M., Norgard, M.V., Plevy, S.E., Smale, S.T., Brennan, P.J., Bloom, B.R., Godowski, P.J., and Modlin, R.L. 1999. Host defense mechanisms triggered by microbial lipoproteins through toll-like receptors. Science 285: 732-736.

Calmette, A., Guerin, C., Negre, L., and Bocquet, A. (1927). Sur la vaccination préventive des enfants nouveau-nés contre la tuberculose par le BCG. Ann. Inst. Pasteur 3: 201.

Chambers, M.A., Williams, A., Gavier-Widen, D., Whelan, A., Hall, G., Marsh, P.D., Bloom, B.R., Jacobs, W.R., and Hewinson, R.G. 2000. Identification of a *Mycobacterium bovis* BCG auxotrophic mutant that protects guinea pigs against *M. bovis* and hematogenous spread of *Mycobacterium tuberculosis* without sensitization to tuberculin. Infect. Immun. 68: 7094-7099.

Colditz, G.A., Brewer, T.F., Berkey, C.S., Wilson, M.E., Burdick, E., Fineberg, H.V., and Mosteller, F. 1994. Efficacy of BCG vaccine in the prevention of tuberculosis. Meta-analysis of the published literature. JAMA 271: 698-702.

Cole, S.T., Brosch, R., Parkhill, J., Garnier, T., Churcher, C., Harris, D., Gordon, S.V., Eiglmeier, K., Gas, S., Barry, C.E., Tekaia, F., Badcock, K., Basham, D., Brown, D., Chillingworth, T., Connor, R., Davies, R., Devlin, K., Feltwell, T., Gentles, S., Hamlin, N., Holroyd, S., Hornsby, T., Jagels, K., and Barrell, B.G. 1998. Deciphering the biology of *Mycobacterium tuberculosis* from the complete genome sequence. Nature 393: 537-544.

Cole, S.T. 1999. Learning from the genome sequence of *Mycobacterium tuberculosis* H37Rv. FEBS Lett. 452: 7-10.

Connell, N.D., Medina-Acosta, E., McMaster, W.R., Bloom, B.R., and Russell, D.G. 1993. Effective immunization against cutaneous leishmaniasis with recombinant bacille Calmette-Guerin expressing the *Leishmania* surface proteinase Gp63. Proc. Natl. Acad. Sci. USA 90: 11473-11477.

Conradt, P., Hess, J., and Kaufmann, S.H.E. 1999. Cytolytic T-cell responses to human dendritic cells and macrophages infected with *Mycobacterium bovis* BCG and recombinant BCG secreting listeriolysin. Microbes Infect. 1: 753-764.

Edelman, R., Palmer, K., Russ, K.G., Secrest, H.P., Becker, J.A., Bodison, S.A., Perry, J.G., Sills, A.R., Barbour, A.G., Luke, C.J., Hanson, M.S., Stover, C.K., Burlein, J.E., Bansal, G.P., Connor, E.M., and Koenig, S. 1999. Safety and immunogenicity of recombinant Bacille Calmette-Guerin (rBCG) expressing *Borrelia burgdorferi* outer surface protein A (OspA) lipoprotein in adult volunteers: a candidate Lyme disease vaccine. Vaccine 17: 904-914.

Falero-Diaz, G., Challacombe, S., Banerjee, D., Douce, G., Boyd, A., and Ivanyi, J. 2000. Intranasal vaccination of mice against infection with *Mycobacterium tuberculosis*. Vaccine 18: 3223-3229.

Fine, P.E.M., Carneira, I.A.M., Milstien, J.B., and Clements, C.J. 1999. Issues relating to the use of BCG in immunization programmes. World Health Organization, Geneva.

Fine, P.E. 2001. BCG: the challenge continues. Scand. J. Infect. Dis. 33: 243-245.

Flynn, J.L., Goldstein, M.M., Triebold, K.J., Koller, B., and Bloom, B.R. 1992. Major histocompatibility complex class I-restricted T cells are required for resistance to *Mycobacterium tuberculosis* infection. Proc. Natl. Acad. Sci. USA. 89: 12013-12017.

Gheorghiu, M., Lagranderie, M.R., Gicquel, B.M., and Leclerc, C.D. 1994. *Mycobacterium bovis* BCG priming induces a strong potentiation of the antibody response induced by recombinant BCG expressing a foreign antigen. Infect. Immun. 62: 4287-4295.

Guleria, I., Teitelbaum, R., McAdam, R.A., Kalpana, G., Jacobs, W.R., Jr, and Bloom, B.R 1996. Auxotrophic vaccines for tuberculosis. Nat. Med. 2: 334-337.

Hess, J., Miko, D., Catic, A., Lehmensiek, V., Russell, D.G., and Kaufmann, S.H. 1998. *Mycobacterium bovis* Bacille Calmette-Guerin strains secreting listeriolysin of *Listeria monocytogenes*. Proc. Natl. Acad. Sci. USA. 95: 5299-5304.

Himmelrich, H., Lo-Man, R., Winter, N., Guermonprez, P., Sedlik, C., Rojas, M., Monnaie, D., Gheorghiu, M., Lagranderie, M., Hofnung, M., Gicquel, B., Clement, J.M., and Leclerc, C. 2000. Immune responses induced by recombinant BCG strains according to level of production of a foreign antigen: malE. Vaccine 18: 2636-2647.

Honda, M., Matsuo, K., Nakasone, T., Okamoto, Y., Yoshizaki, H., Kitamura, K., Sugiura, W., Watanabe, K., Fukushima, Y., and Haga, S. 1995. Protective immune responses induced by secretion of a chimeric soluble protein from a recombinant *Mycobacterium bovis* bacillus Calmette-Guerin vector candidate vaccine for human immunodeficiency virus type 1 in small animals. Proc. Natl. Acad. Sci. USA. 92: 10693-10697.

Horwitz, M.A., Lee, B.W., Dillon, B.J., and Harth, G. 1995. Protective immunity against tuberculosis induced by vaccination with major extracellular proteins of *Mycobacterium tuberculosis*. Proc. Natl. Acad. Sci. USA. 92: 1530-1534.

Horwitz, M.A., Harth, G., Dillon, B.J., and Maslesa-Galic, S. 2000. Recombinant bacillus calmette-guerin (BCG) vaccines expressing the *Mycobacterium tuberculosis* 30-kDa major secretory protein induce greater protective immunity against tuberculosis than conventional BCG vaccines in a highly susceptible animal model. Proc. Natl. Acad. Sci. USA. 97: 13853-13858.

Huebner, R.E. 1996. BCG vaccination in the control of tuberculosis. In: Current Topics in Microbiology and Immunology 215 AD. Division of Tuberculosis Elimination, Centers for Disease Control and Prevention, Atlanta 30333, USA. p. 263-282.

Inaba, K., Inaba, M., Naito, M., and Steinman, R.M. 1993. Dendritic cell progenitors phagocytose particulates, including bacillus Calmette-Guerin organisms, and sensitize mice to mycobacterial antigens *in vivo*. J. Exp. Med. 178: 479-488.

Jabbar, I.A., Fernando, G.J., Saunders, N., Aldovini, A., Young, R., Malcolm, K., and Frazer, I.H. 2000. Immune responses induced by BCG recombinant for human papillomavirus L1 and E7 proteins. Vaccine 18: 2444-2453.

Jungblut, P., Schaible, U., Mollenkopf, H.-J., Zimny-Arndt, U., Raupach, B., Mattow, J., Halada, P., Lamer, S., Hagens, K., and Kaufmann, S.H.E. 1999. Comparative proteome analysis of *Mycobacterium tuberculosis* and *Mycobacterium bovis* BCG strains: towards functional genomics of microbial pathogens. Mol. Microbiol. 33:1103-1117.

Kameoka, M., Nishino, Y., Matsuo, K., Ohara, N., Kimura, T., Yamazaki, A., Yamada, T., and Ikuta, K. 1994. Cytotoxic T lymphocyte response in mice induced by a recombinant BCG vaccination which produces an extracellular alpha antigen fused with the human immunodeficiency virus type 1 envelope immunodominant domain in the V3 loop. Vaccine 12: 153-158.

Kaufmann, S.H.E. 1998. Immunity to intracellular bacteria. In: Fundamental Immunology. W.E. Paul, ed. Lippincott-Raven, Philadelphia. 4: 1335-1371.

Kremer, L., Riveau, G., Baulard, A., Capron, A., and Locht, C. 1996. Neutralizing antibody responses elicited in mice immunized with recombinant bacillus Calmette-Guerin producing the *Schistosoma mansoni* glutathione S-transferase. J. Immunol. 156: 4309-4317.

Kremer, L., Dupre, L., Riveau, G., Capron, A., and Locht, C. 1998. Systemic and mucosal immune responses after intranasal administration of recombinant *Mycobacterium bovis* bacillus Calmette-Guerin expressing glutathione S-transferase from *Schistosoma haematobium*. Infect. Immun. 66: 5669-5676.

Ladel, C.H., Hess, J., Daugelat, S., Mombaerts, P., Tonegawa, S., and Kaufmann, S.H.E. 1995. Contribution of alpha/beta and gamma/delta T lymphocytes to immunity against *Mycobacterium bovis* bacillus Calmette Guerin: studies with T cell receptor-deficient mutant mice. Eur. J. Immunol. 25: 838-846.

Langermann, S., Palaszynski, S., Sadziene, A., Stover, C.K., and Koenig, S. 1994a. Systemic and mucosal immunity induced by BCG vector expressing outer-surface protein A of *Borrelia burgdorferi*. Nature 372: 552-555.

Langermann, S., Palaszynski, S.R., Burlein, J.E., Koenig, S., Hanson, M.S., Briles, DE, and Stover, C.K. 1994b. Protective humoral response against pneumococcal infection in mice elicited by recombinant bacille Calmette-Guerin vaccines expressing pneumococcal surface protein A. J. Exp. Med. 180: 2277-2286.

Leung, N.J., Aldovini, A., Young, R., Jarvis, M.A., Smith, J.M., Meyer, D., Anderson, D.E., Carlos, M.P., Gardner, M.B., and Torres, J.V. 2000. The kinetics of specific immune responses in rhesus monkeys inoculated with live recombinant BCG expressing SIV Gag, Pol, Env, and Nef proteins. Virology 268: 94-103.

Lim, E.M., Lagranderie, M., Le Grand, R., Rauzier, J., Gheorghiu, M., Gicquel, B., and Winter, N. 1997. Recombinant *Mycobacterium bovis* BCG producing the N-terminal half of SIVmac251 Env antigen induces neutralizing antibodies and cytotoxic T lymphocyte responses in mice and guinea pigs. AIDS Research & Human Retroviruses 13: 1573-1581.

Luo, Y., Chen, X., Han, R., and O'Donnell, M.A. 2001. Recombinant bacille Calmette-Guerin (BCG) expressing human interferon-alpha 2B demonstrates enhanced immunogenicity. Clin. Exp. Immunol. 123: 264-270.

Murray, P.J., Aldovini, A., and Young, R.A. 1996. Manipulation and potentiation of antimycobacterial immunity using recombinant bacille Calmette-Guerin strains that secrete cytokines. Proc. Natl. Acad. Sci. USA. 93: 934-939.

Nascimento, I.P., Dias, W.O., Mazzantini, R.P., Miyaji, E.N., Gamberini, M., Quintilio, W., Gebara, V.C., Cardoso, D.F., Ho, P.L., Raw, I., Winter, N., Gicquel, B., Rappuoli, R., and Leite, L.C. 2000. Recombinant *Mycobacterium bovis* BCG expressing pertussis toxin subunit S1 induces protection against an intracerebral challenge with live *Bordetella pertussis* in mice. Infect. Immun. 68: 4877-4883.

Neyrolles, O., Gould, K., Gares, M.P., Brett, S., Janssen, R., O'Gaora, P., Herrmann, J.L., Prevost, M.C., Perret, E., Thole, J.E., and Young, D. (2001). Lipoprotein access to MHC class I presentation during infection of murine macrophages with live mycobacteria. J. Immunol. 166:447-457.

Parrish, N.M., Dick, J.D., and Bishai, W.R. 1998. Mechanisms of latency in *Mycobacterium tuberculosis*. Trends Microbiol. 6: 107-112.

Pelicic, V., Jackson, M., Reyrat, J.M., Jacobs, W.R., Jr, Gicquel, B., and Guilhot, C. 1997. Efficient allelic exchange and transposon mutagenesis in *Mycobacterium tuberculosis*. Proc. Natl. Acad. Sci. USA. 94: 10955-10960.

Power, C.A., Wei, G., and Bretscher, P.A. 1998. Mycobacterial dose defines the Th1/Th2 nature of the immune response independently of whether immunization is administered by the intravenous, subcutaneous, or intradermal route. Infect. Immun. 66: 5743-5750.

Stewart, G.R., Snewin, V.A., Walzl, G., Hussell, T., Tormay, P., O'Gaora, P., Goyal, M., Betts, J., Borwn, I.N., and Young, D.B. 2001. Overexpression of heat-shock proteins reduces survival of *Mycobacterium tuberculosis* in the chronic phase of infection. Nat. Med. 7: 732-737.

Stover, C.K., de, l.C., V, Fuerst, T.R., Burlein, J.E., Benson, L.A., Bennett, LT, Bansal, G.P., Young, J.F., Lee, M.H., and Hatfull, G.F. 1991. New use of BCG for recombinant vaccines. Nature 351: 456-460.

Stover, C.K., Bansal, G.P., Hanson, M.S., Burlein, J.E., Palaszynski, S.R., Young, JF, Koenig, S., Young, D.B., Sadziene, A., and Barbour, A.G. 1993. Protective immunity elicited by recombinant bacille Calmette-Guerin (BCG) expressing outer surface protein A (OspA) lipoprotein: a candidate Lyme disease vaccine. J. Exp. Med. 178: 197-209.

The World Health Report. 2001. World Health Organization, Geneva.

Verbon, A., Hartskeerl, R.A., Schuitema, A., Kolk, A.H., Young, D.B., and Lathigra, R. 1992. The 14,000-molecular-weight antigen of *Mycobacterium tuberculosis* is related to the alpha-crystallin family of low-molecular-weight heat shock proteins. J. Bacteriol. 174: 1352-1359.

Wiker, H.G., and Harboe, M. 1992. The antigen 85 complex: a major secretion product of *Mycobacterium tuberculosis*. Microbiol. Rev. 56: 648-661.

Winter, N., Lagranderie, M., Gangloff, S., Leclerc, C., Gheorghiu, M., and Gicquel 1995. Recombinant BCG strains expressing the SIVmac251nef gene induce proliferative and CTL responses against nef synthetic peptides in mice. Vaccine 13: 471-478.

Yasutomi, Y., Koenig, S., Haun, S.S., Stover, C.K., Jackson, R.K., Conard, P., Conley, A.J., Emini, E.A., Fuerst, T.R., and Letvin, N.L. 1993. Immunization with recombinant BCG-SIV elicits SIV-specific cytotoxic T lymphocytes in rhesus monkeys. J. Immunol. 150: 3101-3107.

Yasutomi, Y., Koenig, S., Woods, R.M., Madsen, J., Wassef, N.M., Alving, C.R., Klein, H.J., Nolan, T.E., Boots, L.J., and Kessler, J.A. 1995. A vaccine-elicited, single viral epitope-specific cytotoxic T lymphocyte response does not protect against intravenous, cell-free simian immunodeficiency virus challenge. J. Virol. 69: 2279-2284.

Yeremeev, V.V., Lyadova, I.V., Nikonenko, B.V., Apt, A.S., Abou-Zeid, C., Inwald, J., and Young, D.B. 2000a. The 19-kD antigen and protective immunity in a murine model of tuberculosis. Clin. Exp. Immunol. 120: 274-279.

Yeremeev, V.V., Stewart, G.R., Neyrolles, O., Skrabal, K., Avdienko, V.G., Apt, A.S., and Young, D.B. 2000b. Deletion of the 19-kDa antigen does not alter the protective efficacy of BCG. Tuber. Lung Dis. 80: 243-247.

Young, D.B. 2001. A post-genomic perspective. Nat. Med. 7:11-13.

Yuan, Y., Crane, D.D., Simpson, R.M., Zhu, Y.Q., Hickey, M.J., Sherman, D.R., and Barry, C.E. 3rd. 1998. The 16-kDa alpha-crystallin (Acr) protein of *Mycobacterium tuberculosis* is required for growth in macrophages. Proc. Natl. Acad. Sci. USA. 95: 9578-9583.

From: *Vaccine Delivery Strategies*
Edited by: Guido Dietrich and Werner Goebel

Chapter 12

Delivery of Protein Antigens and DNA Vaccines by *Listeria monocytogenes*

Guido Dietrich, Ivaylo Gentschev
and Werner Goebel

ABSTRACT

In recent years, the facultative intracellular bacterium *Listeria monocytogenes* has been employed for the delivery of subunit vaccines. Due to its ability to gain access to the cytosol of infected host cells, *L. monocytogenes* is an ideally suited carrier for the introduction of protein antigens or DNA vaccines to the cytosol of professional antigen presenting cells (APC). *L. monocytogenes* was attenuated by the deletion of virulence genes or by the construction of auxotrophic mutant strains. Such attenuated recombinant strains of *L. monocytogenes* have proven to be highly suitable for the elicitation of cell-mediated immunity.

INTRODUCTION: *LISTERIA MONOCYTOGENES* – A MODEL INTRACELLULAR PATHOGEN

Listeria monocytogenes is a gram-positive facultative intracellular microorganism which has been used for decades as a model pathogen for the study of cell-mediated immunity (Kaufmann, 1998). Immunization of mice with a sublethal *L. monocytogenes* infection results in the generation of immunity (Mackaness, 1962) which is largely major histocompatibility complex (MHC) class I mediated. Such infections generate CD8+ T cells, which can adoptively transfer immunity and specifically recognize and kill *Listeria*-infected target cells (Brunt *et al.*, 1990; Harty and Bevan, 1992).

In recent years, the cell biology of *L. monocytogenes* intracellular growth has been defined (Figure 1) (Portnoy *et al.*, 1992). Listerial invasion into nonphagocytic mammalian cells is mainly determined by internalins A and B, encoded by *inlA* and *inlB*, respectively, which form an operon, the regulation of which is partially under the control of the transcription factor PrfA (Lecuit *et al.*, 2001). The two internalins seem to be determining the specificity of the cell type being infected to some extent (Dramsi *et al.*, 1993; Mengaud *et al.*, 1996; Braun *et al.*, 1998; Kuhn and Goebel, 2000). Subsequent to internalization, the bacteria escape from the phagocytic vacuole into the host cell cytosol by lysis of the phagosomal membrane. The bacteria replicate in the cytosol and move by polymerization of host cell actin, they can even spread to neighbouring cells without entering the extracellular milieu. Several virulence factors of *L. monocytogenes* are involved in these processes. Intracellular replication and intra- and intercellular motility of *L. monocytogenes* are mainly determined by virulence genes present in the listerial genome in the form of a virulence gene cluster consisting of the genes *prfA, plcA, hly, mpl, actA* and *plcB* (Portnoy *et al.*, 1992). The transcription of these virulence genes is strictly controlled by PrfA, ensuring that the gene products are only synthesized when the bacteria indeed need them in the phagosome or cytosol of infected cells (Bohne *et al.*, 1996; Dietrich *et al.*, 1998; Renzoni *et al.*, 1999). The crucial step for the listerial infection pattern, the disruption of the phagosomal membrane, is achieved by means of listeriolysin O (encoded by *hly*), a member of the cholesterol-binding, sulfhydryl-activated cytolysin group and a phospholipase C (*plcA*). Once inside the cytosol, the bacteria polymerize the host cell actin, resulting in intracellular movement. The actin polymerization is mediated by the *actA* gene product (Tilney and Portnoy, 1989). Actin-mediated formation of cellular protrusions containing the bacterium and lysis of these protrusions by listeriolysin and the *plcB*-encoded phospholipase C leads to direct infection

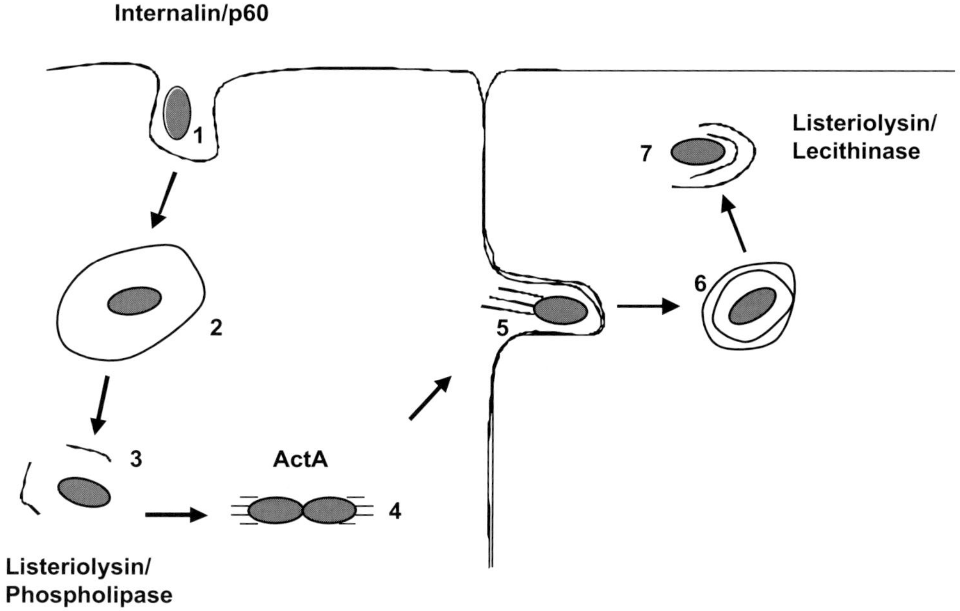

Internalin/p60

Listeriolysin/ Lecithinase

Listeriolysin/ Phospholipase

ActA

Figure 1. Infection of professional antigen presenting cell (APC) by *L. monocytogenes* and intracellular life style of the bacterium. (1) *L. monocytogenes* adheres to APC and is phagocytosed. Internalins and the p60 protein are involved in these processes. (2) *L. monocytogenes* inside the phagosome of the APC. (3) *L. monocytogenes* escapes from the phagosomal compartment by lysis of the phagosomal membrane due to the production of listeriolysin and phospholipase C. (4) *L. monocytogenes* bacteria replicate in the host cell cytosol. Synthesis of the ActA protein results in polymerization of host cell actin and intracellular movement of the bacteria. (5) Spreading to neighbouring cells by formation of pseudopod-like structures. (6) *L. monocytogenes* in a neighbouring cell inside a double membrane-bound vacuole. (7) Direct spreading to the cytosol of neighbouring cells due to lysis of the double membrane of the vacuole by listeriolysin and lecithinase.

of neighbouring cells (Portnoy *et al.*, 1992). This phopholipase is finally processed posttranslationally by the metalloprotease encoded by the *mpl* gene (Ravenau *et al.*, 1992).

The natural properties of *L. monocytogenes* make this bacterium particularly attractive as a potential live vaccine vector for the induction of cell-mediated immunity to foreign antigens. Secreted proteins of *L. monocytogenes* are introduced directly into the phagocytic and cytosolic compartments of APC and hence they have access to both the MHC class II and MHC class I antigen processing and presentation pathways (Figure 2) (Weiskirch and Paterson, 1997; Pamer, 1998; Kerksiek and Pamer, 1999). *L. monocytogenes* strains

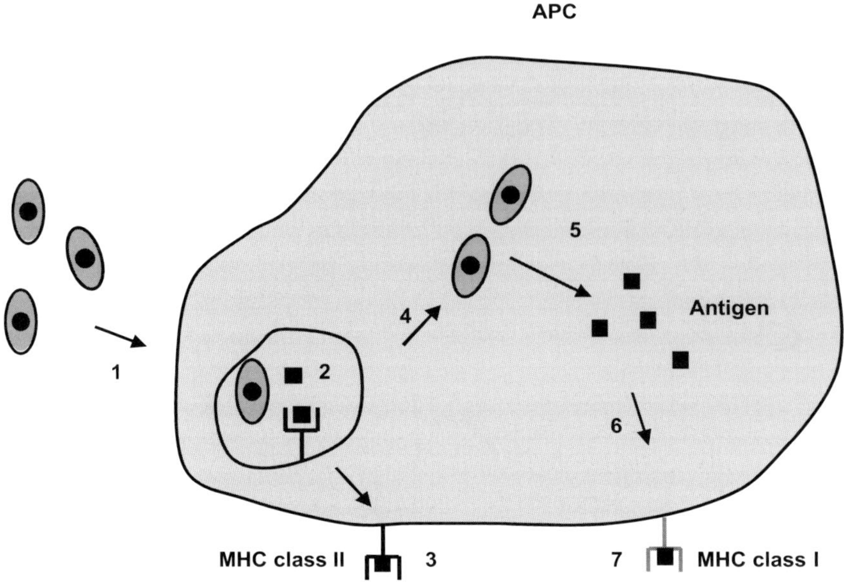

Figure 2. Delivery of heterologous antigens to APC by *L. monocytogenes*. (1) Recombinant *L. monocytogenes* infect an APC. (2) Expression of heterologous antigens in the phagosome leads to processing and (3) presentation together with MHC class II molecules. (4) Escape of recombinant *L. monocytogenes* into the host cell cytosol (5) Antigen expression in the cytosol (6) Processing of antigens by the proteasome and presentation in the context of MHC class I molecules

are therefore ideal candidates for the elicitation of a cell-mediated immune response (Busch *et al.*, 1998). Mutants of *L. monocytogenes* which are unable to enter the cytosol are absolutely avirulent, immunization with such strains does not result in antigen presentation in the context of MHC class I (Hiltbold *et al.*, 1996) and fails to induce protective immunity against wild-type *L. monocytogenes* (Barry *et al.*, 1992; Brunt *et al.*, 1990, Michel *et al.*, 1990). Because it is transmitted by oral exposure, *L. monocytogenes* should be especially suitable for generating mucosal immunity.

INTERACTION OF *L. MONOCYTOGENES* WITH APC

Moreover, *L. monocytogenes* preferentially infects monocytes (Kaufmann, 1998). Phagocytic cells like macrophages and dendritic cells (DCs) are the key APC, and the interaction of *L. monocytogenes* with both cell types has been analysed in great detail. *L. monocytogenes* can infect macrophages with high efficiency, and depending on the receptor the macrophage uses to engulf the bacteria and the amount of cell-surface interleukin 10, the microorganisms are either rapidly killed within the phagosome or can escape into the host cell cytosol, where they can replicate (Fleming and Campbell, 1997). Macrophages respond to infection with *L. monocytogenes* by the transient or persistent activation of host cell signal transduction pathways. In addition, *L. monocytogenes* infection influences expression of various macrophage genes, some of which may hinder or favour bacterial replication (Kuhn and Goebel, 1994, 1998). The production of different proinflammatory cytokines by *L. monocytogenes*-infected macrophages may not only provide important adjuvant effects for vaccination purposes, but may also allow modulation of the immune response as desired.

Dendritic cells (DCs) are the most potent APC known and play a crucial role in initiation and modulation of a specific immune response (Bancherau and Steinman, 1998). *L. monocytogenes* is efficiently internalized by DCs. Some authors found the listeriae to be localized mostly in the phagosomal compartment of DCs and rarely free in the cytosol (Kolb-Mäurer *et al.*, 2000; Gentschev *et al.*, 2000). This predominantly phagosomal localization of *L. monocytogenes* in DCs results in a rapid lysis of the majority of the intracellular bacteria in this cell type, in contrast to the situation in macrophage cells (Kolb-Mäurer *et al.*, 2000, Gentschev *et al.*, 2000 and 2001). In another study, however, the bacteria were observed to be escaping rapidly from the phagosomal compartment of DCs into the host cell cytosol cytosol and listeriolysin was found not to be essential for this phagosomal escape (Paschen *et al.*, 2000).

Infection by *L. monocytogenes* causes maturation of the immature DCs and strong upregulation of CD83, CD25, MHC class II, and the costimulatory molecule B7-2. The lipoteichoic acid (LTA) of *L. monocytogenes* seems to be responsible for this effect (Kolb-Mäurer *et al.*, 2000; Gentschev *et al.*, 2000 and 2001; Paschen *et al.*, 2000). DC maturation is known to correlate with enhanced antigen presentation capacity and strong stimulation of listeriolysin-specific CD4+ T cells by *L. monocytogenes*-infected DCs was observed (Paschen *et al.*, 2000). Attenuated *L. monocytogenes* strains could hence become a valuable tool for subunit vaccine delivery to macrophages as well as DCs.

ATTENUATION OF *L. MONOCYTOGENES*

L. monocytogenes is a human pathogen which can cause disease in even mildly immunocompromised hosts, including pregnant women and neonates, and can not be used as such for vaccination purposes. Two different approaches have been pursued for attenuation of *L. monocytogenes*: inactivation of listerial virulence factors or construction of auxotrophic mutant strains. Reduction of the virulence of *L. monocytogenes* has mainly been achieved by deletion of genes responsible for intracellular motility and cell-to-cell spreading (Barry *et al.*, 1992; Goossens *et al.*, 1992, Paglia *et al.*, 1997; Dietrich *et al.*, 1998). Mutations of the *hly* gene were shown to result in an attenuated phenotype of *L. monocytogenes* (Brunt *et al.*, 1990; Michel *et al.*, 1990). By transposon mutagenesis, Barry *et al.* (1992) identified mutations in the *hly* or *plcB* genes leading to reduced hemolytic and phospholipase C activities, respectively, as attenuating the virulence of *L. monocytogenes*. Inactivation of these genes significantly increased the lethal dose 50 (LD$_{50}$) 10^3- to 10^5-fold. Infection with a sublethal dose of the mutants induced protection in mice against a later challenge with a normally lethal challenge inoculum of wildtype *L. monocytogenes*. While bacteria carrying mutations in the *hly* gene are certainly avirulent, this attenuation comes at the prize of failure to present antigens for CD8+ T cell-activation (Brunt *et al.*, 1990; Michel *et al.*, 1990). A more targeted attenuation was performed by mutation of the *actA* gene (Goosens *et al.*, 1992). This mutant exhibited an LD$_{50}$ which was increased by 1000-fold and induced long-lasting immunity against *L. monocytogenes* challenge infections. Similarly, a deletion of the *mpl* gene encoding the metalloprotease leads to attenuation of *L. monocytogenes* (Paglia *et al.*, 1997). Finally, a triple mutant was constructed, lacking the *mpl*, *actA* and *plcB* genes (Dietrich *et al.*, 1998). This mutant is able to infect APC and to escape from the phagosomal compartment with equal efficiency as wildtype *L. monocytogenes*, but once located in the host cell cytosol, the bacteria are unable to polymerize host cell actin and to spread to neighbouring cells. This mutant therefore exhibited a highly attenuated phenotype and the LD$_{50}$ was 10^3-fold higher as that of wildtype bacteria (Dietrich *et al.*, 1998).

As an alternative to the deletion of virulence genes, auxotrophic mutant strains have been constructed (Alexander *et al.*, 1993; Thompson *et al.*, 1998; Friedman, 2000; Rayevskaya and Frankel, 2001). A transposon insert mutant of *L. monocytogenes* was shown to be deficient in prephenate dehydratase, an enzyme acting in the late pathway for phenylalanine biosynthesis. (Alexander *et al.*, 1993). This mutant strain exhibited a reduced virulence in the murine model and mice vaccinated with the mutant were protected against subsequent challenge with *L. monocytogenes*. D-Alanine is required for the synthesis of the mucopeptide component of the cell walls of virtually all bacteria and is found almost exclusively in the microbial world. A *L. monocytogenes* strain requiring D-alanine for growth was constructed by deleting large portions of the genes for D-alanine biosynthesis, alanine racemase (*dal*) and D-amino acid aminotransferase (*dat*) (Thompson *et al.*, 1998). This mutant strain can be grown *in vitro* when supplemented with D-alanine but is unable to grow outside the laboratory, particularly in the cytoplasm of eukaryotic host cells, the natural habitat of *L. monocytogenes* during infection. In mice, the double-mutant strain was attenuated. The LD_{50} of the double mutant was 7×10^7 when inoculated with D-alanine and 8×10^8 when given without D-alanine, as compared to 10^4 for wildtype *L. monocytogenes*. The double mutant strain was able to induce a cytotoxic T-lymphocyte response and to generate protective immunity against lethal challenge by wild-type *L. monocytogenes* (Thompson *et al.*, 1998) if D-alanine is provided after inoculation (Friedman *et al.*, 2000). This is due to the fact that the double mutant is unable to escape from the phagolysosome of infected cells in the absence of exogenous D-alanine (Friedman *et al.*, 2000). In contrast to reduction of listerial pathgogenicity by deletion of virulence factors, the construction of auxotrophic mutant strains allows controlling the release of recombinant bacteria to the environment.

The adaptation of signature-tagged mutagenesis (STM, Autret *et al.*, 2001) and the utilization of fluorescence technologies to find *in vivo*-induced genes (Wilson *et al.*, 2001) recently allowed the identification of novel attenuating mutations, several of which were found to be localized in previously unknown genes (Autret *et al.*, 2001; Wilson *et al.*, 2001).

ANTIGEN DELIVERY BY *LISTERIA MONOCYTOGENES*

The first report on successful delivery of heterologous antigens by recombinant *L. monocytogenes* was published in 1992 (Schafer *et al.*, 1992). β-galactosidase was expressed in *L. monocytogenes* and immunization of mice resulted in a β-galactosidase-specific CTL response and an only weak humoral response against the recombinant antigen. Since the cell-mediated immune response is particularly important for the clearance of viruses and tumors, *L. monocytogenes* has been exploited for the expression of a wide range of viral (Ikonomidis *et al.*, 1994 and 1997; Frankel *et al.*, 1995; Shen *et al.*, 1995) as well as tumor antigens (Schafer *et al.*, 1992; Pan *et al.*, 1995a, 1995b, and 1999; Paglia *et al.*, 1997). Additionally, an antigen from the parasite *Leishmania major* has recently been cloned in *L. monocytogenes* (Soussi *et al.*, 2000). Here, we will focus on the expression of antigens from viral and parasitic pathogens in *L. monocytogenes* while tumor vaccination is covered by Gunn, Zubair and Paterson in chapter 14 of this volume.

L. monocytogenes was used for the expression and secretion of antigens from influenza virus (Ikonomidis *et al.*, 1994), human immunodeficiency virus (HIV, Frankel *et al.*, 1995), lymphocytic choriomeningitis virus (LCMV, Shen *et al.*, 1995) and cottontail rabbit papilloma virus (Jensen *et al.*, 1997). For stable expression, the antigen-encoding genes were inserted into the listerial genome in most cases except for the study by Ikonomidis *et al.* (1994). In that case, the heterologous antigen was encoded on a plasmid vector.

The influenza virus nucleoprotein was expressed in *L. monocytogenes* fused with the N-terminal secretion signal of listeriolysin (Ikonomidis *et al.*, 1994), as it is generally assumed that secreted bacterial antigens have enhanced access to the immune system (Kaufmann, 1998). Expression of the fusion protein in addition to native listeriolysin ensured direct antigen delivery into the host cell cytosol (Figure 2). Consequently, infection by the recombinant *L. monocytogenes* strain secreting the listeriolysin-NP fusion protein targeted cells for lysis by NP-specific class I-restricted T cells (Ikonomidis *et al.*, 1994). A listeriolysin-negative recombinant *L. monocytogenes* strain expressing the fusion protein was able to present in a MHC class II-dependent manner, failed, however, to introduce the recombinant antigen into the MHC class I-dependent pathway for antigen processing and presentation (Ikonomidis *et al.*, 1994), emphasizing the crucial role of listeriolysin for cytosolic antigen delivery. Immunization of mice expressing either full-length influenza NP or a Kd-restricted epitope (NP147-154), induced a NP-specific CTL response and led to protection against influenza virus infection equalling the efficacy of recombinant vaccinia expressing NP (Ikonomidis *et al.*, 1994).

While initial attempts to control human immundeficiency virus (HIV) infection and development of acquired immune deficiency syndrome (AIDS) were based on elicitation of a humoral immune response, the elicitation of a CTL-response against AIDS experiences increasing appreciation (Shen and Siliciano, 2000). Delivery of HIV antigens by *L. monocytogenes* may provide a promising approach for HIV-vaccination (Mata and Paterson, 2000). HIV Gag, Nef and Env proteins were expressed and secreted by *L. monocytogenes*. Immunization of mice with *L. monocytogenes* engineered to express the p55 HIV Gag gene product led to a strong antigen-specific CTL response (Frankel *et al.*, 1995; Mata *et al.*, 1998; Guzman *et al.*, 1998). In addition, recombinant *L. monocytogenes* expressing Gag were shown to induce Th1-type CD4+ T cells (Mata and Paterson, 1999). These Gag-specific CD8+ and CD4+ T cell responses were able to protect mice against a challenge infection with recombinant vaccinia virus expressing HIV Gag (Mata *et al.*, 2001). Recombinant *L. monocytogenes* are also suitable for antigen delivery in human cells. Infection of human macrophages and DCs with recombinant *L. monocytogenes* expressing an Env T helper epitope demonstrated that heterologous antigen expression in recombinant *L. monocytogenes* results in the presentation of this epitope together with MHC class II molecules and proliferation of an Env-specific T cell line (Guzman *et al.*, 1998). Infection of human monocytes by recombinant *L. monocytogenes* expressing and secreting either HIV Gag or Nef leads to antigen presentation in the context of MHC class I and the *in vitro* induction of CD8+ T cells of HIV-infected donors. This is also true for the attenuated mutant strain lacking alanine racemase (*dal*) and D-amino acid aminotransferase (*dat*). A *daldat* double mutant expressing HIV-Gag is as efficient as virulent recombinant *L. monocytogenes* at boosting Gag-specific human CTLs under *in vitro* conditions (Friedman *et al.*, 2000). Similarly, immunization of mice via the parenteral and oral route with attenuated recombinant *L. monocytogenes daldat* mutants expressing Gag induced a strong CTL response and protection against challenge with recombinant vaccinia virus expressing HIV-Gag (Rayevskaja and Frankel, 2001). However, while the parenteral immunization induced a long-lasting, memory CTL response as well as systemic and mucosal immunity, oral delivery resulted in a transient CTL response and provided protection only against mucosal challenge (Rayevskaja and Frankel, 2001).

Recombinant *L. monocytogenes* are also suitable for vaccination against lymphocytic choriomeningitis virus (LCMV). The interaction between LCMV and its natural host, the mouse, has been used extensively for the analysis of an antiviral CD8+ T cell response and provides an excellent model system to investigate the utility of recombinant *L. monocytogenes* strains for CTL-mediated protection. Recovery from and protection against acute infections with LCMV are almost exclusively dependent on CD8+ T cells, and antibodies initially play only a role for long-term viral control. Protection against intravenous reinfection or reinfection via mucosal surfaces is mediated by neutralizing antibodies. In contrast, activated CTLs that can migrate immediately into infected tissues appear crucial for protection against direct secondary infection (Zinkernagel *et al.*, 1996). In recombinant *L. monocytogenes*, the LCMV nucleoprotein or a CTL epitope thereof was expressed under the control of the listerial *actA* and *hly* promoters and the respective signal sequences were employed for efficient secretion of the antigens (Shen *et al.*, 1995; Goossens *et al.*, 1995). Mice immunized with these recombinant *L. monocytogenes* strains mounted vigorous anti-viral CD8+ T cell and CD4+ T cell responses and controlled and cleared LCMV infection through CD8+ T cell-mediated mechanisms (Shen *et al.*, 1995; Goossens *et al.*, 1995). However, single immunization with recombinant

L. monocytogenes induced memory T cells that first required reactivation before they were able to protect against LCMV (Ochsenbein *et al.*, 1999). This may be due to short persistence of the recombinant *L. monocytogenes* bacteria which are detectable only until day 8 after infection (Ochsenbein *et al.*, 1999). Booster immunizations may provide a means of enhancing these long-term immune responses. A memory CTL response induced by recombinant *L. monocytogenes* strains can interestingly be boosted by a second recombinant *L. monocytogenes* vaccination (Slifka *et al.*, 1996). With live vaccines, one of the inherent difficulties for multiple vaccinations is that the immunity induced against the vector itself often limits its usefulness for revaccination (Cooney *et al.*, 1991).

L. monocytogenes has also been employed for the delivery of antigens from the parasite *Leishmania major* (Soussi *et al.*, 2001). In this experimental setting, the main goal was the elicitation of a strong Th1 type CD4+ T cell response. Infection of mice with *L. major* results, depending on the mouse strain, either in localized self-healing lesions in *L. major* resistant mice (strain B10.D2) or in nonhealing lesions in susceptible animals (strain BALB/c). Resistance and susceptibility have been shown to rely on the preferential expansion of *Leishmania*-reactive Th1 and Th2 type CD4+ T lymphocytes, respectively. In susceptible mice, efficient immunization has been obtained by coadministration of leishmanial antigens together with IL-12 as an adjuvant (Alfonso *et al.*, 1994). Immunization with *L. monocytogenes* recombinantly expressing leishmanial antigens may be a promising approach due to the inherent IL-12 inducing adjuvant activity of the bacterium itself (Mielke *et al.*, 1997). The *L. major* LACK antigen (*Leihmania* homologue of receptors for activated C kinase) was cloned in frame with the listeriolysin secretion signal under the control of the *hly* promoter. (Soussi *et al.*, 2001). The plasmid vector was transformed into a *L. monocytogenes actA* mutant strain where it was maintained in an episomal form rather than inserted into the listerial genome. *In vitro*, these bacteria were shown to efficiently express and secrete the LACK antigen. BALB/c as well as B10.D2 mice were immuniced with the recombinant *L. monocytogenes*-LACK bacteria. The LACK-dependant T lymphocyte stimulation was very brief due to rapid plasmid loss of the bacteria, 24 h post immunization, only 1% of the injected bacteria still harbored the plasmid vector. Nevertheless, in both mouse strains, a short-lived, LACK-specific T cell response was detected. The cytokine profile was consistent with expansion of Th1 CD4+ T cells secreting IFN-γ and IL-2, but not IL-4. This response was much stronger in the *L. major*-resistant B10.D2 mice than in the BALB/c mouse strain. Accordingly, after challenge infection with *L. major*, control of lesion progression could be observed in B10.D2 mice, but only after the mice had received two injections of recombinant *L. monocytogenes*-LACK. In BALB/c-mice, in contrast, the progressive form of the disease could not be restrained (Soussi *et al.*, 2001). The reason may be that the IL-12 secretion after listerial infection with the *actA* mutant strain is short-lived due to the attenuated phenotype of the bacteria resulting in short *in vivo* persistence (Soussi *et al.*, 2001). Another reason may be the rapid plasmid shedding of the listerial carriers, which may result in a very weak antigen delivery.

As an alternative to antigen expression in the bacterial carrier, *L. monocytogenes* can also be employed to promote translocation of soluble exogenous antigens into the cytosolic compartment of APC. Infection of macrophage cells with wild-type *L. monocytogenes* in the presence of soluble ovalbumin resulted in efficient presentation of ovalbumin-derived epitopes together with MHC class I molecules. This was not the case when a listerial strain lacking listeriolysin was used or when TAP$^{-/-}$ macrophage cells were infected (Mazzaccaro *et al.*, 1996).

COMPARTMENTALIZATION OF ANTIGEN DELIVERY

For heterologous antigens delivered by recombinant carriers, expression level, stability, localization and subcellular site of antigen delivery are expected to have significant impact on the development of an antigen-specific CTL response and protective immunity. In most recombinant *L. monocytogenes* strains, the heterologous antigens were fused with the N-terminal secretion signals of listeriolysin or ActA, since it is believed that antigen secretion by intracellular pathogens is required for the elicitation of an efficient CTL response (Hess *et al.*, 1996, 1997). Interestingly, recent studies have shown that secretion of the heterologous antigens by recombinant *L. monocytogenes* is not essential for the elicitation of a T cell response (Paglia *et al.*, 1997; Shen *et al.*, 1998; Guzman *et al.*, 1998; Tvinnereim and Harty, 2000). Immunizations with a listerial strain expressing either secreted or cytoplasmic forms of a CTL epitope of β-galactosidase resulted in equal protective efficacies against challenge with a β-gal-expressing fibrosarcoma (Paglia *et al.*, 1997). Similarly, a pair of recombinant *L. monocytogenes* strains was constructed which express a LCMV nucleoprotein CTL epitope in the context of carrier proteins which are either exported or restricted to the listerial cyotoplasm (Shen *et al.*, 1998). Immunizing doses of as little as 10^3 recombinant *L. monocytogenes* bacteria induced almost equal magnitudes of T cell reactivity against the heterologous antigen and the listerial antigens p60 and listeriolysin. Both strains elicited LCMV-NP-specific memory and protective immunity against LCMV. Finally, recombinant *L. monocytogenes* strains expressing a HIV gp120 helper T cell epitope in either secreted, surface-bound or cytoplamsic form resulted in similar efficiency of antigen presentation in the context of MHC class II molecules (Guzman *et al.*, 1998). This is in contrast to antigen delivery by recombinant *Salmonella* strains (Hess *et al.*, 1996, and 1997). In the case of recombinant *Salmonella*, heterologous antigens like the listerial antigens p60, listeriolysin and superoxide dismutase (SOD) need to be secreted by the vaccine delivery strains for the induction of an efficient CTL response and protective immunity against *L. monocytogenes* infection. An explanation for this differential importance of antigen compartimentalization in the recombinant carriers might be that a substantial fraction (about 90%) of *L. monocytogenes* bacteria is killed in the phagosome of macrophages prior to *L. monocytogenes* escape into the cytosol (de Chastellier and Berche, 1994). At this stage of infection the bacteria are already producing high amounts of listeriolysin, so they are able to break the phagosomal membrane despite being lysed themselves by the host cell. The contents of the bacterial cytoplasm released into the phagosome might thus be able to enter the host cell cytosol. However, the antimicrobial activities of gamma interferon are interestingly not required for the CTL response of IFN-γ knockout mice against LCMV-NP expressed by *L. monocytogenes* in a nonsecreted form (Tvinnereim and Harty, 2000). As an alternative, listeriae escaping from the phagosome of the infected cell may nevertheless undergo lysis in the cytosol, releasing the nonsecreted antigens directly to this host cell compartment.

Correct compartimentalization of antigen delivery within the host cell instead seems to be more important for delivery by recombinant *L. monocytogenes*. Expression of the fusion proteins under the control of either the *hly*- or the *actA*-promotor warrants antigen expression in the infected host cell. In addition, efficient delivery into the host cell cytosol is of equal importance for recombinant *L. monocytogenes* and recombinant *Salmonella*. Listeriolysin-negative mutant strains fail to induce protection against wild-type *L. monocytogenes* (Barry *et al.*, 1992; Brunt *et al.*, 1990, Michel *et al.*, 1990). Hence, the expression of active listeriolysin is a key determinant for the efficacy of listerial vaccine strains. Therefore, direct heterologous antigen expression and secretion into the cytosol of the infected cell seems to be optimal for effcient processing and presentation by the MHC class I pathway and the induction of a CTL response, as shown for influenza-NP (Ikonomidis *et al.*, 1994). Similar to recombinant *L. monocytogenes*, recombinant *Salmonella* having access to the cytosol of infected cells by secretion of hemolytically active listeriolysin induce a greatly enhanced CTL response and protection in comparison to isogenic strains expressing and secreting a hemolytically inactive version of listeriolysin (Hess *et al.*, 2000). While the escape of recombinant *L. monocytogenes* strains into the host cell cytosol is very important for antigen presentation in the context of MHC class I molecules, the expression of listeriolysin seems to have a minor impact on presentation together with MHC class II. *L. monocytogenes hly* and *actA* deletion mutants were constructed which express a MHC class II-restricted epitope of HIV Env. Infection of human APC (macrophages and DCs) with these two strains - which are retained either in the phagosome (*hly* mutant) or in the cytosol (*actA* mutant) of infected cells - resulted in similar efficacy of presentation of the HIV Env T helper cell epitope in the context of MHC class II (Guzman *et al.*, 1998).

In future studies, the importance of optimal antigen compartmentalization for the outcome of vaccinations should be addressed for a wide range of antigens. While the secretion of LCMV-NP did not seem to be crucial for elicitation of protection in this particular model, this may not hold true for all antigens. In addition, many proteins that may be attractive antigens for generating cellular immune responses may not be efficiently secreted by recombinant *L. monocytogenes*. While the influence of antigen compartmentalization within the delivery vehicle itself is not clear, it is with no doubt, however, that the delivery of the vaccines to the cytosol of the infected cells is absolutely crucial for an efficient CTL response. The expression of hemolytically active listeriolysin is one of the most important features of recombinant *L. monocytogenes* for vaccine delivery and should therefore not be altered.

DNA Vaccine Delivery By *L. monocytogenes*

L. monocytogenes can not only be employed for the delivery of heterologous antigens expressed by the bacterium, but also for delivery of DNA vaccine vectors leading to antigen expression by infected host cells. A strain attenuated by deletion of the genes *mpl*, *actA* and *plcB* was employed (Dietrich *et al.*, 1998). Delivery of the plasmid DNA into the cytosol was achieved by specific autolysis of the bacteria in this compartment (Figure 3). To this end, a gene encoding the lysis protein of a *Listeria*-specific bacteriophage was cloned under the control of the listerial *actA*-promoter, which is preferentially active in the host cell cytosol. Bacteria harbouring this transcription unit undergo rapid lysis upon entering the cytosol of the host cell (Dietrich *et al.*, 1998). This attenuated suicide strain of *L. monocytogenes* was used as a vehicle for the delivery of plasmid vectors carrying either the *gfp*-gene (coding for the

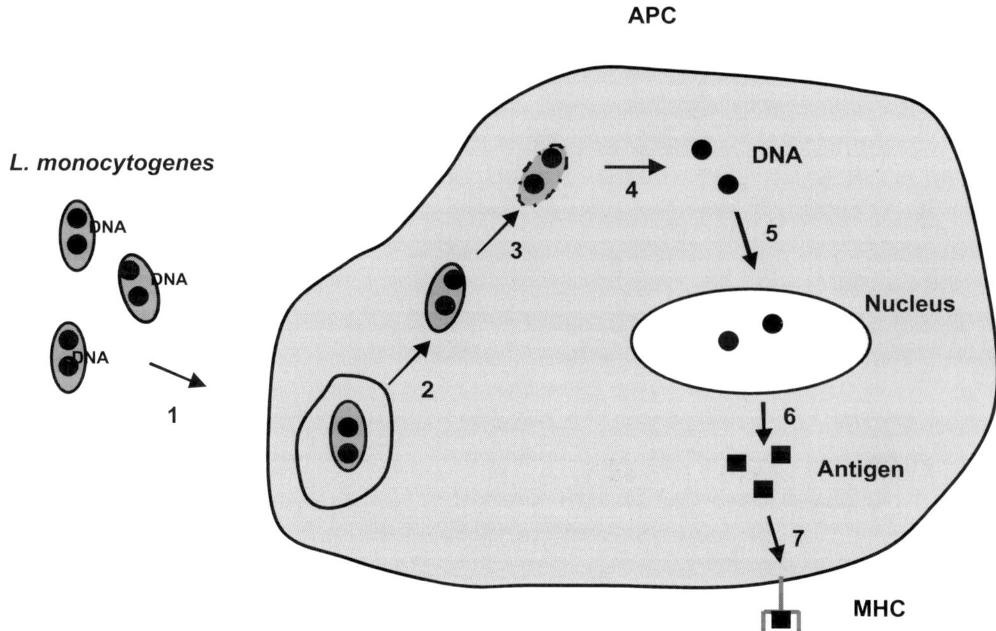

Figure 3. Delivery of DNA vaccines to APC by *L. monocytogenes*. (1) Recombinant *L. monocytogenes* carrying DNA vaccine vectors infect an APC. (2) Escape of recombinant *L. monocytogenes* into the host cell cytosol. (3) Autolysis of the bacteria due to expression of phage lysin under the control of P_{actA}. (4) Release of plasmid DNA into the cytosol of APC. (5) Plasmid DNA enters host cell nucleus. (6) Antigen expression by APC. (7) Processing of antigens and presentation together with MHC molecules.

green fluorescent protein, GFP) or the *cat*-gene (encoding chloramphenicol acetyl tranferase, CAT) under the control of the CMV-promoter. Efficient plasmid delivery and subsequent GFP- and CAT-expression were obtained in a murine macrophage-like cell line (Dietrich *et al.*, 1998) as well as in murine fibroblast cells (G. Dietrich, S. Gfrörer and I. Gentschev, unpublished data).

Attenuated suicide *L. monocytogenes* are also suitable for the delivery of plasmid DNA in primary APC. Infection of bone marrow-derived macrophages (BMM) from BALB/c mice with bacteria harbouring a eukaryotic GFP-expression vector led to strong GFP-expression by the macrophage cells (Spreng *et al.*, 2000). The expression of heterologous antigens after listerial plasmid delivery results in efficient processing and presentation together with MHC class I molecules. This could be shown with a DNA vaccine vector encoding the major H-2K^b T cell epitope from chicken ovalbumin (OVA$_{257-264}$). When this plasmid was delivered to BMM by attenuated suicide *L. monocytogenes*, the T cell epitope was presented efficiently together with MHC class I molecules, as shown by the activation of a OVA$_{257\text{-}264}$-specific T cell hybridoma (Dietrich *et al.*, 1998). Attenuated suicide *L. monocytogenes* can also deliver eukaryotic expression vectors into dendritic cells. Infection of immature human blood dendritic cells with attenuated suicide *L. monocytogenes* carrying a GFP-expression vector resulted in a significant portion of the infected cells expressing GFP (Kolb-Mäurer *et al.*, 2000; Gentschev *et al.*, 2000 and 2001). Interestingly, the rapid lysis of the listeriae in the host cell phagosome of DCs is not detrimental for plasmid delivery to this cell type. *L. monocytogenes* strains could therefore become a valuable tool for subunit vaccine delivery to DC.

An alternative to the autolysis of intracellular listeriae due to expression of a phage lysin is the killing of the bacteria by the addition of antibiotics for plasmid release. Employing tetracyclin-mediated lysis of intracytosolic *L. monocytogenes*, Hense *et al.* (2001) could achieve delivery of eukaryotic β-galactosidase- and GFP-expression vectors to a wide range of cell types *in vitro*, including human larynx and lung carcinoma cells, mouse macrophages, hamster and Kangaroo rat kidney cells. In several cell lines, this strategy was superior to conventional means of transfection like $CaPO_4$-mediated plasmid transfer (Hense *et al.*, 2001). However, in a direct comparison of phage lysin-mediated plasmid delivery and killing of intracellular bacteria by treatment with the antibiotics penicillin and streptomycin, the latter was demonstrated to result in the transfection of a markedly lower proportion of cells (Dietrich *et al.*, 1998).

Efficient invasion of the bacteria is an important prerequisite for plasmid delivery by *L. monocytogenes* to nonphagocytic cell types like human nasopharyngeal and lung epithelial cells as well as Kangaroo rat kidney cells. Deletion of *inlA* and *inlB* impaired the plasmid delivery drastically (Hense *et al.*, 2001). In addition, the phagosomal escape function mediated by listeriolysin and the phospholipases PlcA and PlcB is crucial for plasmid transfer to the cytosol of infected cells. *L. monocytogenes* mutant strains lacking listeriolysin, PlcA and PlcB are virtually unable to transfect cell lines *in vitro* (Hense *et al.*, 2001).

Recently, *in vivo* delivery of eukaryotic antigen expression vectors by attenuated suicide *L. monocytogenes* was demonstrated. Intraperitoneal (i.p.) injection of attenuated suicide *L. monocytogenes* results in delivery of a GFP-expression vector to peritoneal macrophages (Spreng *et al.*, 2000). Hence, the *in vivo* delivery of DNA vaccines by attenuated suicide *L. monocytogenes* should be suitable for the elicitation of a strong humoral and cellular immune response against plasmid-encoded antigens. The suitability of the antibiotics-mediated delivery strategy for *in vivo* plasmid delivery remains to be addressed. Additionally, this method may not be suitable for general vaccination purposes due to the need to apply antibiotics in order to achieve optimal vaccine potency.

Whereas the spreading-negative mutant strain of *L. monocytogenes* lacking the *mpl*, *actA* and *plcB* genes is highly attenuated due to its inability to move intra- and intercellularly, the intracellular expression of the *Listeria*-specific phage lysin further increases the attenuation of the bacteria. This may offer an additional containment measure, which is important especially for the use of such live vaccines in clinical settings (Spreng *et al.*, 2000).

An important issue concerning the safety of DNA vaccines is their possible integration into the host cell genome, which might potentiate oncogenesis (Donnelly *et al.*, 1997). Integration of DNA vacine vectors is hence not acceptable in vaccine settings. For both modes of listerial plasmid delivery, chromosomal integration was found at least *in vitro* (Dietrich *et al.*, 1998; Hense *et al.*, 2001). These findings may be due to the high plasmid copy numbers which are delivered to each single cell by the bacterial carriers, furthermore they still await an *in vivo* evaluation. Additionally, the cells carrying genomic integrations should ultimately be destroyed by the CTL response against plasmid encoded antigens (Davis *et al.*, 1998) and antigens derived from the carrier bacteria (Kaufmann, 1998).

ADJUVANT EFFECT OF *L. MONOCYTOGENES*

Infection with *L. monocytogenes* induces the production of a variety of cytokines; among these, IL-12, IL-2, IL-1, IFN-γ and TNF-α have significant protective roles during primary or secondary listerial infection in the mouse (Kaufmann, 1998, Kuhn and Goebel, 1994 and 1998). Development of CD4+ T cells is influenced by the cytokines present in the local microenvironment. The listerial cell wall component lipoteichoic acid (LTA) stimulates IL-12 expression by macrophages through a CD14-mediated pathway (Cleveland *et al.*, 1996). IL-12 in turn is well-known to stimulate the production of IFN-γ by NK cells and T cells which leads to a TH1 type CD4+ T cell development, activates the microbicidal activities of phagocytic cells and promotes the generation of a cell mediated immune response. The listerial LTA additionally induces the maturation of human DCs (Gentschev *et al.*, 2000).

Several virulence factors of *L. monocytogenes*, including listeriolysin and the two phospholipases, have been shown to have significant impact on the responses of host cells on listerial infections. Macrophages, DCs, epithelial and endothelial cells respond to listerial infection by the transient or persistent activation of host cell signal transduction pathways. This, in turn, results in the differential regulation of several cytokines, cytokine receptors and components of the MHC complexes (Kuhn and Goebel, 1994 and 1998). In general, listerial infection results in the induction of a strong cellular response including CTL and T helper type 1 immunity to the carrier itself, but also to passenger antigens and vaccines delivered by recombinant *L. monocytogenes*.

REQUIREMENTS FOR APPLICATION OF RECOMBINANT *L. MONOCYTOGENES* IN HUMANS

Intriguingly, most studies on recombinant *L. monocytogenes*-based vaccine delivery have been performed in the murine model, with the exception of one single study, in which rabbits were immunized (Jensen *et al.*, 1997). While recombinant *L. monocytogenes* are certainly an excellent tool to study vaccination approaches resulting in cellular immunity, vaccine researchers are apparently hesitating to employ them in a clinical setting. Only tests in primates and especially clinical studies with rationally designed attenuated mutant strains of *L. monocytogenes* which have been shown to be safe in appropriate animal models will reveal whether recombinant *L. monocytogenes* strains have a general value for vaccination purposes aiming at the elicitation of a CTL response. There are, however, several aspects of recombinant *L. monocytogenes* as vaccine delivery vehicles which have to be addressed in more detail before such clinical studies should be started.

First of all, the safety of *L. monocytogenes* as vaccine vehicle has to be assessed. Attenuated live vaccines have to strike a delicate balance, in which they must retain their immunostimulatory capacity without having pathogenic effects. While bacterial live vaccines like attenuated *Salmonellae* and *Mycobacterium bovis* BCG have been used in humans for decades and have been shown to be sufficiently safe, this is not clear for *L. monocytogenes*. Several attenuating mutations have been identified for *L. monocytogenes* (Barry *et al.*, 1992; Alexander *et al.*, 1993; Goosens *et al.*, 1995; Paglia *et al.*, 1997; Dietrich *et al.*, 1998; Thompson *et al.*, 1998). Promising novel mutations have been found by STM (Autret *et al.*, 2001). These attenuated strains must be evaluated very carefully in a wide range of experimental animals before clinical trials can be envisaged, especially in the case of immunocompromization. Appropriate mutations of the listerial invasins (like InlA and InlB) may increase the tropism for professional APC, thereby decreasing the side-effects and risks associated with the infection of other cell types. While the attenuated strains have to be sufficiently safe, at the same time, they have to retain the favorable immunological proterties of wild-type *L. monocytogenes*. Rather than attenuating *L. monocytogenes*, the addition of specific virulence genes to non-pathogenic *Listeria* species such as *L. innocua* may offer an attractive alternative approach (Darji *et al.*, 1995). Another obstacle to the general employment of recombinant *L. monocytogenes* vaccine carriers may be the inherent plasmid instability in the absence of selection (Ikonomidis *et al.*, 1994). While for the recombinant expression of heterologous antigens, the integration of the expression cassettes into the listerial genome proved to be a sufficient approach, for the delivery of DNA vaccine vectors, alternative modes have to be found for stable episomal replication. In recombinant *Salmonella* strains, this problem has been solved by the construction of vectors containing an essential gene which was deleted from the bacterial genome, leading to stable maintenance of the plasmid vector without antibiotic selection even under *in vivo* conditions (Curtiss *et al.*, 1990). For *L. monocytogenes* it has been shown that the placement of the *prfA* gene on a plasmid construct enforces retention of this vector in a *prfA*-negative *L. monocytogenes* mutant strain even under *in vivo* conditions (Ikonomidis *et al.*, 1994).

In addition, the influence of preexisting immunity against *L. monocytogenes* on the efficacy of recombinant *L. monocytogenes* for vaccination purposes has to be evaluated. Healthy adults are immune to *L. monocytogenes* and this immunity may compromise the capacitiy of recombinant *L. monocytogenes* to reach the imunologically relevant organs and sites after vaccination. On the other hand, boosting of the CTL response by a second immunization with recombinant *L. monocytogenes* strains has been shown to be possible in the murine model (Slifka *et al.*, 1996; Bouwer *et al.*, 1999; Tvinnereim and Harty, 2000), indicating that efficient immunization may be achieveable in spite of the presence of anti-*Listeria* immunity. However, in this scenario the optimal display of the T cell antigen seems to be crucial, since only secondary immunizations with recombinant *L. monocytogenes* strains secreting the heterologous T cell antigen led to an effcicient CTL response (Tvinnereim and Harty, 2000).

CONCLUSIONS

The rational design of efficacious bacterial carrier strains for the development of live vaccines requires the detailed knowledge of the nature of the carrier to be used and the quality of the immune response elicited in different hosts. The advanced knowledge of the genetic basis of *L. monocytogenes* virulence allows the rational design for suitable carrier strains for different immune responses. *L. monocytogenes* has clearly been demonstrated to be a very efficient vehicle for the delivery of protein antigens and DNA vaccines and for the elicitation of cellular immune responses. The most attractive features of recombinant *L. monocytogenes* for the development of live vaccines include the applicability via the mucosal route, the preferred replication in cells adherent to the inductive sites of the immune system, the capacitiy to enter the cytosol of infected cells and the inherent adjuvant effect of the bacteria. Recombinant *L. monocytogenes* are suitable live vaccines for the protection against a wide range of intracellular pathogens including viruses, bacteria and parasites, but also against tumors. It will be very instructive to compare in future studies the efficacy of recombinant *L. monocytogenes* directly to alternative vaccines which allow the elicitation of a cellular immune response, like *M. bovis* BCG, attenuated *Salmonellae* and *Shigellae* as well as viral systems.

ACKNOWLEDGEMENTS

We would like to thank Y. Paterson for helpful comments during the preparation of the manuscript and M. Dietrich for critical reading.

REFERENCES

Alexander,J.E., Andrew, P.W., Jones, D., and Roberts, I.S. 1993. Characterization of an aromatic amino acid-dependent *Listeria monocytogenes* mutant: attenuation, persistence, and ability to induce protective immunity in mice. Infect. Immun. 61: 2245-2248.

Alfonso, L.C., Scharton, T.M., Vieira, L.Q., Wysocka, M., Trinchieri, G., and Scott, P. 1994. The adjuvant effect of interleukin-12 in a vaccine against *Leihmania major*. Science 263: 235-237.

Autret, N., Dubail, I., Trieu-Cuot, P., Berche, P., and Charbit, A. 2001. Identification of new genes involved in the virulence of *Listeria monocytogenes* by signature-tagged transposon mutagenesis. Infect. Immun. 69: 2054-2065.

Banchereau, J., and Steinman. R.M. 1998. Dendritic cells and the control of immunity. Nature 392, 245–252.

Barry, R.A., Bouwer, H.G., Portnoy, D.A., and Hinrichs, D.J. 1992. Pathogenicity and immunogenicity of *Listeria monocytogenes* small-plaque mutants defective for intracellular growth and cell-to-cell spread. Infect. Immun. 60: 1625-1632.

Bohne, J., Kestler, H., Übele, C., Sokolovic, Z., and Goebel, W. 1996. Differential regulation of the virulence genes of *Listeria monocytogenes* by the transcriptional activator PrfA. Mol. Microbiol. 20: 1189-1198

Bouwer, H.G., Shen, H., Fan, X., Miller, J.F., Barry, R.A., and Hinrichs, D.J. 1999. Existing antilisterial immunity does not inhibit the development of a *Listeria monocytogenes*-specific primary cytotoxic T-lymphocyte response. Infect. Immun. 67: 253-258.

Braun, L., Ohayon, H., and Cossart, P. 1998. The InlB protein of *Listeria monocytogenes* is sufficient to promote entry into mammalian cells. Mol. Microbiol. 27: 1077-1087.

Brunt, L.M., Portnoy, D.A., and Unanue, E.R. 1990. Presentation of *Listeria monocytogenes* to CD8+ T cells requires secretion of hemolysin and intracellular bacterial growth. J. Immunol. 145: 3540-3546.

Busch, D.H., Pilip, I.M., Vijh, S., and Pamer, E.G. 1998. Coordinate regulation of complex T cell populations responding to bacterial infection. Immunity 8: 353-362.

Cleveland, M.G., Gorham, J.D., Murphy, T.L., Tuomanen, E., and Murphy, K.M. 1996. Lipoteichoic acid preparations of gram-positive bacteria induce interleukin-12 through a CD14-dependent pathway. Infect. Immun. 64:1906-1912.

Cooney, E.L., Collier, A.C., Greenberg, P.D., Coombs, R.W., Zarling, J., Arditti, D.E., Hoffman, M.C., Hu, S.L., and Corey, L. 1991. Safety of and immunological response to a recombinant vaccinia virus vaccine expressing HIV envelope glycoprotein. Lancet. 337: 567-572.

Curtiss, R. 3rd, Galan, J.E., Nakayama, K., and Kelly, S.M. 1990. Stabilization of recombinant avirulent vaccine strains *in vivo*. Res. Microbiol. 141: 797-805.

Darji, A., Chakraborty, T., Niebuhr, K., Tsonis, N., Wehland, J., and Weiss, S. 1995. Hyperexpression of listeriolysin in the nonpathogenic species *Listeria innocua* and high yield purification. J. Biotechnol. 43: 205-212.

Davis, H.L., Brazolot Millan, C.L., and Watkins, S.C. 1997. Immune-mediated destruction of transfected muscle fibers after direct gene transfer with antigen-expressing plasmid DNA. Gene Ther. 4: 181-188.

de Chastellier, C., and Berche, P. 1994. Fate of *Listeria monocytogenes* in murine macrophages: evidence for simultaneous killing and survival of intracellular bacteria. Infect. Immun. 62: 543-553.

Dietrich, G., Bubert, A., Gentschev, I., Sokolovic, Z., Simm, A., Catic, A., Kaufmann, S.H.E., Hess, J., Szalay, A.A., and Goebel W. 1998. Delivery of antigen-encoding plasmid DNA into the cytosol of macrophages by attenuated suicide *Listeria monocytogenes*. Nat. Biotechnol. 16: 181-185.

Dietrich, G., Kolb-Mäurer, A. Spreng, S., Schartl, M., Goebel, W., and Gentschev, I. 2001. Gram-positive and Gram-negative bacteria as carrier systems for DNA vaccines, Vaccine 19: 2506-2512.

Dramsi, S., Kocks, C., Forestier, C., and Cossart, P. 1993. Internalin-mediated invasion of epithelial cells by *Listeria monocytogenes* is regulated by the bacterial growth state, temperature, and pleiotropic activator *prfA*. Mol. Microbiol. 9: 931-941.

Fleming, S.D., and Campbell, P.A. 1997. Some macrophages kill *Listeria monocytogenes* while others do not. Immunol. Rev. 158: 69-77.

Frankel, F.R., Hegde, S., Lieberman, J., and Paterson, Y. 1995. Induction of cell-mediated immune responses to human immunodeficiency virus type 1 Gag protein by using *Listeria monocytogenes* as a live vaccine vector. J. Immunol. 155: 4775-4782.

Friedman, R.S., Frankel, F.R., Xu, Z., and Lieberman, J. 2000. Induction of human immunodeficiency virus (HIV)-specific CD8 T-cell responses by *Listeria monocytogenes* and a hyperattenuated *Listeria* strain engineered to express HIV antigens. J. Virol. 74: 9987-9993.

Gentschev, I., Dietrich, G., Spreng, S., Kolb-Mäurer, A., Daniels, J., Hess, J., Kaufmann, S.H.E., and Goebel, W. 2000. Bacterial antigen and DNA delivery systems. J. Biotechnol. 83: 19-26.

Gentschev, I., Dietrich, G., Spreng, S., Kolb-Mäurer, A., Brinkmann, V., Grode, L., Kaufmann, S.H.E., Hess, J., and Goebel, W. 2001. Recombinant attenuated bacteria for the delivery of subunit vaccines. Vaccine 19: 2621-2628.

Goossens, P.L., and Milon, G. 1992. Induction of protective CD8+ T lymphocytes by an attenuated *Listeria monocytogenes actA* mutant. Int. Immunol. 4: 1413-1418.

Goossens, P.L., Milon, G., Cossart, P., and Saron, M.F. 1995. Attenuated *Listeria monocytogenes* as a live vector for induction of CD8+ T cells *in vivo*: a study with the nucleoprotein of the lymphocytic choriomeningitis virus. Int. Immunol. 7: 797-805.

Guzman, C.A., Saverino, D., Medina, E., Fenoglio, D., Gerstel, B., Merlo, A., Li Pira, G., Buffa, F., Chakraborty, T., and Manca, F. 1998. Attenuated

Listeria monocytogenes carrier strains can deliver an HIV-1 gp120 T helper epitope to MHC class II-restricted human CD4+ T cells. Eur. J. Immunol. 28: 1807-1814.

Harty, J.T., and Bevan, M.J. 1992. CD8+ T cells specific for a single nonamer epitope of *Listeria monocytogenes* are protective *in vivo*. J. Exp. Med. 175: 1531-1538.

Hense, M., Domann, E., Krusch, S. Wacholz, P., Dittmar, K.E.J., Rohde, M., Wehland, J., Chakraborty, T., and Weiss, S. 2001. Eukaryotic expression plasmid transfer from the intracellular bacterium *Listeria monocytogenes* to host cells. Cell. Microbiol. 3: 599-609.

Hess, J., Gentschev, I., Miko, D., Welzel, M. Ladel, C., Goebel, W., and Kaufmann, S.H.E. 1996. Superior efficacy of secreted over somatic antigen display in recombinant *Salmonella* vaccine induced protection against listeriosis. Proc. Natl. Acad. Sci. USA. 93: 1458-1463.

Hess, J., Dietrich, G., Gentschev, I., Miko, D., Goebel, W., and Kaufmann, S.H.E. 1997. Protection against murine listeriosis by an attenuated recombinant *Salmonella typhimurium* vaccine strain that secretes the naturally somatic antigen superoxide dismutase. Infect. Immun. 65: 1286-1292.

Hess, J., Grode, L., Gentschev, I., Hellwig, J., Fensterle, J., Brinkmann, V., Dietrich, G., Krohne, G.F., Goebel, W., and Kaufmann, S.H.E. 2000. Secretion of different listeriolysin cognates by recombinant attenuated *Salmonella typhimurium*: superior efficacy of haemolytic over non-haemolytic constructs after oral vaccination, Microbes Infect. 2: 1799-1806.

Hiltbold, E.M., Safley, S.A., and Ziegler, H.K. 1996. The presentation of class I and class II epitopes of listeriolysin O is regulated by intracellular localization and by intracellular spread of *Listeria monocytogenes*. J. Immunol. 157: 1163-1175.

Ikonomidis, G., Paterson, Y., Kos, F.J., and Portnoy, D.A. 1994. Delivery of a viral antigen to the class I processing and presentation pathway by *Listeria monocytogenes*. J. Exp. Med. 180: 2209-2218.

Ikonomidis, G., Portnoy, D.A., Gerhard, W., and Paterson, Y. 1997. Influenza-specific immunity induced by recombinant *Listeria monocytogenes* vaccines. Vaccine 15: 433-440.

Jensen, E.R., Selvakumar, R., Shen, H., Ahmed, R., Wettstein, F.O., and Miller, J.F. 1997. Recombinant Listeria monocytogenes vaccination eliminates papillomavirus-induced tumors and prevents papilloma formation from viral DNA. J. Virol. 71: 8467-8474.

Jeyasekaran, G., Karunasagar, I., and Karunasagar, I. 1996. Incidence of *Listeria spp.* in tropical fish. Int. J. Food Microbiol. 31: 333-340.

Kaufmann, S.H.E. 1998. Immunity to intracellular bacteria. In: Fundamental Immunology, W.E. Paul, ed. Lippincott-Raven, Philadelphia. p. 1335-1371.

Kerksiek, K.M., and Pamer, E.G. 1999. T cell responses to bacterial infection. Curr. Opin. Immunol. 11: 400-405.

Kolb-Mäurer, A., Gentschev, I., Fries, H.W., Fiedler, F., Bröcker, E.B., Kämpgen, E., and Goebel, W. 2000. *Listeria monocytogenes*-infected human dendritic cells: invasion and host cell response. Infect. Immun. 66: 3680-3688.

Kuhn, M., and Goebel, W. 1994. Induction of cytokines in phagocytic mammalian cells infected with virulent and avirulent *Listeria strains*. Infect. Immun. 62: 348-356.

Kuhn, M., and Goebel, W. 1998. Host cell signalling during *Listeria monocytogenes* infection. Trends Microbiol. 6: 11-15.

Kuhn, M., and Goebel, W. 2000. Internalization of *Listeria monocytogenes* by nonprofessional and professional phagocytes. Subcell. Biochem. 33: 411-436.

Lecuit, M., Vandormael-Pournin, S., Lefort, J., Huerre, M., Gounon, P., Dupuy, C., Babinet, C., and Cossart, P. 2001. A transgenic model for listeriosis: role of internalin in crossing the intestinal barrier. Science 292:1722-1725.

Mackaness, GB. 1962. Cellular resistance to infection. J. Exp. Med. 116: 381-406.

Mata, M., Travers, P.J., Liu, Q., Frankel, F.R., and Paterson, Y. 1998. The MHC class I-restricted immune response to HIV-gag in BALB/c mice selects a single epitope that does not have a predictable MHC-binding motif and binds to Kd through interactions between a glutamine at P3 and pocket D. J. Immunol. 161: 2985-2993.

Mata, M., and Paterson, Y. 1999. Th1 T cell responses to HIV-1 Gag protein delivered by a *Listeria monocytogenes* vaccine are similar to those induced by endogenous listerial antigens. J. Immunol. 163: 1449-1456.

Mata, M., and Paterson, Y. 2000. *Listeria monocytogenes* as an alternative vaccine vector for HIV. Arch. Immunol. Ther. Exp. (Warsz) 48: 151-162.

Mata, M., Yao, Z., Zubair, A., Syres, K., and Paterson, Y. 2001 Evaluation of a recombinant *Listeria monocytogenes* expressing an HIV protein that protects mice against viral challenge. Vaccine 19: 1435-1445.

Mazzaccaro, R.J., Gedde, M., Jensen, E.R., van Santen, H.M., Ploegh, H.L., Rock, K.L., and Bloom, B.R. 1996. Major histocompatibility class I presentation of soluble antigen facilitated by *Mycobacterium tuberculosis* infection. Proc. Natl. Acad. Sci. USA. 93: 11786-11791.

Mengaud, J., Ohayon, H., Gounon, P., Mége, R.M., and Cossart, P. 1996. E-cadherin is the receptor for internalin, a surface protein required for entry of *Listeria monocytogenes* into epithelial cells. Cell 84: 923-932.

Michel, E., Reich, K.A., Favier, R., Berche, P., and Cossart, P. 1990. Attenuated mutants of the intracellular bacterium *Listeria monocytogenes* obtained by single amino acid substitutions in listeriolysin O. Mol. Microbiol. 1990 4: 2167-2178.

Mielke, M.E., Peters, C., and Hahn, H. 1997. Cytokines in the induction and expression of T-cell-mediated granuloma formation and protection in the murine model of listeriosis. Immunol. Rev. 158: 79-93.

Ochsenbein, A.F., Karrer, U., Klenerman, P., Althage, A., Ciurea, A., Shen, H., Miller, J.F., Whitton, J.L., Hengartner, H., and Zinkernagel, R.M. 1999. A comparison of T cell memory against the same antigen induced by virus versus intracellular bacteria. Proc. Natl. Acad. Sci. USA. 96: 9293-9298.

Paglia, P., Arioli, I., Frahm, N., Chakraborty, T., Colombo, M.P., and Guzman, C.A. 1997. The defined attenuated *Listeria monocytogenes* delta mp12 mutant is an effective oral vaccine carrier to trigger a long-lasting immune response against a mouse fibrosarcoma. Eur. J. Immunol. 27: 1570-1575.

Pamer, EG. 1998. Cell-mediated immunity: the role of bacterial protein secretion. Curr. Biol. 8: R457-460.

Pan, Z.K., Ikonomidis, G., Lazenby, A., Pardoll, D., and Paterson, Y. 1995a. A recombinant *Listeria monocytogenes* vaccine expressing a model tumour antigen protects mice against lethal tumour cell challenge and causes regression of established tumours. Nat. Med. 1: 471-477.

Pan, Z.K., Ikonomidis, G., Pardoll, D., and Paterson, Y. 1995b. Regression of established tumors in mice mediated by the oral administration of a recombinant *Listeria monocytogenes* vaccine. Cancer Res.55: 4776-4779.

Pan, Z.K., Weiskirch, L.M., and Paterson, Y. 1999. Regression of established B16F10 melanoma with a recombinant *Listeria monocytogenes* vaccine. Cancer Res. 59: 5264-5269.

Paschen, A., Dittmar, K.E., Grenningloh, R., Rohde, M., Schadendorf, D., Domann, E., Chakraborty, T., and Weiss, S. 2000. Human dendritic cells infected by *Listeria monocytogenes*: induction of maturation, requirements for phagolysosomal escape and antigen presentation capacity. Eur. J. Immunol. 30: 3447-3456.

Portnoy, D.A., Chakraborty, T., Goebel, W., and Cossart, P. 1992. Molecular determinants of *Listeria monocytogenes* pathogenesis. Infect. Immun. 60: 1263-1267.

Ravenau, J., Geoffroy, C., Beretti, J.L., Gaillard, J.L., Alouf, P., Berche, P. 1992. Reduced virulence of a *Listeria monocytogenes* phospholipase-deficient mutant obtained by transposon insertion into the zinc metalloprotease gene. Infect. Immun. 60: 916-921.

Rayevskaya, M.V., and Frankel, F.R. 2001. Systemic immunity and mucosal immunity are induced against human immunodeficiency virus Gag protein in mice by a new hyperattenuated strain of *Listeria monocytogenes*. J. Virol. 76: 2786-2791.

Renzoni, A., Cossart, P., and Dramsi, S. 1999. PrfA, the transcriptional activator of virulence genes, is upregulated during interaction of *Listeria monocytogenes* with mammalian cells and in eukaryotic cell extracts. Mol. Microbiol. 34: 552-561.

Schafer, R., Portnoy, D.A., Brassell, S.A., and Paterson, Y. 1992. Induction of a cellular immune response to a foreign antigen by a recombinant Listeria monocytogenes vaccine. J. Immunol. 149: 53-59.

Shen, H., Slifka, M.K., Matloubian, M., Jensen, E.R., Ahmed, R., and Miller, J.F. 1995. Recombinant *Listeria monocytogenes* as a live vaccine vehicle for the induction of protective anti-viral cell-mediated immunity. Proc. Natl. Acad. Sci. USA. 92: 3987-3991.

Shen, H., Miller, J.F., Fan, X., Kolwyck, D., Ahmed, R., and Harty, J.T. 1998. Compartmentalization of bacterial antigens: differential effects on priming of CD8 T cells and protective immunity. Cell 92: 535-545.

Shen, X., and Siliciano, R.F. 2000. Preventing AIDS but not HIV-1 infection with a DNA vaccine. Science 290: 463-465.

Slifka, M.K., Shen, H., Matloubian, M., Jensen, E.R., Miller, J.F., Ahmed, R. 1996. Antiviral cytotoxic T-cell memory by vaccination with recombinant *Listeria monocytogenes*. J. Virol. 70: 2902-2910.

Soussi, N., Milon, G., Colle, J.H., Mougneau, E., Glaichenhaus, N., Goossens, P.L. 2000. *Listeria monocytogenes* as a short-lived delivery system for the induction of type 1 cell-mediated immunity against the p36/LACK antigen of *Leishmania major*. Infect. Immun. 68: 1498-1506.

Spreng, S., Dietrich, G., Niewiesk, S., ter Meulen, V., Gentschev, I., and Goebel, W. 2000. Novel bacterial systems for the delivery of recombinant protein or DNA, FEMS Immunol. Med. Microbiol. 27: 299-304.

Thompson, R.J., Bouwer, H.G., Portnoy, D.A., and Frankel, F.R. 1998. Pathogenicity and immunogenicity of a *Listeria monocytogenes* strain that requires D-alanine for growth. Infect. Immun. 66: 3552-3361.

Tilney, L.G., and Portnoy, D.A. 1989. Actin filaments and the growth, movement, and spread of the intracellular parasite, *Listeria monocytogenes*. J. Cell Biol. 109: 1597-1608.

Tvinnereim, A.R., and Harty, J.T. 2000. CD8(+) T-cell priming against a nonsecreted *Listeria monocytogenes* antigen is independent of the antimicrobial activities of gamma interferon. Infect. Immun. 68: 2196-2204.

Weiskirch, L.M., and Paterson, Y. 1997. *Listeria monocytogenes*: a potent vaccine vector for neoplastic and infectious disease. Immunol. Rev. 158: 159-169.

Wilson, R.C., Tvinnereim, A.R., Jones, B.D., and Harty, J.T. 2001. Identification of *Listeria monocytogenes in vivo*-induced genes by fluorescence-activated cell sorting. Infect. Immun. 69: 5016-5024.

Zinkernagel, R.M., Bachmann, M.F., Kundig, T.M., Oehen, S., Pirchet, H., and Hengartner, H. 1996.On immunological memory. Annu. Rev. Immunol. 14: 333-367.

From: *Vaccine Delivery Strategies*
Edited by: Guido Dietrich and Werner Goebel

Chapter 13

Transfer of Eukaryotic Expression Plasmids to Mammalian Host Cells by Gram-negative Bacteria

Siegfried Weiss and Trinad Chakraborty

ABSTRACT

The concept of transkingdom transfer of DNA from bacteria to other organisms has recently been extended to include eucaryotic host cells. Attenuated intracellular bacteria or non-pathogenic bacteria equipped with adhesion and invasion properties have now been demonstrated to transfer eukaryotic expression plasmids to mammalian host cells *in vitro* and *in vivo*. Here, we review the use of Gram-negative bacteria for induction of immune responses towards protein antigens encoded by the plasmid, their use to complement genetic defects or deliver immunotherapeutic proteins. Plasmid transfer is effected by bacterial death within the host cell usually resulting from metabolic attenuation. It is also possible that bacterial macromolecule secretion machineries direct DNA transfer to the infected host cell. Plasmid transfer has been reported for *Shigella flexneri, Salmonella typhimurium* and *S. typhi, S. choleraesuis, Yersinia pseudotuberculosis* and *Escherichia coli,* but clearly this property can be extended to include any bacterial species as has recently been demonstrated with *Agrobacterium tumefaciens.* Gene transfer *in vivo* attempts were mainly directed towards vaccination strategies using *Shigella* and *Salmonella* as carrier where this type of immunization was more efficacious than either direct application of antigen, using the same bacterium as a heterologous carrier expressing the antigen via a prokaryotic promoter, or vaccination with naked DNA. The efficacy of induction of protective immune responses by such DNA carriers and ease of generating these vehicles for gene transfer using technology validated for mass vaccination programs makes this a highly attractive area for further research and development.

INTRODUCTION

Transkingdom DNA transfer from bacterial carriers to mammalian host cells is now well established. Several bacterial species with different invasive properties were show to be able to transfer eukaryotic expression plasmids. *Shigella flexneri, Salmonella typhimurium, S. typhi, S. cholerasuis, Listeria monocytogenes, Yersinia pseudotuberculosis, Agrobacterium tumefaciens,* recombinant *Escherichia coli* as well as a laboratory strain of *E. coli* have been tested successfully so far (Sizemore *et al.*, 1995; Courvalin *et al.*, 1995; Powell *et al.*, 1996; Darji *et al.*, 1997; Dietrich *et al.*, 1998, Fennelly *et al.*, 1999; Dietrich *et al.*, 2001; Kunik *et al.*, 2001; Shiau *et al.*, 2001a, and 2001b). Conceptually, the use of bacteria to transfer DNA into mammalian host cells was not unexpected. Transfer of plasmids has been observed between Gram-negative and Gram-positive bacteria as well as between bacteria and yeast (Heinemann and Sprague, 1989; Trieu-Cuot *et al.*, 1993; Charpentier *et al.*, 1999). Furthermore, bacteria-mediated plasmid transfer is standard methodology for the generation of recombinant plants (Lessl and Lanka, 1994) and has been in industrial use for more than fifteen years. Finally, low level detection of transfer of recombinant plasmid/SV40 virus hybrids from a non-pathogenic *E. coli* strain to mammalian cells via protoplast fusion was reported in 1980 (Schaffner, 1980). Thus, exploiting the ability of bacteria to transfer expression plasmids directly to mammalian host cells *in vitro* and *in vivo* was a logical consequence.

PATHWAYS OF BACTERIA-MEDIATED GENE TRANSFER

Two major pathways of bacteria-mediated DNA transfer to mammalian host cells have become obvious from the experiments reported so far. They can be classified according to whether the bacterium escapes from the phagolysosome after invasion or not. Thus, the first pathway can be characterized as follows: the carrier bacterium enters the target cell which is either phagocytic or phagocytosis is induced by the microorganism itself. Subsequently, the bacterium escapes from the phagocytic vacoule which requires dedicated factors produced by the microorganism. Following escape from the vacuole into the cytosol, bacterial lysis occurs because of an attenuation that is achieved by rendering the carrier bacteria auxotrophic for an essential physiological component that can not be supplied by the host cell. Alternatively, inducible autolytic mechanisms or antibiotics have been used to kill the carrier bacteria inside the host cell. The death of the bacteria leads to liberation of the expression plasmid and transfer into the nucleus of the host cell, where the encoded protein is expressed. This transfer process is likely to be very efficient since the plasmids released from the bacterial cell are probably still associated with DNA-binding proteins that might protect the plasmids from degradation and enhance nuclear import.

The second major pathway was discovered when *S. typhimurium*, a bacterium that remains in the phagocytic vesicle and dies there due to a metabolic attenuation, was also shown to be able to transfer expression plasmids (Darji *et al.*, 1997). Here, transfer *in vitro* has only been documented for primary murine and human macrophages and dendritic cells (Darji *et al.*, 1997; Xiang *et al.*, 2000; Paglia *et al.*, 2000; Montosi *et al.*, 2000, Dietrich *et al.*, 2001). However, the efficiency of plasmid transfer into some of these host cells under certain conditions *in vitro* is surprisingly high, occasionally reaching close to 100%. Thus far, no tissue culture cell lines have yet been found into which *Salmonella* were able to transfer DNA. For dendritic cells and activated bone marrow derived macrophages, pathways have been reported that lead to transport of macromolecules from the endocytic vesicle to the cytosol (Norbury *et al.*, 1995; Rodriguez *et al.*, 2000). Whether such cellular pathways are involved in DNA transport across the vesicular membrane or whether secretion systems of the carrier bacteria themselves are capable of introducing macromolecules into the cytosol of the host cell can not be answered at the moment.

Interestingly, attenuated *E. coli* was found to be able to transfer expression plasmids into mammalian cell lines. In this case, the bacteria were engineered to become invasive and to be able to escape from the phagocytic vacuole (Courvalin *et al.*, 1995). Several established cell lines of epithelial origin could be transfected this way. In a follow up of this study, it could be shown that, although escape from the vacuole improved the transfer efficiency, it was not essential for DNA transfer *per se* (Grillot-Courvalin *et al.*, 1998). Thus, as previously observed with *Salmonella*, eukaryotic expression plasmids can also be transferred by *E. coli* without leaving the vacuole. However, the respective mechanisms involved seem to be distinct since DNA transfer by *Salmonella* is restricted to primary macrophages and dendritic cells while *E. coli* appears to have a much broader spectrum. Recently, Shiau *et al.* (2001a) have shown that intramuscular application of a laboratory strain of *E. coli* carrying an antigen encoding expression plasmid elicited a specific immune response in the vaccinated mice. This suggests that non-pathogenic unmodified *E. coli* can also transfer DNA into phagocytic cells *in vivo*. Whether the DNA transfer mechanisms of these two bacteria are specific for the particular bacterial species is unclear. Without direct comparisons of the bacterial vehicles in use and the immune response generated it is difficult to discern such transfer mechanisms.

A third pathway has recently been discovered. *Agrobacterium tumefaciens*, a bacterium that is known to transfer expression cassettes into plant cells, was shown to transfer also expression cassettes into HeLa cells (Kunik *et al.*, 2001). No invasion of the host cell was required in order to achieve DNA transfer. Thus, this pathway will only be used by bacteria that are specialized for such a DNA transfer and possess the appropriate transfer apparatus.

APPLICATIONS OF BACTERIA-MEDIATED GENE TRANSFER

Applications for bacteria-mediated expression plasmid transfer can be classified into two types: genetic vaccination and gene therapy. Currently, genetic vaccination protocols deliver either naked or chemically packaged DNA by the intramuscular, intradermal, or oral route using expression plasmids that encode the antigen. Antigen is expressed by the vaccinated host and results in the induction of an immune response. This type of vaccination offers tremendous flexibility with regard to antigen modification and targeting and includes the possibility of modulating the induced immune response e.g. by co-expression of cytokines. To date, considerable information has been accumulated on the molecular and cellular details that are involved during induction of immune responses by genetic vaccination (Gurunathan *et al.*, 2000). Nevertheless, genetic vaccination is besotted with problems of low efficiency. Often multiple administrations are required to raise significant immune reactions or prime boost schedules have to be employed. In addition, a general goal in vaccinology is to mucosally, i.e. orally or nasally, apply all of the possible vaccines since this represents the easiest way of administration (Levine and Dougan, 1998).

The use of bacteria as carriers for mucosal application of DNA vaccines addresses some of the problems of naked DNA vaccination and provides additional benefits. A) Many bacteria target inductive sites and cells of the immune system, meaning that the antigen is expressed in immunologically relevant cells. B) Bacterial cell wall components and unmethylated DNA motifs of the bacterial genome provide adjuvant activity and will enhance immune reactions (Wagner, 1999; Aderem and Ulevitch, 2000). C) The bacterial carrier and the antigen encoding plasmid are different entities. Therefore, modulation and specific targeting of the immune response should be possible by either modifying the expression vector (e.g. by co-expression of cytokines or costimulatory molecules) or by choosing an appropriate bacterial carrier strain. D) Finally, bacteria are cost effective to produce, easy to store and transport, controllable by common antibiotics and the coding capacity of some plasmids is virtually unlimited which will be useful for the design of multi-component vaccines. So far, attempts to use Gram-negative bacteria as carrier for mucosal genetic vaccination have been concentrating on *S. typhimurium, S. typhi, S. cholerasuis* and *S. flexneri.*

At first, gene therapy has raised great enthusiasm with respect to treatment of monogenic disorders. However, there has been little success so far. Part of the problem is the lack of efficient vectors that target transgene expression to the right cells *in vivo* but at the same time do not induce adverse effects. The non-replicative vectors that are usually employed in these procedures are derived either from modified replication-defective viruses or standard expression plasmids. Here, bacteria-mediated gene transfer offers a simple alternative to the commonly used methods as it exhibits some unique properties. A) Bacteria are controllable by common antibiotics. B) The intrinsic tissue tropism of some bacteria can be used to target genes to certain organs and their mucosal port of entry might facilitate their administration. C) Some bacteria are able to spread from cell-to-cell and are thus able to target tissue layers unaccessible to non-replicating transfer vehicles. D) The almost unlimited coding capacity of bacterial plasmids should allow transfer of large genomic fragments and by using appropriate recombinant bacterial carriers might even promote homologous recombination. Therefore, the development of bacteria as efficient transfer vehicles for the therapy of monogenic defects appears to be a desirable goal.

To date, many experiments using bacteria as vectors for gene therapy were mainly directed towards transfer of reporter genes or therapeutic DNA *in vitro* (Courvalin *et al.*, 1995; Grillot-Courvalin *et al.*, 1998; Montosi *et al.*, 2000; Hense *et al.* 2001). However, data from *in vivo* experiments are accumulating where *S. typhimurium* has successfully been used to transfer expression plasmids encoding either cytokines or therapeutic ligands (Urashima *et al.* 2000; Paglia *et al.* 2000; Yuhua *et al.*, 2001). Such results, as a proof of principle, are extremely promising and more than justify further exploration of this approach.

ATTENUATED *SALMONELLA TYPHIMURIUM* AS DNA CARRIER

Most of the data on bacteria-mediated gene transfer have been accrued using attenuated *S. typhimurium* as carrier. Mice are a natural host of these bacteria, thus, experiments can be performed under physiological conditions. In addition, *S. typhimurium* is also applicable to humans as vaccine carrier and several strains have proved to be safe for administration (Mastroeni *et al.*, 2000). Two metabolically attenuated strains have been employed as DNA carrier so far: *S. typhimurium aroA* that is unable to synthesize aromatic amino acids (Hoiseth and Stocker, 1981) but retains a certain pathogenic potential since it is still lethal in mice deficient in the production of IFNγ (Paglia *et al.*, 2000; Darji *et al.*, unpublished) and *S. typhimurium* 22-11 that is defective in its purine metabolism (Leung and Finlay, 1991; Brunham and Zhang, 1999). Mainly commercially available vectors such as pCMVβ (Clonetec) or pCDNA3 (Invitrogen) have been used as eukaryotic expression plasmids.

Gene transfer experiments leading either to induction of an immune response against pathogens for prophylactic vaccination or tumor therapy or to expression of therapeutic proteins have been described. Originally, genes encoding listeriolysin and ActA (two virulence factors of *L. monocytogenes*) and β-galactosidase (β-gal) of *E. coli* were successfully tested (Darji *et al.*, 1997). Cytotoxic and helper T cells (mainly Th1cells) as well as specific antibodies could be detected against these antigens even after oral application of a single dose of the recombinant *Salmonella*. This type of administration was by far superior to oral application of the same number of *Salmonella* that expressed high amounts of antigen as heterologous protein. In addition, T cell memory could only be induced under these circumstances by the oral application of recombinant *Salmonella* that carried the eukaryotic expression plasmid and not by the *Salmonella* expressing the antigen themselves (Darji *et al.*, 2000). In addition, immunization with *Salmonella* carrying the listeriolysin encoding expression plasmid elicited a protective response against a lethal challenge with *L. monocytogenes*. These findings were obtained in BALB/c mice which are highly susceptible to *Salmonella* infection. Extension to strains of a more resistant phenotype and to outbred mice revealed that cytotoxic and helper T cell responses could be induced in all of these strains after only a single application. However, several administrations of the recombinant *Salmonella* were required to elicit specific antibodies to the antigens studied (Darji *et al.*, 2000 and unpublished). This indicates that with the present carrier, mainly T cell responses are elicited while more improvements will be required to generate strong general antibody responses.

Nasal application of antigen often results in a general mucosal immune reponse. Therefore, nasal and oral application of *Salmonella* based DNA vaccines encoding β-gal or a fusion antigen of the outer membrane protein and the fimbriae derived from *Pseudomonas aeroginosa* were compared. To observe a T cell response in the spleen, several nasal administrations were necessary as compared to a single dose for oral administration (Darji *et al.*, 2000 and unpublished). Antibodies could also be observed, but they were peculiar to the route of application (oral: gut, saliva and serum; nasal: lung, saliva and serum) and were mainly of the IgG class with hardly any antigen specific IgA (Darji *et al.*, 2000 and unpublished). We interpreted these results as being a dose dependent phenomenon, whereby antigen might be limiting under these conditions since 500-fold less bacteria were applied to the nostrils of the mice than to the mouth. In addition, bacteria or antigen expressing cells might disseminate quickly from the port of entry, thus preventing the induction of a local mucosal antibody response.

Four more infection systems have been tested so far using *S. typhimurium* as DNA vaccine carrier. A codon optimized expression cassette for gp120 of HIV was tested as oral DNA vaccine (Shata *et al.*, 2001). Strong induction of IFN-γ in CD8 T cells could be demonstrated when cells were isolated from Peyer's Patches or spleen. In contrast, such activity could only be revealed in the spleen when the naked expression plasmid was applied intramuscularly.

Partial protective responses could be obtained against *Chlamydia trachomatis* using an expression plasmid encoding the major outer membrane protein as antigen (Brunham and Zhang, 1999). Interestingly, this protection was observed in the lung, although the vaccine was administered orally. Similarly, oral transgene vaccination using the glycoprotein D of Herpes simplex virus-2 as antigen resulted in induction of cytotoxic and helper T cells (Fló *et al.*, 2001). In addition, such mice were protected against a lethal intravaginal challenge with virus and local IFN-γ production could be observed in this organ after the challenge. These findings are in agreement with the recent observation that T cells disseminate into the tissue after activation in inductive lymphoid organs (Reinhardt *et al.*, 2001) and might explain the discrepancy with our findings on local antibody production (Darji *et al.*, 2000).

T cells and antibody responses could also be observed using the surface protein of hepatitis B virus as antigen (Woo *et al.*, 2001). In this case, *Salmonella* based oral DNA vaccination proved to be superior over intramuscular application of the naked expression plasmid or the recombinant subunit vaccine. *In vitro* transfection of macrophages using the recombinant *Salmonella* allowed the quantitation of antigen expression. Obviously, only low protein expression is obtained under these circumstances in macrophages when compared with conventional transfectants. Nevertheless, the direct expression of the antigen in inductive cells of the immune system might more than compensate for such low expression levels of antigen. On the other hand, this could also explain why antibody production is generally low in this system and some mouse strains require more than one application in order to respond in this way. When such *in vitro* transfected macrophages were administered intraperitoneally or intramuscularly, an immune response of the same quality was induced as with the normal oral application of the recombinant *Salmonella* (Zheng *et al.*, 2001).

Extremely promising results have been obtained with *S. typhimurium* mediated oral DNA vaccination in tumor models. Using β-gal as surrogate tumor antigen in an aggressive fibrosarcoma, partial protective immunity could be induced by orally administering *Salmonella* carrying β-gal encoding plasmids (Paglia *et al.*, 1998). Similarly, using the β-gal-expressing murine renal cell carcinoma line RENCA-ß-Gal, Zöller and Christ (2001) have demonstrated superior efficacy in inducing tumor protection when the antigen encoding plasmids were delivered in bacterial carriers as opposed to injecting naked DNA.

Even more promising are the results obtained by the group of Reisfeld using autologous tumor antigens. First, they used *Salmonella* that carried minigenes encoding epitopes of the tumor antigens gp100 and TRP2 fused to ubiquitin for immunization. This resulted in retardation of growth of the melanoma B16 (Xiang *et al.*, 2000). Since gp100 and TRP2 are self-antigens, this might suggest that *Salmonella*-mediated DNA vaccination is able to break tolerance towards autologous tumor antigens. These findings were extended by using a murine neuroblastoma and minigenes encoding epitopes derived of tyrosine hydroxylase fused with ubiquitin as antigen (Lode *et al.*, 2000). Further extension of this work showed that complete antigens without the ubiquitin fusion partner can also be used as antigens. In a mouse strain that was transgenic for human carcinoembryonic antigen (hCEA), whereby hCEA functioned as self antigen, oral immunization with *S. typhimurium* carrying an expression plasmid that encoded hCEA resulted in induction of specific cytotoxic T cells (Xiang *et al.*, 2001). In addition, the growth of a colon carinoma expressing hCEA as tumor antigen was retarded. This response could be strongly improved by applying a fusion protein between IL-2 and an antibody that targeted the recombinant cytokine to the tumor. When the same treatment was applied to a lung metastasis model using the same recombinant tumors and mice, most animals remained metastasis-free (Niethammer *et al.*, 2001a).

A similar improvement of the protective immune response was reported recently by the same group using the original B16 melanoma model and the epitopes of gp100 and TRP2 fused to ubiquitin as antigens. Targeting of IL-2 to the tumor shortly after the challenge via a fusion to an anti-ganglioside antibody resulted in complete protection against the melanoma in most mice (Niethammer *et al.*, 2001b). By these experiments it could also be shown that during the induction phase of the immune response, no help from CD4 T cells was required to induce tumor specific CD8 cytotoxic T cells. This is in agreement with the strong adjuvant capacity of the bacterial plasmid carrier.

The obvious efficiency of *S. typhimurium* in transferring eukaryotic expression plasmids to host cells *in vivo* and *in vitro* has prompted its use also for applications different than genetic vaccination. Human dendritic cells have been shown to be susceptible to transfection by *Salmonella* (Dietrich *et al.*, 2001), although the percentage of transfectants obtained is still low. Our original finding that primary macrophages can be transfected to a high degree *in vitro* using *S. typhimurium* has been further extended. Percentages of transfectants close to 100% have been obtained with murine as well as human macrophages (Paglia *et al.*, 2000; Montosi *et al.*, 2000). The latter system was used to complement a monogenic defect in macrophages from patients with hereditary hemochromatosis by transferring a plasmid encoding the cDNA of the hemochromatosis gene *HFE* (Montosi *et al.*, 2000). In addition, several applications *in vivo* have been reported. Mice defective in IFN-γ would normally succumb to a challenge with *S. typhimurium aroA*. However, when these bacteria carried an expression plasmid encoding IFN-γ and thus were able to transfer DNA that leads to a complementation of the genetic defect, at least in some cells, the mice were able to resist the bacterial challenge (Paglia *et al.*, 2000). Similarly, transfer of human or murine IL-12 and GM-CSF encoding cDNA via *S. typhimurium* in mice resulted in measurable levels of the particular recombinant cytokine in the serum of such mice and caused the retardation of subcutaneously applied tumors (Yuhua *et al.*, 2001).

In a murine B cell lymphoma model, *Salmonella* were used to transfer a soluble form of the human CD40 ligand (CD40L) orally. Stimulation of normal antigen presenting cells with CD40L results in up-regulation of MHC class I and class II as well as co-stimulatory molecules. In B cell lymphomas, stimulation via CD40L leads to growth suppression *in vitro* and *in vivo*. Oral administration of *S. typhimurium* that carried an expression plasmid encoding a soluble form of CD40L protected mice against a simultaneous challenge with the B cell lymphoma (Urashima *et al.*, 2000). This treatment was still partially effective when the recombinant *Salmonella* were applied one week after the challenge and still retarded the tumor growth when administered two to three weeks after tumor application. CD40L was detectable for several weeks in the serum of these mice. Histological examination showed that after oral administration of the recombinant *Salmonella* many cells expressed CD40L in Peyer's Patches, while only few of such cells could be found in spleen.

DNA TRANSFER BY RECOMBINANT ATTENUATED *S. TYPHIMURIUM* EXPRESSING LISTERIOLYSIN

The restriction of DNA transfer via *S. typhimurium* to primary macrophages and dendritic cells could limit the applicability of this system. To overcome this limitation and to allow plasmid transfer also into established cell lines *in vitro* and possibly also to improve *in vivo* performance, *Salmonella* that were engineered to secrete listeriolysin - the pore-forming toxin listeriolysin of *L. monoctogenes* - have been used (Gentschev *et al.*, 1995). These bacteria are able to escape from the phagocytic vacuole into the cytosol of the host cell. Co-infection of primary macrophages with *Salmonella* secreting listeriolysin and *Salmonella* carrying an ovalbumin encoding expression plasmid considerably enhanced antigen expression in these host cells (Catic *et al.*, 1999). Similar enhancements of reporter gene expression were observed *in vivo* in the peritoneum of mice three days after oral administration of *Salmonella* secreting listeriolysin and carrying a green fluorescent protein (GFP) encoding expression plasmid at the same time (Dietrich *et al.*, 2000).

ATTENUATED *SALMONELLA TYPHI* AS DNA CARRIER

S. typhi is not pathogenic in mice, therefore, studies with these bacteria as DNA carrier are limited to nasal or intra-peritoneal administration in these animals. However, a proof of principle using these bacteria is very important since approved vaccine strains already exist. Thus, clinical trials would be facilitated using such strains. The strain commonly used for immunization is *S. typhi* Ty21a, a *galE* mutant that lacks a component essential for cell wall synthesis. Recently developed improved strains like CVD 915 are attenuated by a mutation in *guaBA* encoding an essential enzyme of the guanine synthesis pathway (Wang *et al.*, 2001).

Applying intraperitoneally the Ty21a *galE* strain that carried an expression plasmid encoding the nucleoprotein of measles virus as a DNA vaccine resulted in specific cytotoxic T cell responses (Fennelly *et al.*, 1999). Low antibody responses have also been observed when ampicillin treated mice were orally immunized with *S. typhi* Ty21a carrying a plasmid encoding a fragment of tetanus toxin (Woo *et al.*, 2000).

A comprehensive study has been performed using the same tetanus toxin fragment and comparing nasally applied *S. typhi* CVD915 Δ *guaBA* carrying either a eukaryotic expression plasmid or a plasmid with a prokaryotic intracellular inducible promoter (Pasetti *et al.*, 1999). In addition, intramuscular injections of the eukaryotic expression plasmid were also carried out in these experiments. With regard to antibody responses, both immunizations involving bacteria were superior to direct application of the expression plasmid, but bacteria carrying the eukaryotic expression plasmid induced still higher antibody levels than bacteria carrying the inducible prokaryotic expression plasmid. Interestingly, despite the presence of antibodies against LPS after primary immunization, a booster reaction was observed using either of the two recombinant bacteria. This suggests that *Salmonella*-mediated DNA vaccination should also be possible in individuals that have encountered *Salmonella* previously.

ATTENUATED *SALMONELLA CHOLERASUIS* AS DNA CARRIER

Recently, an additional member of the *Salmonella spp.* has proved to be functional as carrier for oral DNA vaccination. A vaccine strain of *S. cholerasusuis* was shown to be able to transfer expression plasmids *in vitro* and *in vivo* (Shiau *et al.*, 2001b). Interestingly, in these experiments co-tranfer of two plasmids by the same bacterium was successfully attempted. One vector was based on a plasmid containing a colE1 origin of replication and encoding the glycoprotein C of the pseudorabies virus. The second vector contained a p15a ori and encoded prothymosin as an immunmodulatory cytokine to enhance the immune response. Primary peritoneal macrophages from mice could be shown to express both proteins after *in vitro* transfer using *S. cholerasuis*. Co-transfer *in vivo* resulted in superior induction of helper and killer T cells and enhanced antibody responses when compared to administration of *Salmonella* carrying only the glycoprotein C encoding plasmid. Improved protection against a lethal dose of the pseudorabies virus could also be demonstrated when the mice were vaccinated with bacteria that carried both plasmids compared to bacteria carrying either one of them. These results suggest that most likely many different *Salmonella* species can be used as DNA carrier. Thus, the system of oral transgene vaccination can be most likely adapted to many different species by using the appropriate invasive DNA carrier. In addition, co-transfer of two plasmid containing different origins of replication offers a very simple and versatile way of modulating immune responses.

ATTENUATED *SHIGELLA FLEXNERI* AS DNA CARRIER

S. flexneri is able to enter intestinal epithelial cells from which it spreads into phagocytic cells lining the gut mucosa. Following entry, it escapes from the endocytic vacuole into the cytosol of the host cell where it uses proteins of the actin-based microfilament system to effect intracellular motility and cell-to-cell spread. This bacterium represents the prototype of a bacterial DNA transfer vehicle and first experiments on bacteria-mediated expression plasmid transfer were carried out using attenuated *S. flexneri* as vector (Sizemore *et al.*, 1995; Courvalin *et al.*, 1995; Powell *et al.*, 1996). Several attenuated mutants are available that variously lack the ability to synthesize aromatic amino acids (*aroA* - Noriega *et al.*, 1994), have a block in cell wall synthesis (*asd* - Sizemore *et al.*, 1995; *dapB* - Courvalin *et al.*, 1995) or are deficient in producing guanine nucleotides (*guaBA* - Noriega *et al.*, 1996).

Using such mutants, the gene encoding β-gal was transferred from the bacterial carrier into various cell lines of epithelial origin.

In vivo DNA transfer was shown directly in the cornea of mice (Sizemore *et al.*, 1995) and in mucosal tissue (Powell *et al.*, 1996). *Shigella* are potential carriers for oral DNA vaccinations since their port of entry into the human host is the gastrointestinal tract. However, mice are not susceptible to gastrointestinal infections with these bacteria. Therefore, nasal immunization is used to investigate potential DNA vaccines transferred by this carrier. Intranasal administration of recombinant *Shigella* carrying plasmids that encoded one of several antigens including β-gal and the fusion, hemagglutinin and nucleoprotein of measles virus has been carried out. Cytotoxic and helper T cells as well as a moderate antibody response could be revealed after repeated vaccination with the recombinant bacteria (Sizemore *et al.*, 1995; 1997; Fennelly *et al.*, 1999).

Shigella harboring the same plasmid encoding a fragment of tetanus toxin as had been used for *S. typhi* above were assessed for their protective capacities (Anderson *et al.*, 2000). In guinea pigs, their efficacy was compared to both *Shigella* carrying the same tetanus fragment either transcribed from an inducible prokaryotic promoter or the naked eukaryotic expression plasmid injected intramuscularly. Intranasal immunization with bacteria carrying eukaryotic expression plasmids was superior with regard to antibody responses when compared to bacteria containing inducible prokaryotic promoters or the isolated expression plasmid. Again, a booster reaction was observed even when the mice contained antibodies against the carrier bacteria. Interestingly, neutralizing antibodies were only induced by the tetanus toxin fragment expressed in the bacterium. This suggests that the appropriate conformation is only obtained in the microorganism and not in the mammalian host. However, this should not influence the T cell response by the bacteria-mediated DNA vaccination.

A similar comparative study between *Shigella* mediated DNA vaccination and vaccination with naked DNA was performed in mice using the codon optimized vector encoding *env* of HIV (Shata and Hone, 2001). Induction of *env* specific IFN-γ producing CD8 T cells was comparable for both routes and also similar to immunization with a recombinant vaccinia virus. However, in a vaccinia virus based protection model, *Shigella*-mediated DNA vaccination was clearly superior to naked DNA. Interestingly, a prime/boost schedule was possible. Priming with the recombinant *Shigella* and boosting with recombinant vaccinia virus led to high levels of IFN-γ producing CD8 T cells in the spleen.

LABORATORY STRAINS OF *ESCHERICHIA COLI* AS DNA CARRIERS

Surprisingly, laboratory strains of *E. coli* K12 can also be used as transfer vector for mammalian cells. Originally, auxotrophic bacteria deficient in *dapB* that is required for cell wall synthesis were shown to transfer expression plasmids into cells of epithelial origin. Although the auxotrophy was not essential for DNA transfer to occur, it resulted in a strong enhancement. Since normal *E. coli* are not invasive for these epithelial cells, they needed to be engineered in order to be able to infect such host cells *in vitro*. In the first report, the virulence plasmid of *S. flexneri* was introduced into these bacteria, which not only enabled them to infect the mammalian cells but also allowed them to escape from the phagosome into the cytosol. Thus, conditions were ideal for gene transfer to occur (Courvalin *et al.*, 1995). In a follow up study, *E. coli* were generated that expressed the invasin gene of *Yersinia pseudotuberculosis*. These bacteria were still able to invade host cells but remained in the vacuole. Nevertheless, they could transfer expression plasmids encoding GFP as reporter gene (Grillot-Courvalin *et al.*, 1998). Bacteria were generated which co-expressed the invasin and intracellularly listeriolysin. The idea was that bacterial lysis in the vacuole would liberate the plasmids and listeriolysin would allow egress to the cytosol following destruction of the membrane of the vesicle. However, only moderately improved transfer rates at low multiplicities of infection (MOIs) were observed with such bacteria (Grillot-Courvalin *et al.*, 1998). At high MOIs, hardly any difference in transfer rates was found between bacteria expressing listeriolysin or not. This indicates that the laboratory strain *E. coli* K12 is able to generate a port for expression plasmids to efficiently cross the phagosomal membrane for delivery into the nucleus of the host cell. Besides transfer of expression plasmids into epithelial cells, transfer into the macrophage line J774 was also reported (Grillot-Courvalin *et al.*, 1998) suggesting that appropriately modified *E. coli* might also have the potential to act as carrier for DNA vaccines.

This suggestion was confirmed by a recent report using the unmodified laboratory strain TG1 as DNA carrier (Shiau *et al,*. 2001a). Transfer of GFP and glycoprotein G of pseudorabies virus encoding expression plasmids into primary peritoneal murine macrophages could be demonstrated *in vitro*. Intramuscular injection of large doses of *E. coli* carrying the glycoprotein G encoding plasmid ($4x10^7$- $4x10^9$) resulted in induction of specific cytotoxic and helper T cells. In addition, partial protection against a lethal challenge with pseudorabies virus was achieved with the higher doses of the recombinant bacteria. Co-injection of *E. coli* that carried a eukaryotic expression plasmid for the cytokine prothymosin enhanced the specific T cell responses and led to improved protection against the virus challenge. Some protection was already observed at the lowest dose of the recombinant bacteria. These promising results were however hampered by the fact that the vaccination procedure resulted in the death of some of the immunized mice as a result of toxic effects of the carrier bacteria. However, such problems might be overcome in the future by selecting appropriate variant strains and using different routes of application.

DNA Transfer By *Yersinia pseudotubercolosis*

With the increasing number of invasive bacteria that can possibly be used as carriers for expression plasmid transfer to host cells, it was not too surprising that also *Yersinia* are able to do so. Using an attenuated strain of *Y. pseudotubercolosis*, GFP could be transferred as reporter gene into human dendritic cells (Dietrich *et al.*, 2001). Although the frequency was rather low, the results are extremely promising since dendritic cells are notoriously difficult to transfect and negative findings have been reported for other systems (Grillot-Courvalin *et al.*, 1998).

DNA Transfer To Mammalian Cells By *Agrobacterium tumefaciens*

Recently it was shown that *A. tumefaciens,* a bacterium that is known to transfer expression cassettes into plant cells without invading them, can be used to transfer expression plasmids into human cell lines (Kunik *et al.*, 2001). *A. tumefaciens* contains the Ti plasmid that encodes the eukaryotic expression cassette as well as the genes necessary for DNA transfer. To be able to transfer DNA, the bacteria adhere to the plant cells via cellulose fibrills. Such fibrills could also be observed when the bacteria adhered to HeLa cells. Subsequent DNA transfer was dependent on the intact transfer apparatus of the Ti plasmid that is also required for DNA transfer to plant cells. Using this system, HeLa, a human embryonic kidney cell line HEK 393 and the neuronal cell line PC12 could be transfected. DNA transferred via *A. tumefaciens* normally integrates into random sites of the genome. Southern blot analysis as well as PCR amplification and sequence analysis revealed that plasmids had integrated into random sites of the genome of HeLa cells similar to integration into the genome of plants.

INDUCTION OF IMMUNE RESPONSES BY ORAL DNA VACCINATION

The immune response that is achieved by oral DNA vaccination using Gram-negative bacteria as carrier is surprisingly strong. Often, single applications resulted in responses that could be increased only marginally by additional applications (Darji *et al.*, 1997, Niethammer *et al.*, 2001a). On the other hand, it was possible to enhance the induction of immune reactions by co-tranfer of cytokine encoding expression plasmids (Shiau *et al.*, 2001 a, 2001b) or to boost the effector phase by parenterally supplying supporting cytokines (Xiang *et al.*, 2001, Niethammer *et al.*, 2001b). In addition, cotransfer of expression plasmids encoding modulatory cytokines could redirect immune reactions regardless of the responses dictated by the bacterial carrier or predetermined by the host. Thus, in order to manipulate this in a rational way, it will be necessary to understand the sequence of events that take place during DNA transfer and characterize the cell typess that are involved during both the transfer process as well as during the immune induction phase.

To be able to follow the initial events of immune induction, we designed a sensitive reporter system that would allow the measurement of cells that express or at least bear antigen expression. Thus, use of antigen presentation and T cell reactivity was used as sensitive indirect read out for the presence of antigen since T cell reactivity would reveal even low amounts of antigen present in a small number of cells. This reporter system revealed several interesting features of *Salmonella*-mediated DNA vaccination. Antigen presentation could be observed already 8 hrs after oral administration of the vaccine bacteria in Peyer's Patches, mesenteric lymph nodes (mLN) and spleen and it remained detectable for at least 35 days in mLN and spleen, whereas at this time point antigen was barely detectable in Peyer's Patches (Darji *et al.*, 2000). Thus, antigen is transported very quickly to deep lymphoid

Figure 1. Schematic representation of the likely sequence of events that lead to antigen expression and subsequent induction of immune responses after oral/mucosal DNA vaccination using bacterial vectors. Bacteria that carry the eukaryotic expression plasmids cross the barrier of the gut or bronchial epithelium and invade preferentially either macrophages or epithelial cells depending on the primary target of the particular carrier bacterium. They remain in the phagocytic vacuole (like *Salmonella*) or escape into the cytosol of the target cell (like *Shigella*). The metabolic attenuation results in bacterial lysis causing liberation, transfer and expression of the plasmid. Cell death occurs in some of the antigen expressing cells and the apoptotic bodies or the debris of such cells are taken up by neighboring dendritic cells which re-present the antigen derived from such cells. Dendritic cells themselves might also be infected and express antigen directly (not shown here).

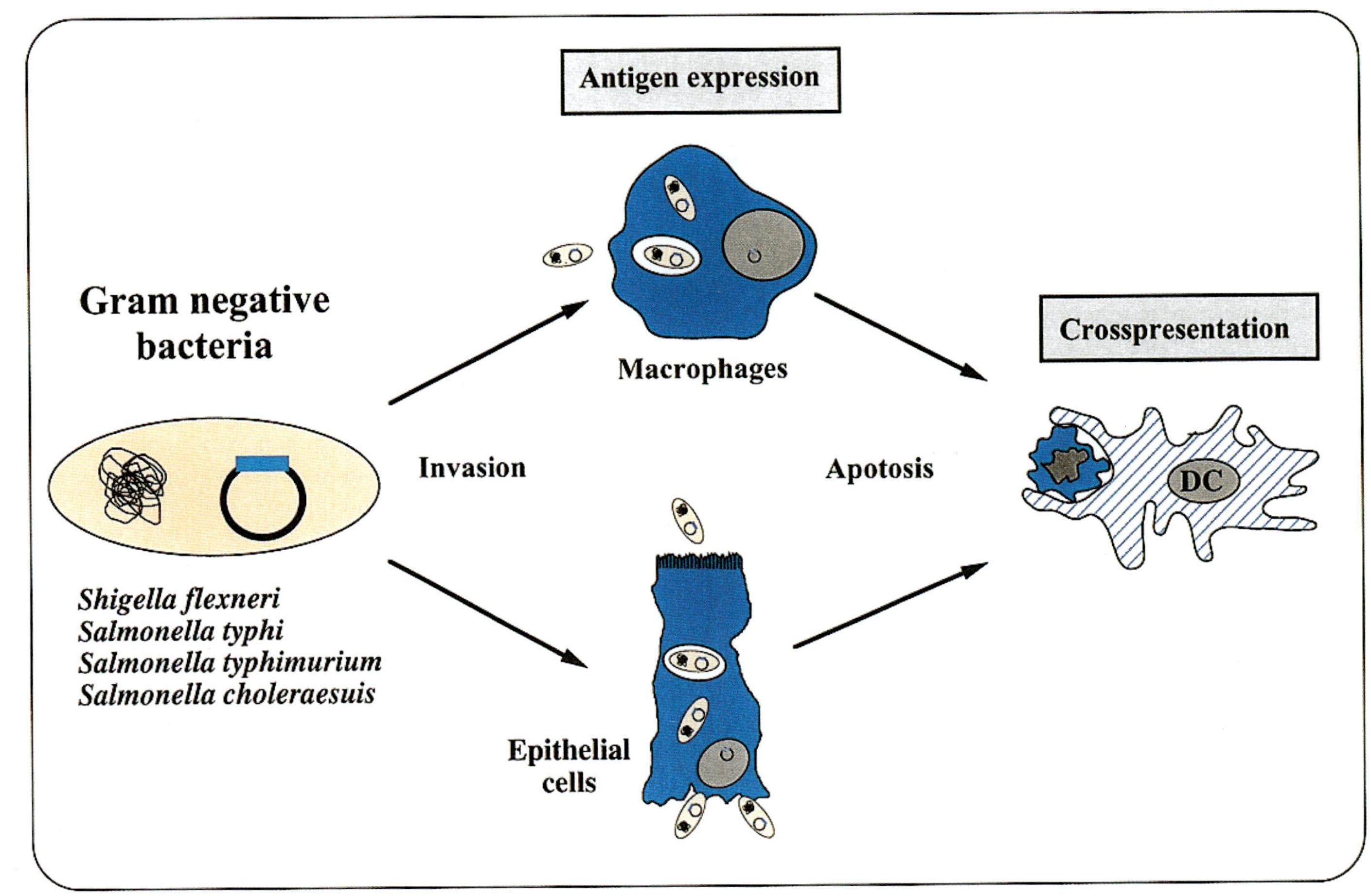

Antigen expression
Crosspresentation
Gram negative
bacteria
Macrophages
Invasion
Apotosis
DC
Shigella flexneri
Salmonella typhi
Salmonella typhimurium
Salmonella choleraesuis
Epithelial
cells

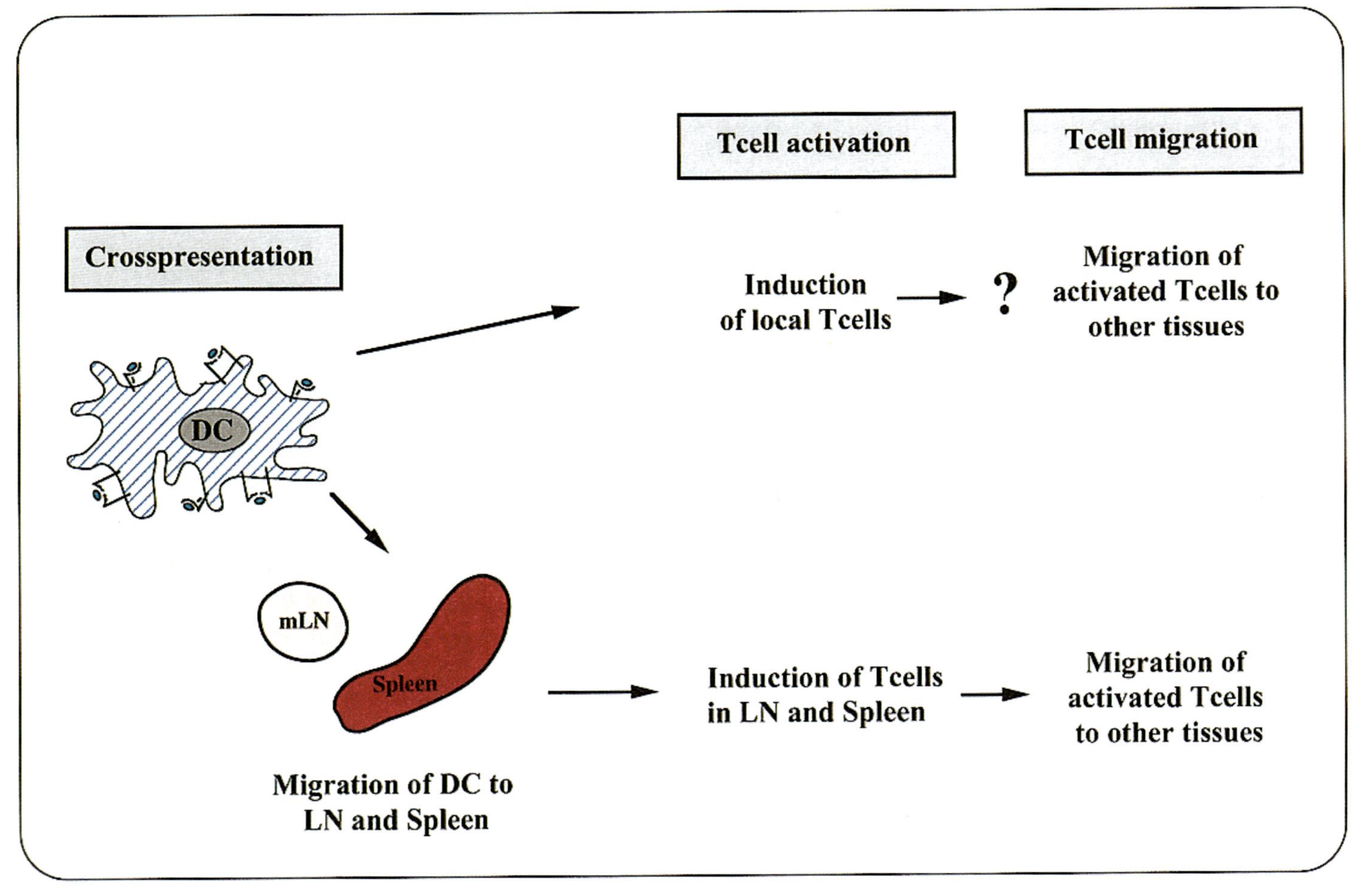

Crosspresentation
Tcell activation
Tcell migration
DC
Induction of local Tcells
? Migration of activated Tcells to other tissues
mLN
Spleen
Migration of DC to LN and Spleen
Induction of Tcells in LN and Spleen
Migration of activated Tcells to other tissues

Figure 2. Schematic representation of the likely sequence of events that lead to antigen expression and subsequent induction of immune responses after oral/mucosal DNA vaccination using bacterial vectors. Cross-presentation of antigens derived from the phagocytosis of dying cells results in the presentation of these antigens by MHC class I and class II molecules. Therefore, these dendritic cells are now able to activate CD4 helper T cells as well as CD8 cytotoxic T cells. Such T cells are activated either locally like in the Peyer's Patch or the antigen is transported to the deep lymphoid organs and T cells are activated there. Activated T cells then disseminate to the various tissues of the body including mucosal tissue.

organs which might explain the systemic response that is usually observed with oral DNA vaccination. In addition, the long lasting antigen presentation in mLN and spleen might explain the efficient induction of immune responses seen with even a single dose of the recombinant vaccine. Finally, the relatively rapid loss of T cell stimulatory capacity in Peyer's Patches and therefore the quick loss of antigen in this lymphoid organ might explain why we detected very little local antibody production (Darji *et al.*, 2000).

Characterization of the cells and the class of molecules that were involved in the presentation of antigen in Peyer's Patches and spleen allowed additional conclusions (Darji *et al.*, to be published). Macrophages in Peyer's Patches were able to present antigen only via MHC class I, indicating direct expression of antigen by these cells, since cytosolic antigens (like β-gal in the experiments described here) are normally only presented via MHC class I. No macrophages in the spleen were found to present antigen. In contrast, dendritic cells in Peyer's Patches as well as in the spleen were able to present antigen via MHC class I and class II. Only at the earliest time point (8 hrs) were dendritic cells found in spleen that exclusively present antigen via MHC class I. A possible interpretation of these experiments is that some of the dendritic cells express antigen directly. Immune modulation should aim to target such cells. On the other hand, most dendritic cells might acquire antigen via cross-presentation, i.e. uptake of apototic antigen expressing cells. This is in accordance with the fact that *Salmonella* are known to induce apotosis in activated macrophages. Under cross-presentation conditions, cytosolic antigens can also be presented via MHC class II (Heath and Carbone, 2001). This should add to the efficiency of oral *Salmonella*-mediated DNA vaccination. Early presentation via MHC class II should lead to induction of helper T cells in the initial phase of the immune response which in turn should amplify cytotoxic T cells and help to trigger B cells. Additional experiments revealed that a subpopulation of dendritic cells was responsible for the transport of antigen from Peyer's Patches to the deep lymphoid organs. No viable bacteria were detected under these conditions. Thus, rapid dissemination of the antigen might be exclusively due to migrating dendritic cells. The hypotheical sequence of events is summarized in Figures 1 and 2.

Due to the lack of an appropriate animal model at present little is known about the mechanisms that lead to the induction of an immune response when *Shigella* is used as a carrier. In analogy to the events found for *S. typhimurium* and taking into consideration the preference of *S. flexneri* for intestinal epithelial cells, a possible mechanism is suggested in Figures 1 and 2. We assume that the bacterium in some of the infected epithelial cells induces apoptosis. Transport of apoptotic epithelial cells to mesenteric lymph nodes by dendritic cells has recently been shown (Huang *et al.*, 2000). Thus, strong cross-presentation might be triggering the induction of the immune response, similar to what has been observed for *S. typhimurium*.

CONCLUSIONS

The results described here were obtained with a first generation of bacterial carrier systems to transfer eukaryotic expression plasmids into host cells *in vitro* and *in vivo*. Plasmids were usually derivatives of commercially available expression plasmids and most of the attenuated bacteria were previously designed as carriers for heterologous expression of antigens. Thus, the results obtained so far are highly encouraging and suggest that further development of this system is desirable.

Multiple improvements should be possible for the carrier as well as for the plasmids. Thus, enhancing infectivity by manipulating culture conditions of the bacterial carrier resulted in higher antibody responses (Darji *et al.*, 2000). Therefore, it should be possible to select variant carrier strains that constitutively display such properties. Other improvements might be introduced into the carrier bacteria themselves, such as altered tissue tropism etc. Similarly, the expression plasmids might be modified e.g. with tissue specific promoters or co-stimulatory molecules but also signals for nuclear transfer and stability and the use of different high copy replicons (e.g. Sindbis, Polyoma) could improve efficacy.

An area of potential application has to date remained largely unexplored. Bermudez and colleagues have shown by using hyperinvasive *Salmonella* that accumulation of these bacteria to high levels in individual organs and solid tumours can be achieved (Zheng *et al.*, 2000). Other bacteria have similar properties (Lemmon *et al.*, 1997, Yazawa *et al.*, 2001). On the other hand, high transfection rates have been detected in macrophages following plasmid transfer from bacteria (Darji *et al.*, 1997, Xiang *et al.*, 2000, Paglia *et al.*, 2000, Montosi *et al.*, 2000). However, transfer was restricted to such cells so far. The use of *Salmonella* that are modified to secrete listeriolysin might enable these bacteria to also transfer transgenes into other cell types Thus, it should be possible, by judicious use of cell-specific promoter elements and different replicons, to direct high levels of organotropic protein production in normal and neoplastic cells.

The ease of manipulating bacteria as transfer vehicles, an increased understanding of the subtle ways bacteria ursurp and manipulate functions of eucaryotic cells, and the genomic information that is becoming available for a wide variety of bacteria species provides the strong impetus for further development of this technology.

ACKNOWLEDGMENT

We would like to thank A. Darji and S. zur Lage for providing unpublished data. This work was supported in part by grants of the BMBF and the DFG to S.W and T.C.

REFERENCES

Aderem, A., and Ulevitch, R.J. 2000. Toll-like receptors in the induction of the innate immune response. Nature 406: 782-787.

Anderson, R.J., Pasetti, M.F., Sztein, M.B., Levine, M.M., and Noriega, F.R. 2000. Δ*guaBA* attenuated *Shigella flexneri* 2a strain CVD 1204 as a *Shigella* vaccine and as a live mucosal delivery system for fragment C of tetanus toxin. Vaccine 18: 2193-2202.

Brunham, R.C., and Zhang, D. 1999. Transgene as vaccine for chlamydia. Am. Heart J. 138: 519-522.

Catic, A., Dietrich, G., Gentschev, I., Goebel, W., Kaufmann, S.H., and Hess, J. 1999. Introduction of protein or DNA delivered via recombinant *Salmonella typhimurium* into the major histocompatibility complex class I presentation pathway of macrophages. Microbes. Infect. 1: 113-121.

Charpentier, E., Gerbaud, G., and Courvalin, P. 1999. Conjugative mobilization of the rolling-circle plasmid pIP823 from *Listeria monocytogenes* BM4293 among gram-positive and gram-negative bacteria. J. Bacteriol. 181: 3368-3374.

Courvalin, P., Goussard, S., and Grillot-Courvalin, C. 1995. Gene transfer from bacteria to mammalian cells. C. R. Acad. Sci. III 318: 1207-1212.

Darji, A., Guzman, C.A., Gerstel, B., Wachholz, P., Timmis, K.N., Wehland, J., Chakraborty, T., and Weiss, S. 1997. Oral somatic transgene vaccination using attenuated *S. typhimurium*. Cell 91: 765-775.

Darji, A., zur Lage, S., Garbe, A.I., Chakraborty, T., and Weiss, S. 2000. Oral delivery of DNA vaccines using attenuated *Salmonella typhimurium* as carrier. FEMS Immunol. Med. Microbiol. 27: 341-349.

Dietrich, G., Bubert, A., Gentschev, I., Sokolovic, Z., Simm, A., Catic, A., Kaufmann, S.H., Hess, J., Szalay, A.A., and Goebel, W. 1998. Delivery of antigen-encoding plasmid DNA into the cytosol of macrophages by attenuated suicide *Listeria monocytogenes*. Nat. Biotechnol. 16: 181-185.

Dietrich, G., Spreng, S., Gentschev, I., and Goebel, W. 2000. Bacterial systems for the delivery of eukaryotic antigen expression vectors. Antisense Nucleic Acid Drug Dev. 10: 391-399.

Dietrich, G., Kolb-Mäurer, A., Spreng, S., Schartl, M., Goebel, W., and Gentschev, I. 2001. Gram-positive and gram-negative bacteria as carrier systems for DNA vaccines. Vaccine 19: 2506-2512.

Fennelly, G.J., Khan, S.A., Abadi, M.A., Wild, T.F., and Bloom, B.R. 1999. Mucosal DNA vaccine immunization against measles with a highly attenuated *Shigella flexneri* vector. J. Immunol. 162: 1603-1610.

Fló, J., Tisminetzky, S., and Baralle, F. 2001. Oral transgene vaccination mediated by attenuated *Salmonellae* is an effective method to prevent Herpes simplex virus-2 induced disease in mice. Vaccine 19: 1772-1782.

Gentschev, I., Sokolovic, Z., Mollenkopf, H.J., Hess, J., Kaufmann, S.H., Kuhn, M., Krohne, G.F., and Goebel, W. 1995. *Salmonella* strain secreting active listeriolysin changes its intracellular localization. Infect. Immun. 63: 4202-4205.

Grillot-Courvalin, C., Goussard, S., Huetz, F., Ojcius, D.M., and Courvalin, P. 1998. Functional gene transfer from intracellular bacteria to mammalian cells. Nat. Biotechnol. 16: 862-866.

Gurunathan, S., Klinman, D.M., and Seder, R.A. 2000. DNA vaccines: immunology, application, and optimization. Annu. Rev. Immunol. 18: 927-974.

Heath, W.R., and Carbone, F.R. 2001. Cross-presentation, dendritic cells, tolerance and immunity. Annu. Rev. Immunol. 19: 47-64.

Heinemann, J.A., and Sprague, G.F., Jr. 1989. Bacterial conjugative plasmids mobilize DNA transfer between bacteria and yeast. Nature 340:205-209.

Hense, M., Domann, E., Krusch, S., Wachholz, P., Dittmar, K.E.J., Rohde, M., Wehland, J., Chakraborty, T., and Weiss, S. 2001. Eukrayotic expression plasmid transfer from the intracellular bacterium *Listeria monocytogenes* to host cells. Cell. Microbiol. 3: 599-609.

Hoiseth, S.K., and Stocker, B.A. 1981. Aromatic-dependent *Salmonella typhimurium* are non-virulent and effective as live vaccines. Nature 291: 238-239.

Huang, F.P., Platt, N., Wykes, M., Major, J.R., Powell, T.J., Jenkins, C.D., and MacPherson, G.G. 2000. A discrete subpopulation of dendritic cells transports apoptotic intestinal epithelial cells to T cell areas of mesenteric lymph nodes. J. Exp. Med. 191:435-444.

Kunik, T., Tzfira, T., Kapulnik, Y., Gafni, Y., Dingwall, C., and Citovsky, V. 2001. Genetic transformation of HeLa cells by *Agrobacterium*. Proc Natl Acad Sci USA. 98: 1871-1876.

Lemmon, M.J., v. Zijl, P., Fox, M.E., Mauchline, M.L., Giaccia A.J., Minton, N.P., and Brown, J.M. 1997. Anaerobic bacteria as a gene delivery system that is controlled by the tumor microenvironment. Gene Ther. 4: 791-796.

Lessl, M., and Lanka, E. 1994. Common mechanisms in bacterial conjugation and Ti-mediated T-DNA transfer to plant cells. Cell 77: 321-324.

Leung, K.Y., and Finlay, B.B. 1991. Intracellular replication is essential for the virulence of *Salmonella typhimurium*. Proc. Natl. Acad. Sci. USA. 88: 11470-11474.

Levine, M.M., and Dougan, G. 1998. Optimism over vaccines administered via mucosal surfaces. Lancet 351: 1375-1376.

Lode, H.N., Pertl, U., Xiang, R., Gaeldicke, G., and Reisfeld, R.A. 2000. Tyrosine Hydroxylase-based DNA vaccination is effective against murine neuroblastoma. Med. Ped. Oncol. 35: 641-646.

Mastroeni, P., Chabalgotty, J.A., Dunstan, S.J., Maskell, D.L., and Dougan, G. 2000. *Salmonella*: immune responses and vaccines. Vet. J. 161: 132-164.

Montosi, G., Paglia, P., Garuti, C., Guzmán, C.A., Bastin, J.M. Colombo, M.P., and Pietrangelo, A. 2000. Wild-type HFE protein normalizes transferrin iron accumulation in macrophages from subjects with hereditary hemochromatosis. Blood 96: 1125-1129.

Niethammer, A.G., Primus, F.J., Xiang, R., Dolmann, C.S., Ruehlmann, J.M., Ba, Y., Gillies, S.D., and Reisfeld, R.A. 2001a. An oral DNA vaccine against human carcinoembrionic antigen (CEA) prevents growth and disssemination of Lewis lung carcinoma in CEA transgenic mice. Vaccine 20: 421-429.

Niethammer, A.G., Xiang, R., Ruehlmann, J.M., Lode, H.N. Dolman, C.S., Gillies, S.D., and Reisfeld R.A. 2001b. Targeted Interleukin 2 therapy enhances protective immunity induced by an autologous oral DNA vaccine against murine melanoma. Cancer Res. 61: 6178-6184.

Norbury, C.C., Hewlett, L.J., Prescott, A.R., Shastri, N., and Watts, C. 1995. Class I MHC presentation of exogenous soluble antigen via macropinocytosis in bone marrow macrophages. Immunity 3: 783-791.

Noriega, F.R., Wang, J.Y., Losonsky, G., Maneval, D.R., Hone, D.M., and Levine, M.M. 1994. Construction and characterization of attenuated Δ*aroA* Δ*virG Shigella flexneri* 2a strain CVD 1203, a prototype live oral vaccine. Infect. Immun. 62: 5168-5172.

Noriega, F.R., Losonsky, G., Lauderbaugh, C., Liao, F.M., Wang, J.Y., and Levine, M.M. 1996. Engineered Δ*guaB-A* Δ*virG Shigella flexneri* 2a strain CVD 1205: construction, safety, immunogenicity, and potential efficacy as a mucosal vaccine. Infect. Immun. 64: 3055-3061.

Paglia, P., Medina, E., Arioli, I., Guzman, C.A., and Colombo, M.P. 1998. Gene transfer in dendritic cells, induced by oral DNA vaccination with *Salmonella typhimurium*, results in protective immunity against a murine fibrosarcoma. Blood 92: 3172-3176.

Paglia, P., Terrazzini, N., Schulze, K., Guzman, C.A., and Colombo, M.P. 2000. *In vivo* correction of genetic defects of monocyte/macrophages using attenuated *Salmonella* as oral vectors for targeted gene delivery. Gene Ther. 7:1725-1730.

Pasetti, M.F., Anderson, R.J., Noriega, F.R., Levine, M.M., and Sztein, M.B. 1999. Attenuated Δ*guaBA Salmonella typhi* vaccine strain CVD 915 as a live vector utilizing prokaryotic or eukaryotid expression systems to deliver foreign antigens and elicit immune responses. Clin. Immun. 92:76-89.

Powell, R.J., Lewis, G.K., and Hone, D.M. 1996. Introduction of eukaryotic expression cassettes into animal cells using bacterial vector delivery system. In: Vaccines 96: Molecular Approaches to the Control of Infectious Disease. Cold Spring Harbor Laboratory Press, Cold Spring Harbor,NY, p. 183-187.

Reinhardt, R.L., Khoruts, A., Mercia, R., Zell, T., and Jenkins, M.K. 2001. Visualizing the generation of memory CD4 T cells in the whole body. Nature 410: 101-105.

Rodriguez, A., Regnault, A., Kleijmeer, M., Ricciardi-Castagnoli, P., and Amigorena, S. 1999. Selective transport of internalized antigens to the cytosol for MHC class I presentation in dendritic cells. Nat. Cell Biol. 1: 362-368.

Schaffner, W. 1980. Direct transfer of cloned genes from bacteria to mammalian cells. Proc. Natl. Acad. Sci. USA. 77: 2163-2167.

Shata, M.T., and Hone, D.M. 2001. Vaccination with a *Shigella* DNA vaccine vector induces antigen-specific CD8[+] T cells and antiviral protective immunity. J. Virol. 75:9665-9670.

Shata, M.T., Reitz, M.S.Jr., DeVico, A.L., Lewis, G.K., and Hone, D.M. 2001. Mucosal and systemic HIV-1 Env-specific $CD8^+$ T-cells develop after intragastric vaccination with a *Salmonella* Env DNA vaccine vector. Vaccine 20: 623-629.

Shiau, A.-L., Chu C.-Y., Su, W.C., and Wu, C.-L.2001a. Vaccination with the glycoprotein D gene of pseudorabies virus delivered by nonpathogenic *Escherichia coli* elicits protective immune responses. Vaccine 19: 3277-5467.

Shiau, A-.L., Chen, Y.-L., Liao, C.-Y., Huang, Y.-S., and Wu, C.-L. 2001b. Prothymosin enhances protective immune responses induced by oral DNA vaccination against pseudorabies delivered by *Salmonella choleraesuis*. Vaccine 19: 3947-3956.

Sizemore, D.R., Branstrom, A.A., and Sadoff, J.C. 1995. Attenuated *Shigella* as a DNA delivery vehicle for DNA-mediated immunization. Science 270: 299-302.

Sizemore, D.R., Branstrom, A.A., and Sadoff, J.C. 1997. Attenuated bacteria as a DNA delivery vehicle for DNA-mediated immunization. Vaccine 15: 804-807.

Trieu-Cuot, P., Derlot, E., and Courvalin, P. 1993. Enhanced conjugative transfer of plasmid DNA from *Escherichia coli* to *Staphylococcus aureus* and *Listeria monocytogenes*. FEMS Microbiol. Lett. 109: 19-23.

Urashima, M., Suzuki, H., Yuza, Y., Akiyama, M., Ohno, N., and Eto, Y. 2000. An oral CD40 ligand gene therapy against lymphoma using attenuated *Salmonella typhimurium*. Blood 95: 1258-1263.

Wagner, H. 1999. Bacterial CpG DNA activates immune cells to signal infectious danger. Adv. Immunol. 73:329-368.

Wang, J.Y., Pasetti, M.F., Noriega, F.R., Anderson, R.J., Wassermann, S.S., Galen, J.E., Sztein, M.B., and Levine, M.M. 2001. Construction, genotypic and phenotypic characterization, and immunogenicity of attenuated ΔguaBA *Salmonella enterica* serovar *Typhi* strain CVD 915. Infect. Immun. 69: 4734-4741.

Woo, P.C., Tsoi, H.W., Leung, H.C., Wong, L.P., Wong, S.S., Chan, E., and Yuen, K.Y. 2000. Enhancement by ampicillin of antibody responses induced by a protein antigen and a DNA vaccine carried by live-attenuated *Salmonella enterica* serovar *Typhi*. Clin. Diagn. Lab. Immunol. 7: 596-599.

Woo, P.C.Y., Wong, L.P., Zheng, B.J., and Yuen, K.Y. 2001. Unique immunogenicity of Hepatitis B virus DNAvaccine presented by live-attenuated *Salmonella typhimurium*. Vaccine 19: 2945-2954.

Yazawa, K., Fujimori, M., Nakamura, T., Sasaki, T., Amano, J., Kano, Y. and Taniguchi, S. 2001. *Bifidobacterium longum* as a delivery system for gene therapy of chemically induced rat mammary tumors. Breast Cancer Research and Treatment 66: 165-170.

Yuhua, L., Y, Kunyuan, G., Hui, C., Yongmei, X, Chaoyang, S, Xun, T., and Daming R. 2001. Oral cytokine gene therapy against murine tumor using attenuated *Salmonella typhimurium*. Int. J. Cancer 94: 438-443.

Xiang, R., Lode, H.N., Chao, T.H., Ruehlmann, J.M., Dolman, C.S., Rodriguez, F., Whitton, J.L., Overwijk, W.W., Restifo, N.P., and Reisfeld, R.A. 2000. An autologous oral DNA vaccine protects against murine melanoma. Proc. Natl. Acad. Sci. USA. 97: 5492-5497.

Xiang, R., Silletti, S., Lode, H.N., Dolman, C.S., Ruehlmann, J.M., Niethammer, A.G., Pertl, U., Gillies, S.D., Primus, F.J, and Reisfeld, R.A. 2001. Protective Immunity against human carcinoembryonic antigen (CEA) induced by an oral DNA vaccine in CEA-transgenic mice. Clin. Cancer Res. 7: 856S-864S.

Zheng, B., Woo, P.C.Y., Ng, M., Tsoi, H., Wong, L., and Yuen, K. 2001. A crucial role of macrophages in the immune responses to oral DNA vaccination against hepatitis B virus in a murine model. Vaccine 20: 140-147.

Zheng, L-I., Luo, X., Feng, M., Li, Z., Le, T., Ittensohn, M., Trailsmith, M., Bermudes, D., Lin, S.L. and King, I.C. 2000. Tumor amplified protein expression therapy: *Salmonella* as a tumor-selective protein delivery vector. Oncol. Res. 12: 127-135.

Zöller, M., and Christ, O. 2001. Prophylactic tumor vaccination: comparison of effector mechanisms initiated by protein versus DNA vaccination. J. Immunol. 166: 3440-3450.

From: *Vaccine Delivery Strategies*
Edited by: Guido Dietrich and Werner Goebel

Chapter 14

Recombinant Intra-cellular Bacteria as Carriers for Tumor Antigens

George R. Gunn, III, Abba C. Zubair
and Yvonne Paterson

ABSTRACT

It is about 100 years since William Coley first used bacteria as non-specific stimulators of the immune system for tumor therapy. With the discovery of antigens associated with tumors to which a specific immune response can be directed, bacteria can now be engineered to target antigens to the immune system in addition to providing adjuvant properties. Intra-cellular bacteria are particularly attractive candidate vectors of this class of antigens because of their ability to induce strong cell mediated immunity that can target tumor cells regardless of the cytosolic localization of the tumor antigen. In addition the propensity of intra-cellular bacteria to infect phagocytic cells aids delivery of the antigens directly to professional antigen presenting cells, which express co-stimulatory molecules, and stimulate efficient priming of a T cell response. In addition bacteria may be safer vectors for tumor antigens than viral vectors because of the wide spectrum of antibiotics to which they are susceptible in the event of unforeseen susceptibility by the patient. The potent Th1-type immune response induced by intra-cellular bacteria, the readily available genetic tools to manipulate the bacteria's phenotype, and the potential safety advantages inherent in bacteria provide the rationale for investigating them as potential vaccine vectors for targeting tumor antigens. Here we will review the history, and recent use of three intra-cellular bacterial vectors, *Listeria monocytogenes*, *Salmonella typhimurium,* and the BCG vaccine strain of *Mycobacterium bovis.*

INTRODUCTION

It has long been a goal of immunologists to direct an effective immune response to target tumor cells. However, in order to target an immune response to a tumor it is necessary to overcome self-tolerance. Tumor cells are originally derived from normal cells, and therefore share the majority of their potential antigens with other normal cells in the host. The immune system has developed several levels of control that govern the recognition, and attack of "self" tissue. It is this tolerance to self that must be broken in a selective manner before an effective tumor-specific immune response can be mounted.

Some of the earliest attempts to incite the immune system to target a tumor for destruction were carried out by William B. Coley from 1891-1936. Coley noticed that several sarcoma patients who developed erysipelas (a streptococcal infection of the skin) underwent a regression of their tumors (Coley, 1893). He began injecting preparations of heat-killed, gram-positive streptococci combined with gram-negative *Serratia marcescens* directly into tumors (Coley, 1909). These "Coley's toxins" were also administered as intramuscular injections in the buttocks or in the pectoral region as a supplement to the intratumoral injections (Coley, 1909). Coley claimed a greater than 10% cure rate in patients treated with his bacterial preparations (Wiemann, and Starnes, 1994). Although the mechanism for the regression of the tumors was not understood at the time, and the immune system was not well characterized, Coley, and his contemporaries were pioneers in the field of tumor immunotherapy.

The ultimate goal of tumor immunotherapy is to utilize the power of the immune system to target, and destroy tumor cells both at the primary tumor site as well as distant metastatic sites. Effective tumor immunotherapy holds several potential advantages over traditional surgical, radiotherapy or chemotherapeutic approaches to cancer treatment, including exquisite specificity, and a reduction of the number, and severity of side effects. In order for tumor immunotherapy to be effective, tumors must first express antigens that are in some way specific to the tumor itself, and are accessible to the effectors of the immune response. It is also necessary for responding lymphocytes to receive the proper co-stimulation through cognate interactions with antigen presenting cells (APC), as well as growth factor, and cytokine stimulation.

Although there has been speculation on the existence of tumor antigens since early in the 1900s (Schreiber *et al.*, 1988), it was not until the 1990s that they were actually isolated, and cloned. Tumor antigens can be roughly classified into four groups: mutated self-antigens, shared tumor antigens, tissue specific antigens, and viral antigens (Boon *et al.,* 1994). Mutated self-antigens arise when normal genes undergo mutation as part of the neoplastic process. This yields aberrant proteins that are accessible to the immune system. Mutated self-antigens are commonly the result of mutations in oncogenes such as p53, retinoblastoma or members of the epidermal growth factor (egf) receptor family, but can also arise from genes that encode proteins that have no direct role in the transformed phenotype. Shared tumor antigens are not specific to one tumor, but are expressed by multiple tumors that arise independently. Common examples of shared tumor antigens include the MAGE, BAGE, and GAGE families of antigens originally isolated from human melanoma but now known to be present in other tumors (Chomez *et al.*, 2001). Shared tumor antigens are often expressed at low levels in tissues considered to be immune privileged, such as the testis or the placenta, and may be the products of genes expressed during embryonic development that are silent in normal cells. Tissue specific tumor antigens are expressed by tumors as well as the normal tissue from which they have arisen. For example, the melanoma-associated tumor antigens tyrosinase, and tyrosinase-related protein 1 (TRP-1) are also expressed by normal melanocytes. Immune responses that target TRP-1 can lead to vitiligo as normal melanocytes are also killed by the anti-TRP-1 immune response (Overwijk *et al.*, 1999). Finally, viral infections have been associated with certain types of tumors. Epstein-Barr virus, and human papillomavirus are examples of transforming viruses commonly associated with specific human tumors (Boon *et al.*, 1994). Virally derived proteins expressed by these tumors have the advantage of being immunologically "foreign", and can serve as tumor-associated antigens.

THE IMMUNE RESPONSE TO TUMOR ANTIGENS

It is clear that tumor rejection is largely mediated by a strong cellular immune response (Berd, 1998). It is therefore important that the available tumor antigens are presented to responding T cells by class I and/or class II MHC molecules. Although presentation of antigenic peptides by the tumor cells themselves is ultimately necessary for recognition, and killing by responding CTLs, the initial priming of the anti-tumor response is probably exclusively stimulated by antigen presenting cells (APCs) such as macrophages (Mφ), and dendritic cells (DC). Work by Drew Pardoll and colleagues has shown, in transplantable tumor systems, that bone marrow-derived APCs are responsible for the stimulation necessary to prime a tumor rejection response (Huang *et al.*, 1994). This presentation of tumor antigens by "professional" antigen presenting cells is commonly called cross-priming (Pardoll, 1998). It is therefore necessary for a tumor immunotherapeutic to stimulate such APCs to present tumor antigens, thereby priming a tumor-specific immune response.

Cytokines have also been demonstrated to play a major role in tumor rejection responses. Cytokines of the Th1-type are particularly effective for inducing inflammatory responses within the tumor. The hallmark of a Th1-type cytokine profile includes the interleukins IL-2, and IL-12 as well as TNF-α, and IFN-γ. The cytokine IL-12 is known to be the driving force behind the shift to a Th1-type cytokine profile (Hsieh *et al.*, 1993; Manetti *et al.*, 1993). IL-12, expressed, and secreted by Mφs, DCs, and possibly B cells, stimulates the secretion of IFN-γ. In a positive feedback loop, IL-12 release is boosted by IFN-γ (Boehm *et al.*, 1997; Trinchieri, and Scott 1999). IFN-γ is released from activated, and naive NK cells, and T cells (Boehm *et al.*, 1997; Trinchieri, and Scott, 1999). Activated T cells have also been shown to induce IL-12 secretion by Mφs, and dendritic cells (Germann *et al.*, 1993; Macatonia *et al.*, 1995). This T cell-dependent induction of IL-12 expression is mediated by the interaction of CD40L on the surface of activated T cells that ligate CD40 on the surface of IL-12 producing cells (Cella *et al.*, 1996; Shu *et al.*, 1995). IFN-γ acts to stimulate Mφs to directly kill tumor cells (Pace *et al.*, 1985). It also acts in an anti-angiogenic manner, blocking the formation of new blood vessels within tumors (Maheshwari *et al.*, 1991; Sato *et al.*, 1990; Beatty, and Paterson, 2001). IFN-γ also leads to the upregulation of the expression of MHC class I, and II molecules (Boehm *et al.*, 1997). Mouse models have shown that both TNF-α (Creasey *et al.*, 1986; Haranaka *et al.*, 1984), and IL-2 (Rosenberg, 1984; Rosenberg *et al.*, 1985; Winkelhake *et al.*, 1987) can significantly influence tumor regression. The cytokine granulocyte macrophage-colony stimulating factor (GM-CSF) has been used effectively in tumor immunotherapy as well (Dranoff *et al.*, 1993). GM-CSF expressed in the tumor microenvironment promotes the differentiation of immature DCs which, in turn, very efficiently stimulate virgin T cells to respond to tumor antigens (Pardoll, 1998). Even the Th-2 type cytokine, IL-4, can be important for tumor regression in some tumor models. IL-4 associated regression is largely mediated by a massive influx of eosinophils, which create an inflammatory response within the tumor (Tepper *et al.*, 1992). Antigen presentation, and cytokines work in concert with cognate stimulation through the B7/CD28 co-stimulatory pathway to activate tumor specific T cells (June *et al.*, 1990). It is ultimately the activation of tumor-specific T cells that determines the outcome of the anti-tumor response. These T cells must be able to overcome any tolerance to tumor antigens as well as possible immunosuppressive activities mediated by the tumor itself. Once tumor specific T cells are activated, a race begins between tumor cell replication, and T cell mediated destruction. The outcome of this race determines the survival or demise of the host bearing the tumor.

It is well known that the immune system responds quite effectively to viral, and bacterial infections, yet not very well to tumor associated antigens. Resident T cells that recognize tumor antigens tend to remain ignorant rather than becoming activated. This may be due to a lack of co-stimulation in the tumor site (Melero *et al.*, 1997). It has also been proposed that tumors do not provide the "danger signal" that bacterial, and viral infections do, providing inflammation, and an influx of antigen presenting cells (Fuchs, and Matzinger, 1996). Aside from failing to produce a danger signal, tumors have been shown to actively evade the immune response. Tumors can often downregulate expression of tumor antigens (Urban *et al.*, 1982; Uyttenhove *et al.*, 1983; Wortzel *et al.*, 1983), MHC molecules (Haywood, and McKhann, 1971; Hui *et al.*, 1984; Trowsdale *et al.*, 1980; Wallich *et al.*, 1985), and antigen processing machinery (Restifo *et al.*, 1991). Some tumors even secrete immunosuppressive cytokines such as TGF-β (Torre-Amione *et al.*, 1990). Thus designing effective tumor vaccines poses special problems usually not encountered in conventional vaccine development.

Cellular immune responses to tumor antigens provide another benefit when compared to humoral responses because cellular immune responses are capable of targeting antigens regardless of their compartmentalization within the tumor cell. Tumor antigens can have one of five general locations or destinations within the tumor cell. They can be localized in the nucleus, the mitochondria, the cytoplasm, be expressed on the surface of the cell, or be secreted. Typically, secreted antigens or cell surface antigens are the only types accessible to a humoral immune response. In contrast, peptides derived from proteins, regardless of their cellular or extracellular destination, can be presented by MHC class I molecules to responding CD8[+] T cells (York, and Rock, 1996). MHC class I molecule/peptide complexes give the immune system a means of sampling the autologous proteins expressed by a cell.

It is with these complexities in mind that tumor immunologists attempt to develop therapeutics that overcome natural ignorance to tumor antigens, and provide the necessary co-stimulatory signals, antigen presentation, and cytokines to ensure recognition, and lysis of tumor cells in an antigen-specific manner. Theoretically, the best immunotherapeutic approach would be to induce a cellular immune response with a Th1 type cytokine profile targeting a tumor antigen that is effectively presented by both MHC class I, and II molecules in a cytokine environment that stimulates the development of long-lived adaptive immunity. Intracellular bacteria are attractive vehicles to induce such responses.

LISTERIA MONOCYTOGENES, AND THE CELLULAR IMMUNE RESPONSE

Listeria monocytogenes is a Gram-positive rod that can infect humans, and animals. Soon after entering the blood stream, these bacteria are phagocytosed by MΦs, Kupffer cells, neutrophils, and monocytes. *L. monocytogenes* then escapes from the phagocytic vacuole, largely by the action of the thiol-activated, pore-forming hemolysin, listeriolysin-O (LLO), and enters the cytoplasm of the cell (Gaillard *et al.*, 1987; Tilney, and Portnoy, 1989). The gene *plcA* encodes a phosphatidylinositol-specific phospholipase C (PI-PLC) that improves the efficiency of this vacuole escape (Camilli *et al.*, 1993). The cytoplasm of a cell serves as a rich growth medium for the bacteria allowing *L. monocytogenes* to undergo replication rapidly (Marquis *et al.*, 1993). The listerial virulence gene *actA* encodes a protein, ActA, which is positioned in a polar manner on the outer surface of the bacterium. ActA polymerizes the host cell actin forming a tail of actin that pushes the listeriae around the cytoplasm of the cell (Kocks *et al.*, 1992). This intracellular motility allows *L. monocytogenes* to form pseudopods that extend from the infected cell, and are taken up by neighboring cells. In this manner *L. monocytogenes* can spread from one cell to another without leaving the cytoplasm or contacting the extracellular milieu. Thus, *L. monocytogenes* remains largely sequestered from the humoral arm of the immune system. Through the action of LLO, and a second, broad-range phospholipase C

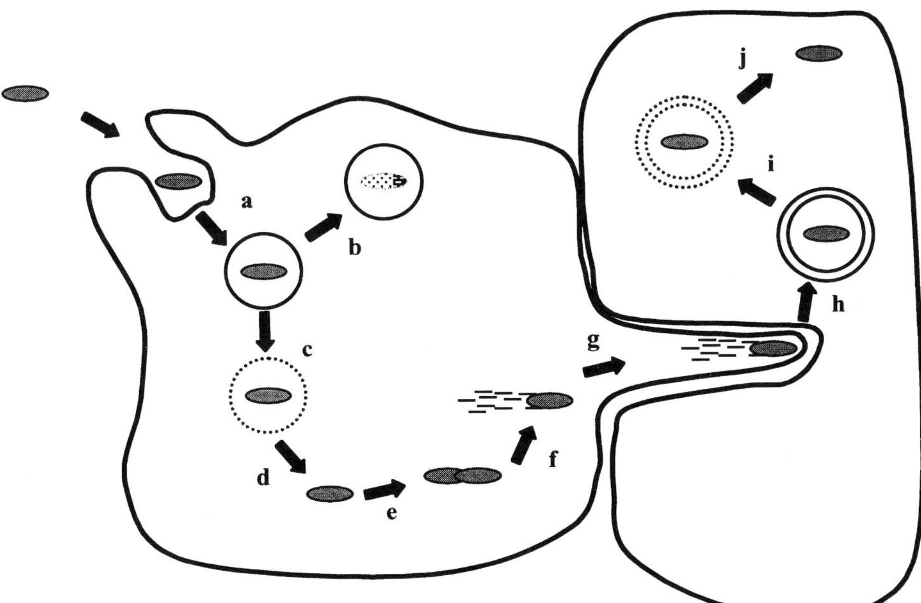

Figure 1. *Listeria monocytogenes* intracellular lifecycle. (a) Blood borne *L. monocytogenes* is rapidly phagocytosed by macrophages, Kupffer cells and neutrophils. (b) The majority of the phagocytosed bacteria are killed in the phagosomal-lysosomal compartment. (c and d) Approximately 10% of the *L. monocytogenes* rupture the phagosome by the action of LLO, a phosphatidylinositol-specific PLC A, and a broad-range phosphatidylcholine specific PLC B, escaping into the cytoplasm. (e) In the cytoplasm the bacteria rapidly replicate. (f and g) The protein Act A polymerizes the host cell actin, pushing the bacteria through the cytoplasm, occasionally resulting in pseudopod-like structures that are phagocytosed by neighboring cells (h), (i) and (j) *Listeria* then perforate this double membrane vacuole with LLO and the broad-range PLC to allow the cycle to begin again.

(PLC), *L. monocytogenes* escapes from the double walled phagosome, and begins the intracellular growth, and replication cycle again (Smith *et al.*, 1995; Vazquez-Boland *et al.*, 1992). The virulence genes encoding the PLCs, *plcA*, and *plcB*, and the other virulence genes, *hly*, and *actA*, are regulated by the pluri-potential transcription factor PrfA, which is encoded by the *prfA* gene (Portnoy *et al.*, 1992). Figure 1 summarizes this intracellular lifecycle. *Listeria monocytogenes* infection in the mouse serves as a classic model of cellular immunity (Mackaness, 1969). Control of the infection is mediated by a complex interaction of Mϕs, NK cells, neutrophils, and T cells (Unanue, 1997). Neutrophils are seen as the first line of defense, and are closely followed by activated Mϕs. These Mϕs secrete IL-12, and TNF-α, which stimulate NK cells to secrete IFN-γ (Unanue, 1997). IL-12 influences the development of the T cell response, which tends to be of the Th1 type (Mata, and Paterson, 1999). The responding T cells also secrete IFN-γ, which in turn stimulates Mϕs to become activated, upregulate class I, and class II

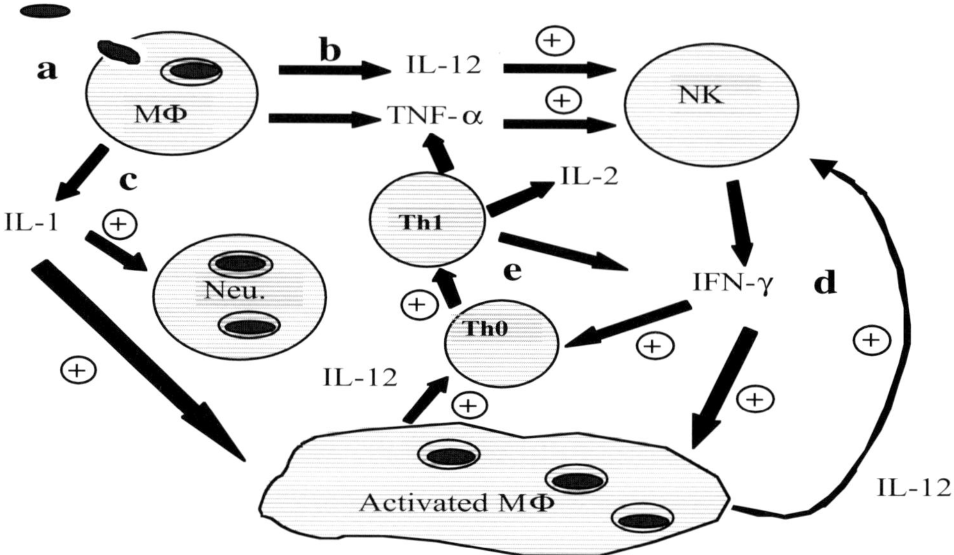

Figure 2. *Listeria monocytogenes* induces a cytokine cascade early in infection. (a) Bacteria are taken up by phagocytic cells including macrophages (Mφ) and neutrophils. Cell wall components activate macrophages to produce (b) IL-12 and TNF-α that activate NK cells, and (c) IL-1 that activates neutrophils. Activated NK cells produce (d) IFN-γ that acts on macrophages to upregulate antigen processing machinery and increase the further production of IL-12 and (e) drives the maturation of Th0 cells to Th1 cells.

MHC molecules, and secrete more IL-12 (Paterson, and Ikonomidis, 1996). Figure 2 summarizes the cytokine cascade, and its influence on innate effector cells early after *L. monocytogenes* infection.

While less is known about the neutrophil response to *L. monocytogenes* than the macrophage response, the early neutrophil response is necessary for control of the initial infection. The neutrophil response is particularly important for control of the bacterial infection in the liver (Unanue, 1997). Neutrophils lyse infected hepatocytes, releasing the *L. monocytogenes* into the extracellular milieu where they can be captured, and lysed (Mocci *et al.*, 1997). Neutrophils possess potent anti-microbial machinery including granular enzymes, anti-microbial peptides, and reactive oxygen intermediates. Neutrophils have also been implicated in keeping the CNS clear of invading *L. monocytogenes* during murine listeriosis (Lopez *et al.*, 2000).

Although innate effectors can limit *Listeria* infection in mice, T cells are necessary for resolution of the infection. In the mouse model CD4[+], and

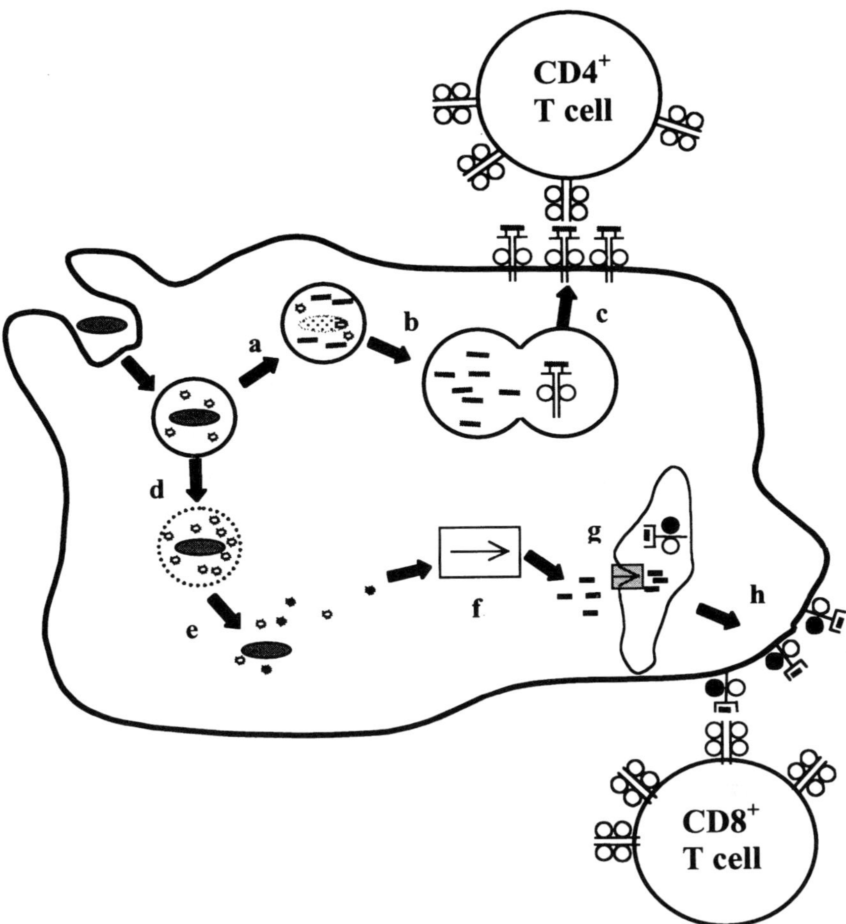

Figure 3. *Listeria monocytogenes* antigens are presented to both CD4+ and CD8+ T cells. (a) Phagocytosed *L. monocytogenes* that are unable to lyse the phagosomal-lysosomal membrane are degraded (b) and their proteins are broken down into peptides that can be loaded onto MHC class II molecules (c) and presented to CD4+ T cells. Alternatively, if the bacteria succeed in lysing the phagosomal membrane (d), they and their secreted virulence factors are released into the cytoplasm (e). These secreted proteins are cleaved by the proteasome (f) and the resulting peptides are transported into the endoplasmic reticulum where they are loaded onto MHC class I molecules (g). The class I MHC molecules egress to the cell membrane (h) where they present the peptides to CD8+ T cells.

CD8$^+$ T cells begin to join the anti-*Listeria* response starting at day 3 of infection (Unanue, 1997). Over the next several days the CD4$^+$, and CD8$^+$ compartments respond, proliferating, and clearing infected cells (Unanue, 1997). Presentation to CD4$^+$ or CD8$^+$ T cells largely depends on whether the bacteria escape from the phagosome (Figure 3). *L. monocytogenes* that are killed in the phagosomal-lysosomal compartment are degraded. Their proteins are broken down into peptides, which can then be loaded onto MHC class II molecules. These class II molecules transit to the cell surface where they present the peptides to CD4$^+$ T cells (Watts, 1997). If *L. monocytogenes* succeeds in perforating the phagosomal membrane, and escapes into the cytoplasm, then secreted proteins are targeted to the proteasome for degradation. The proteasome degrades the proteins into peptides that are transported into the endoplasmic reticulum (ER) via the transporter associated with antigen processing (TAP) system (Stevanovic, and Schild, 1999). In the ER, the peptides are loaded onto MHC class I molecules, which are then transported to the cell surface (Stevanovic, and Schild, 1999). The MHC class I molecules on the surface of the cell present the peptides to responding CD8$^+$ T cells (Figure 3).

Parenthetically, the role of γδ T cells is less clear in the anti-listerial response. γδ T cells are not essential for resolution of *L. monocytogenes* infection in the mouse, though their absence leads to a somewhat slowed clearance of the bacteria (DiTirro *et al.*, 1998). It has been suggested that the role of γδ T cells in the liver is to direct cellular traffic during the early response to the infection, reducing neutrophil infiltration, and recruiting Mϕs by secreting MCP-1 (DiTirro *et al.*, 1998). Ultimately the αβ T cells are responsible for resolving the infection.

As mentioned previously, the most effective anti-tumor immune responses are cellular immune responses with a Th1 type cytokine profile. *L. monocytogenes* infection induces such an immune response (Mata, and Paterson, 1999). *L. monocytogenes* delivers secreted antigens directly to APCs, which express co-stimulatory molecules, and stimulate efficient priming of a T cell response. Additionally, *L. monocytogenes* is susceptible to a wide range of antibiotics, and does not express the endotoxins associated with Gram negative bacteria. The potent Th1-type immune response, the readily available genetic tools to manipulate the bacteria's phenotype, and the potential safety advantages inherent in Gram positive bacteria provide the rationale for investigating *L. monocytogenes* as a potential vaccine vector for targeting tumor antigens.

DEVELOPMENT OF *L. MONOCYTOGENES* AS A VACCINE VECTOR FOR TUMOR ANTIGENS

The potential of recombinant *L. monocytogenes* to serve as a vaccine vector was first explored a decade ago (Schafer *et al.*, 1992). In this initial study, a recombinant *L. monocytogenes* strain, DP-L967, was generated by transposon-mediated insertion of a gene, which resulted in the constitutive expression of *Escherichia coli* β-galactosidase. DP-L967 was used to determine if the anti-listerial immune response would also expand to include this new model antigen. DP-L967 was found to induce β-galactosidase specific CTLs, but induction of delayed-type hypersensitivity was weak, with only 15% of the mice responding. The responding CTLs were shown to be $CD8^+$, $TCR\alpha\beta^+$, $Thy-1.2^+$, and MHC class I $H-2^d$ restricted. These CTLs were a minor sub-population, and needed several rounds of *in vitro* stimulation before they were detectable in a CTL assay. This rather weak CTL response was attributed to the relatively low level of expression of the β-galactosidase antigen, and to its not being secreted by the bacteria. It has since been shown that secretion of an antigen by *L. monocytogenes* is necessary for the efficient induction of protective T cell responses (Darji *et al.*, 1998). The primary lesson of this study was the proof of the concept that recombinant *L. monocytogenes* can deliver a foreign antigen to the immune system in such a way that an immune response is generated that targets the foreign antigen as well as the native listerial antigens.

β-galactosidase was also used as a model antigen to test the ability of an attenuated mutant of *L. monocytogenes* to act as an oral vaccine carrier to induce anti-tumor immunity against a mouse fibrosarcoma that was transduced with this model antigen. The host *L. monocytogenes* lacked the metalloprotease enzyme required to activate PLC B (see Figure 1). To facilitate the secretion of the antigen outside the bacterial cell wall, and in the cytoplasm of the infected cell, only the $H-2^d$ immunodominant epitope of β-gal was used with either PrfA or ActA as carrier proteins. In a prophylactic setting, the β-gal epitope expressing recombinants were able to protect about 40% of mice from lethal tumor challenge after prior immunization (Paglia *et al.*, 1997). This rather modest level of protection may have been due to loss of the plasmid by the host bacteria since no attempt was made to ensure its retention *in vivo* in the absence of antibiotic selection.

Follow up studies in our laboratory, utilizing a new recombinant, DP-L2028, demonstrated the potency of *L. monocytogenes* as a delivery system for secreted antigens (Ikonomidis *et al.*, 1994, and 1997). This secreted antigen, a fusion protein consisting of a truncated, and non-functional virulence factor, LLO, joined to the influenza nucleoprotein (NP), was processed, and presented to NP-specific T cells (Ikonomidis *et al.*, 1994). To guarantee retention of the plasmid *in vivo*, a copy of the *prfA* gene was included on the plasmid, which was then used to transform a *prfA* negative mutant of *L. monocytogenes* that is incapable of *in vivo* replication in the absence of the episomal expression of *prfA*. DP-L2028 efficiently induced NP-specific CD8[+] CTLs in mice following infection (Ikonomidis *et al.*, 1994). It was also demonstrated that escape from the phagosome is necessary for recognition by CD8[+] T cells, but not MHC class II restricted CD4[+] T cells (Ikonomidis *et al.*, 1994). This recombinant strain, DP-L2028 was used to demonstrate the effectiveness of recombinant *L. monocytogenes* as a tumor immunotherapeutic (Pan *et al.*, 1995a). DP-L2028 (referred to in this paper as Lm-NP) was used to target an immune response to the influenza nucleoprotein. This protein was also expressed as a model tumor antigen by the BALB/c mouse-derived tumors CT26-NP, and Renca-NP. Not only did Lm-NP treatment protect mice in a NP-specific manner from subsequent tumor challenge, but Lm-NP treatment also induced the complete regression of macroscopic Renca-NP tumors (Pan *et al.*, 1995a). The studies then showed that Lm-NP treatment induced CTLs that lysed CT26-NP, and Renca-NP *in vitro*, and that CD8[+] T cells are necessary for tumor protection. Lm-NP immunized mice that were depleted of CD4[+] T cells prior to tumor challenge were only able to slow the growth of the CT26-NP tumors, not to reject them. CD4[+] T cells, therefore, are also important for protection from tumor challenge.

L. monocytogenes infects humans, and animals naturally via the oral route. To test this method of delivery, a subsequent study administered Lm-NP orally, and examined the influence on the growth of NP-expressing tumors (Pan *et al.*, 1995b). Oral delivery of Lm-NP induced the regression of established, macroscopic CT26-NP tumors. Lm-NP has also been shown to induce the regression of established, macroscopic B16F10-NP tumors (Pan *et al.*, 1999). B16F10 is a highly tumorigenic, and poorly immunogenic melanoma derived from the C57Bl/6 mouse that shows a very low expression of MHC class I molecules, and no detectable expression of MHC class II molecules (Fidler, 1975). B16F10 has proven to be largely resistant to immunotherapeutic treatments, and as such is a very stringent test of the effectiveness of Lm-NP as a tumor immunotherapeutic.

Taken together, these tumor immunotherapy models demonstrate the ability of *L. monocytogenes* to deliver a model tumor antigen to APCs that stimulate an immune response, which in turn targets the tumor. Though the results of the Lm-NP studies are impressive, there remained a major caveat, the choice of the highly immunogenic influenza nucleoprotein as an antigen. The retrovirally transduced, NP expressing tumor lines mentioned previously express high levels of NP, and that expression is, in some cases, lost under the pressure of the immune response (Pan *et al.*, 1995a). Therefore, it becomes important to test the ability of recombinant *Listeria* to target more appropriate tumor antigens, and to further analyze the tumor rejection response induced by such strains.

RECOMBINANT *L. MONOCYTOGENES* VACCINES AGAINST HPV TRANSFORMED TUMORS

In order to more effectively assess the ability of *L. monocytogenes* to induce anti-tumor immunity targeting a clinically relevant human tumor antigen we chose a tumor antigen which is present in the majority of cervical cancer cells. Human papillomaviruses (HPV) comprise a diverse family of double stranded DNA viruses that infect epithelial tissues. More than 90% of cervical carcinomas have detectable levels of HPV DNA, most commonly of the HPV 16 genotype (Resnick *et al.,* 1990; Van Den Brule *et al.*, 1991). Expression of the HPV 16 early gene products, E6, and E7, is sufficient to immortalize human, and rodent cells (Halbert, *et al.*, 1992; Kanda *et al.*, 1988). These proteins are constitutively expressed by HPV associated tumors, and are necessary for maintenance of the transformed phenotype (Choo, *et al.,* 1994). As such they are ideal candidates for target antigens in tumor immunotherapy.

We developed a model utilizing the HPV 16 E6, and E7 immortalized mouse tumor line to test the anti-tumor effectiveness of the E7-specific immune responses induced by E7 secreting *Listeria* strains. TC-1 is a lung epithelial cell immortalized by HPV-16 E6, and E7, and transformed by pVEJB expressing activated human c-Ha-*ras* (Lin *et al.,* 1996). It is an aggressive tumor, syngeneic with the C57Bl/6 mouse. Like human HPV associated tumors, TC-1 constitutively expresses E6, and E7. We have constructed two *Listeria* strains that secrete E7, but were generated with two very different expression systems. The first strain, Lm-E7, was generated by inserting the E7 gene into a non-essential open reading frame in the *L. monocytogenes* chromosome. Lm-E7 possesses a single copy of the E7 gene, and the expression, and secretion of the recombinant protein is driven by the *hly* promoter, and signal sequence. The second strain, Lm-LLO-E7, was generated with a multi-copy episomal expression system. Lm-LLO-E7 expresses, and secretes a fusion protein consisting of a truncated LLO joined at the C-terminus to E7.

Although both *L. monocytogenes* recombinants secrete the E7 tumor antigen they induce radically different anti-tumor responses. Lm-LLO-E7 treatment effectively cures the majority of tumor bearing mice. *In vivo* antibody depletion studies demonstrated that the anti-tumor response requires $CD4^+$, and $CD8^+$ T cells as well as IFN-γ (Gunn *et al.* 2001). Alternatively, Lm-E7 treatment of tumor bearing mice has little impact on the growth of the tumor. Surprisingly, the depletion of $CD4^+$ T cells greatly improves the effectiveness of the Lm-E7 treatment with approximately 25% of treated mice undergoing complete regression of established TC-1 tumors. The transfer of $CD4^+$ T cells from mice immunized with Lm-E7 can abrogate the anti-TC1 immune response induced by Lm-LLO-E7-treated recipient mice (Gunn *et al.*,2001). This finding led us to further analyze the role of $CD4^+$ T cells in the induction or suppression of tumor immunity.

A subset of $CD4^+$ T cells has been described to possess a suppressive regulatory function. These $CD25^+$ T cells are important for the maintenance of self-tolerance, and their depletion can result in the induction of autoimmunity (Sakaguchi *et al.*, 1995). $CD4^+CD25^+$ regulatory T cells inhibit organ-specific autoimmune diseases induced by $CD4^+CD25^-$ T cells, and are potent suppressors of their activation *in vitro*. However, recently they have been shown to suppress both proliferation, and IFN-γ production by $CD8^+$ T cells (Piccirillo, and Shevach, 2001). $CD4^+$, $CD25^+$ T cells have also been demonstrated to aid tumor growth by suppressing anti-tumor immune responses (Onizuka *et al.*, 1999). The depletion of $CD25^+$ cells in Lm-E7 treated mice greatly improved the anti-tumor response. Although none of the mice were cured, the mice treated with Lm-E7, and anti-CD25 developed tumors much more slowly than mice receiving Lm-E7, and a control antibody (Gunn *et al.*, 2001). Furthermore, transforming growth factor-β (TGF-β) has been reported to be secreted by $CD4^+$, $CD25^+$ suppressive T cells (Read *et al.*, 2000). TGF-β has been demonstrated to protect tumors from immune responses in immune competent hosts (Chang *et al.*, 1993; Torre-Amione *et al.*, 1990). The depletion of TGF-β in Lm-E7-treated, tumor-bearing mice facilitated the regression of over 60% of the TC-1 tumors. However, following the termination of the anti-TGF-β antibody administration, most of the tumors returned, and began to grow (Gunn *et al.*, 2001). These studies demonstrate the potential for effective or suppressive immunity induced by recombinant bacterial vectors.

Using an infectious disease model for HPV, the Cotton Tail Rabbit Papilloma virus (CRPV) model, Jensen, and associates studied the efficacy of recombinant Lm expressing CRPV E1 protein (E1-rLm) as a prophylactic vaccine for CRPV infection, and CRPV DNA-induced papillomas (Jensen *et al.*, 1997). This study showed that E1-rLm immunization of rabbits did not protect against papilloma formation on cutaneous challenge with CRPV but did control papilloma growth in that papillomas regressed in about 77% of rabbits that responded to E1-rLm vaccination. These animals remained papilloma free for at least five months. However, some rabbits had transient, partial or no regression of papillomas. They also demonstrated that the protection observed was cell mediated, and E1-specific antibody was not involved.

LISTERIA MONOCYTOGENES AS A COLEY'S TOXIN

We have noted that *L. monocytogenes* can act in a non-specific manner to slow tumor growth (Pan *et al.,* 1999, Gunn *et al.*, 2001). Thus in the B16F10-NP, and TC-1 studies described above the growth of these tumors was slowed in mice infected with control *Listeria monocytogenes* recombinants that expressed irrelevant antigens. This non-specific slowing or bystander response is thought to be mediated by cytokines induced during the anti-*Listeria* response (Pan *et al.,* 1999). For instance, the cytokines IFN-γ, TNF-α, and IL-12 have been implicated in the blocking of angiogenesis within tumors (Maheshwari *et al.*, 1991; Sato *et al.*, 1990; Voest *et al.*, 1995, Beatty, and Paterson, 2000). Recently, we have shown (Angel Varela-Rohena, and Yvonne Paterson, unpublished) that the non-specific slowing of TC-1 tumors by *L. monocytogenes* is accompanied by a decreased vascularization of the tumor. This phenomenon clearly contributes to the impressive efficacy of *L. monocytogenes* as a tumor immunotherapeutic.

L. monocytogenes, similar to other intra-cellular bacteria as we discuss below, can also promote immunity to unidentified tumor antigens. We have shown that intra-tumoral (i.t.) immunization of the mouse colon carcinoma CT26 with *L. monocytogenes* (that does not carry a tumor antigen) will induce the regression of the tumor, and induce long-lived immunity to further challenge with CT-26 (Christian Peters, and Yvonne Paterson, unpublished). However, the animals must be pre-immunized with the *Listeria* vaccine to induce this effect. We believe that *Listeria* specific T cells infiltrate the tumor, and kill tumor cells infected with the bacterium. This could result in dead tumor cells being processed, and their antigens presented to the immune system with the induction of immunity directed to tumor antigens. In a naive animal, tumor growth during the induction phase of *Listeria* specific T cells after i.t. immunization would not be rapid enough to control the tumor burden, whereas pre-immunization ensures an existing population of *Listeria* specific T cells.

OTHER INTRA-CELLULAR BACTERIA AS VACCINE VECTORS FOR TUMOR ANTIGENS

Many of the properties of *L. monocytogenes* in inducing cell mediated immunity are shared by other intracellular bacteria such as *Salmonella,* and BCG (Bacillus Calmette-Guerin strain of *M. bovis*). *Salmonella typhimurium,* like *Listeria,* has been shown to induce a Th1 type immune response (Everest *et al.,* 1997; Harrison *et al.,* 1997) even when delivered orally (Harrison *et al.,* 1997; George, 1996). In addition IFN-γ, which is a major Th1 type cytokine, is important in inducing immunity to *S. typhimurium* infection through the activation of macrophages (Ramarathinam *et al.*, 1991; Mastroeni *et al.,* 1992). *Salmonella,* unlike *Listeria,* does not escape from the endosomal compartment, instead it survives in the phagocytic cell in a modified phagosome by preventing phagosome/lysosome fusion (Buchmeier, and Heffron, 1991). However, despite its vacuolar localization, it has been demonstrated that antigens derived from *Salmonella* can be processed via the MHC class I pathway with the generation of antigen-specific CD8[+] T cells (Flynn *et al.*, 1990; Hess *et al.*, 1997; Harding, and Pfeifer, 1994; Verma *et al.,* 1995).

BCG, Bacillus Calmette-Guerin, is a human tuberculosis vaccine derived from a strain of *Mycobacterium bovis* that has been attenuated by 230 serial passages *in vitro* (Calmette *et al.,* 1924). BCG, like *Salmonella,* invades, and lives in macrophages in a vacuolar compartment. Unlike *Listeria,* and *Salmonella,* mycobacteria are not usually transmitted by the oral route, but as aerosolized droplets via the respiratory route. CD4[+] T cells are important in resistance to mycobacterial infection. In addition, mycobacterial infections, including BCG, like *Listeria,* and *Salmonella,* induce a predominantly Th1 type immune response (Mutis *et al.,* 1993; Yang, and Mitsuyama, 1997; Erb *et al.,* 1998). There is strong evidence that peptides derived from intracellular mycobacteria can be presented directly to a CD8[+] T cell population via the MHC class I pathway (Flynn *et al.,* 1992; Cooper *et al.,* 1997). Furthermore, only live mycobacteria are efficient in facilitating antigen processing via MHC class I pathway in murine macrophages (Mazzacaro e*t al.,* 1996)

Salmonella, and BCG have been studied for years as possible vaccine vectors for infectious disease (Hone *et al.,* 1999; Aldovini, and Young, 1999). Nevertheless, the use of these bacteria as carriers of passenger tumor antigens for therapeutic vaccines has not been widely exploited.

RECOMBINANT *SALMONELLA* AS A DELIVERY AGENT

The role of recombinant *Salmonella* as a cancer therapeutic against tumors has only been explored by a few investigators. The innate immune response to *Salmonella,* as with *Listeria,* and BCG, acts to slow tumor growth (Eisenstein *et al.,* 1995) suggesting that attenuated strains could be used as an adjuvant in tumor therapy. In addition, an attenuated auxotrophic recombinant strain of *Salmonella* that preferentially accumulates in both human, and murine tumor tissues has been developed for direct therapy of tumors, and to potentially act as a "magic bullet" for the delivery of anti-tumor chemotherapeutic agents (Pawalek *et al.,* 1997; Bermudes *et al.,* 2000; Zheng *et al.,* 2000). Systemic administration of these selected strains can result in up to 1,000 times more bacteria homing to tumors than to other tissues (Bermudes *et al.,* 2000; Zheng *et al.,* 2000). Pawelek, and colleagues demonstrated melanoma regression after immunization of melanoma-bearing mice with a tumor-targeted *Salmonella* strain expressing HSV thymidine kinase, and a prodrug, gancicyclovir (Pawelek *et al.,* 1997). This study demonstrated that attenuated *Salmonella* would be useful both for inherent anti-tumor activity, and delivery of therapeutic proteins to cancer cells *in vivo* (Pawelek *et al.,* 1997).

Salmonella has also been used to deliver biological response modifiers such as cytokines or adhesion molecules. B cell lymphomas express the CD40 molecule. Ligation of this cell surface receptor with CD40L results in the upregulation of Fas, B7-1, and B7-2 rendering the tumor cell a better target for anti-tumor T cell immunity. Urashima, and colleagues transfected the human CD40L gene into *S. typhimurium,* and orally administered the resulting strain (ST40L) to mice prior to challenge with the BCL B-cell lymphoma (Urashima *et al.,* 2000). This prophylactic immunization with ST40L resulted in a significant protection of the mice against BCL challenge.

Salmonella, and *Listeria* infections result in accumulation of these bacteria in the liver. This tropism of *Salmonella* has been harnessed for hepatic malignancies (Saltzman *et al.,* 1996; 1997). An attenuated vaccine strain of *Salmonella* (thi4550) was engineered to secrete IL-2, and secretion of a biologically active cytokine was verified by NK cell activation. Oral delivery of this recombinant resulted in an approximately 60% reduction in twelve day established liver metastases of the MCA-38 murine adenocarcinoma (Saltzman *et al.,* 1996). Depletion of CD8[+] T cells, and NK cells consistently abrogated the anti-tumor efficacy of the thi4550(pIL-2) *Salmonella* recombinant, whereas elimination of CD4[+] T cells, and Kupffer cells had no effect (Saltzman *et al.,* 1997). These studies suggest that the delivery of IL-2 by thi4550 results in activation of both adaptive, and innate anti-tumor immunity.

RECOMBINANT *SALMONELLA* AS A VACCINE VECTOR FOR TUMOR ANTIGENS

The model "tumor" antigen, *E. coli* β-galacosidase (β-gal), has been used to test the efficacy of *Salmonella* as a vector for passenger tumor antigens by a number of investigators. Prophylactic oral immunization with *Salmonella* vaccine strains that express β-gal protected 80% of mice against challenge with a fibrosarcoma transfected with β-gal compared to 50% of mice surviving when the host *Salmonella* strain was used (Medina *et al.,* 2000). This study confirms the strong non-specific anti-tumor effect that *Salmonella* can induce (Eisenstein *et al.,* 1995) as well as demonstrating that adaptive immunity to tumor antigens can be induced by recombinant *Salmonella* through the oral route. This group (Paglia *et al.,* 1998) also used *Salmonella* as a carrier for foreign genes under the control of a CMV promoter to test whether oral immunization could also be used to deliver DNA systemically through the oral route. Using green fluorescent protein as the foreign gene, they found gene expression in macrophages, and dendritic cells in spleens after oral immunization. A similar construct carrying the entire gene for β-gal was used to orally immunize mice prior to tumor challenge with a fibrosarcoma transfected with β-gal, resulting in protection of about 75% of the mice (Paglia *et al.,* 1998).

Zoller, and Christ (2001) used the murine renal carcinoma RENCA transformed with β-gal to compare the efficacy of two different vaccination strategies, and a combined protocol in a prophylactic setting. They compared a DNA vaccine for *lacZ* delivered either alone or by *Salmonella,* and β-gal loaded dendritic cells or a combination of one of the DNA vaccines, and pulsed dendritic cells. Oral delivery of a DNA vaccine with attenuated *Salmonella* had previously been shown to induce an effective immune response against the antigen encoded by the gene under the control of a eukaryotic promoter (Darji *et al.,* 1997). Although all of the protocols tested by Zoller, and Christ (2001) resulted in some protection against tumor challenge, oral vaccination of *Salmonella* carrying the DNA plasmid followed by i.v. transfer with protein pulsed dendritic cells gave the highest survival rates. This combined vaccine therapy was shown to be superior because of the strong CD8$^+$ T cell response induced by the *Salmonella* delivery of the DNA combined with activation of Th cells by protein pulsed dendritic cells.

The delivery of DNA vaccines by intracellular bacteria provides several advantages that will be described in more detail by Weiss, and Chakraborty in this volume. As delivery vehicles for tumor antigens, in addition to the improved delivery of the DNA vaccine to professional antigen presenting cells, oral delivery of the DNA vaccine may overcome peripheral T cell tolerance to tumor self antigens. Reisfeld, and colleagues (Xiang *et al.,* 2000; Niethammer *et al.,* 2001) have exploited the ability of *Salmonella* to invade through the intestinal tract to deliver tumor antigen DNA by this route. Murine, and human melanoma tumors overexpress a number of tissue specific proteins that are involved in the synthesis of melanin from tyrosine that are true "self" antigens. Minigenes encoding the MHC class I immunodominant epitopes in the H-2^b mouse for two of these antigens, gp100, and TRP-2, were fused to the murine ubiquitin gene under the control of the CMV promoter, and delivered by *Salmonella* to C57Bl/6 mice by oral gavage prior to a lethal challenge with the syngeneic murine B16 melanoma tumor (Xiang *et al.,* 2000). Ubiquitination of cellular proteins is thought to enhance their degradation by proteasomes and, therefore, their access to the MHC class I processing pathway. Significant protection against tumor challenge was achieved using this vaccine strategy that correlated with improved CD8$^+$ T cell CTL responses capable of killing B16 tumor cells *in vitro,* and of secreting IFN-γ on stimulation with B16. Since the translation products of the gp100, and TRP-2 minigenes used in the DNA vaccine were CTL epitopes that should not require further processing, it is somewhat surprising that the ubiquitination of the minigenes was required for vaccine efficacy. In a further study (Niethammer *et al.,* 2001) the efficacy of the *Salmonella* delivered gp100/TRP-2 DNA vaccine was enhanced by combining it with IL-2 fused to an antibody specific for the tumor cell surface marker, GD2, to deliver this cytokine directly to the tumor.

Salmonella has also been explored as a vector for HPV antigens but largely as a mucosal delivery vehicle for a prophylactic vaccine against HPV infection rather than a tumor immunotherapeutic against HPV transformed cancer. The L1 major capsid protein of HPV-16 self assembles into virus like particles (VLPs), and is the most appropriate target antigen for a prophylactic vaccine

(Lowy, and Schiller, 1998). A recombinant attenuated *Salmonella* vaccine vector (PhoPc) that expresses the L1 antigen as VLPs has been developed, and used to generate mucosal, and systemic neutralizing antibodies in mice (Nardelli-Haefliger *et al.*, 1997). This was the first demonstration that HPV-16 VLPs can self-assemble in prokaryotes. Using the ability of *Salmonella* to induce mucosal immunity, this approach could provide a most effective prophylactic vaccine against HPV infection in the genital tract. Although an attenuated strain was used (PhoPc), further attenuation of the host strain of *Salmonella* carrying the L1 antigen resulted in less sustained immune responses (Benyacoub *et al.,* 1999). Vaccination of mice intra-nasally with the *Salmonella* recombinant expressing HPV 16 L1 VLPs induced anti-tumor immunity, and significantly slowed the growth of an HPV immortalized mouse tumor in a prophylactic, and therapeutic setting (Revaz *et al.,* 2001). The mouse tumor used, C3, is very similar to the TC-1 tumor described above except that it was immortalized with the entire HPV genome whereas TC-1 was immortalized with E6, and E7 alone. Although L1 is not involved in the transformation process by HPV, C3 obviously continues to express L1 protein, and had previously been shown to be susceptible to immunotherapy with L1 VLP particles (De Bruijn *et al.* 1998). However, vaccination with VLPs containing L1 or L2 alone is unlikely to be effective with human cancer because the capsid proteins have not been detected in naturally arising HPV transformed tumors (Greenstone *et al,* 1998).

Induction of an antibody response in mice against HPV-16 E6, and E7 after immunization with recombinant *aroA⁻ Salmonella* strains expressing E6, and E7 has also been demonstrated (Krul *et al.*, 1996). In another approach, attenuated *Salmonella typhimurium* (*aroA, aroD*) strains were constructed that directed the expression of hepatitis B core antigen particles (HBcAg) or the fusion protein of HBcAg, and HPV 16 E7. These were put under the control of an *in vivo* inducible *nirB* promoter. Mice were immunized orally or intravenously, and humoral, and cellular E7, and HBcAg mediated responses were monitored. The strain expressing the HBcAg-E7 fusion protein induced anti-E7 humoral IgG, and IgA responses in the intestines of orally immunized mice (Londono *et al.*, 1996). This provides evidence that *Salmonella* can induce mucosal immunity against HPV derived antigens. Taken together, these studies demonstrate the potential of *Salmonella* as a vaccine vector for both prophylaxis against HPV infection, and as a therapeutic for HPV associated malignancies.

BCG As A Tumor Immunotherapeutic

Despite the excellent safety record of BCG as a vaccine, and its ability to readily accept large genes, to our knowledge, it has not been used as a vaccine vector for tumor antigens. Because of its inherent immunostimulatory properties, BCG has been explored as an adjuvant for autologous tumor cell vaccines to enhance anti-tumor immune responses for a variety of cancers including prostate cancer (Harris *et al.*, 2000), colorectal cancer (Yip *et al.*, 2000; Habal *et al.*, 2001), melanoma (Mastrangelo, 1996; Leong *et al.*, 1999), renal cell carcinoma (Li *et al*, 2000, Schwaab *et al.*, 2000), and astrocytoma (Wood *et al.*, 2000). In addition, the intravesical adminstration of BCG is established in the clinic for the treatment of superficial bladder cancer (Lamm, 1992; Morales, and Nickel, 1992). However, large, and frequent doses are often required to induce a strong immune response to eradicate tumors, and occasionally this may lead to a disseminated mycobacteriosis. Combination therapy with intravesical BCG plus interferon alpha has been shown to be far more efficacious for bladder cancer than either agent alone. BCG transformed to express human interferon-alpha 2B has been tested for is ability to stimulate the production of IFN-γ, IP-10, and TNF-α by peripheral blood mononuclear cells from bladder cancer patients, and shown to have enhanced effects over BCG alone suggesting that it might provide an improved treatment for the disease (Luo *et al.*, 1999, 2001).

To enhance the immunostimulatory properties of the mycobacterium, BCG has been genetically manipulated to secrete various mammalian cytokines (Murray *et al.*, 1996; Luo *et al.*, 2001). Recombinant BCG strains secreting functional IL-2, IL-4, IL-6, GM-CSF, and IFN-γ have been generated, and characterized (Murray *et al.*, 1996) These recombinant cytokine-secreting BCG strains have demonstrated a more potent induction of cell mediated immune response than the wild-type BCG strain. The most profound effect was induced by IL-2, GM-CSF, and IFNγ secreting BCG strains that exhibited an enhanced antigen-specific T cell response following *in vitro* stimulation with purified protein derivative (PPD). In addition, when administered intravenously in mice to induce CTL, no adverse effects were observed (Murray *et al.*, 1996).

Therefore, the use of recombinant BCG that can secrete cytokine gene products could offer improved cancer immunotherapy with BCG as an adjuvant.

SAFETY ISSUES, AND LIMITATIONS OF BACTERIA-BASED RECOMBINANT VACCINES

Safety is a great concern when using live recombinant vaccines. A good candidate recombinant vaccine vector should have minimal complications in humans. One of the drawbacks for using viral vectors is the concern of their transforming properties, and high risk of mutagenesis in addition to infectious pathology. On the other hand, bacterial vectors have minimal frequency of these properties but do retain the ability to cause serious systemic diseases. BCG has a good safety record, and has been used as a safe vaccine against TB but it still is not free of complications. Side effects of BCG vaccination have been correlated with the amount of dead BCG cells in the vaccine preparations (Milstein, and Gibson, 1990). *Salmonella* causes minor gastroenteritis but can cause serious systemic disease even in healthy individuals. There is a serious safety issue about *Listeria* in humans with impaired immune systems such as immunosuppressed adults, newborn infants, and pregnant women (Gellin, and Broome, 1989). The most likely individuals for vaccination with live recombinant vaccines are cancer patients with advanced disease whose immune systems may have been damaged by prior chemotherapy or radiation treatment. Unfortunately, most if not all live recombinant vaccine vectors are potentially hazardous to immunocompromised individuals. Nevertheless, intracellular bacteria, unlike viral vectors, are readily curable by a wide range of antibiotics that can be administered in the case of adverse reactions to therapy. Use of attenuated strains, even though they have variable efficacy, might be a good option with minimal side effects especially to immunocompromised patients. Finally, the issue of prior exposure to these infectious agents could well limit their efficacy. Both *Listeria*, and *Salmonella* are ubiquitous food borne organisms, and BCG has been used as a vaccine against tuberculosis in a large proportion of the world.

REFERENCES

Aldovini, A., and Young, R. 1999. Recombinant BCG Vaccines. In: Intracellular Bacterial Vaccine Vectors: Immunology, Cell Biology, and Genetics, Y. Paterson, ed. Wiley-Liss, A John Wiley and Sons, Inc. Publication. New York. p. 151-169.

Beatty, G., and Paterson, Y. 2001. IFN-gamma dependent inhibition of tumor angiogenesis by tumor infiltrating CD4$^+$ T cells requires tumor responsiveness to IFN-gamma. J. Immunol. 166: 2276-2282.

Benyacoub, J., Hopkins, S., Potts, A., Kelly, S., Kraehenbuhl, J.P., Curtiss, R. 3rd, De Grandi, P., and Nardelli-Haefliger, D. 1999. The nature of the attenuation of *Salmonella typhimurium* strains expressing human papillomavirus type 16 virus-like particles determines the systemic, and mucosal antibody responses in nasally immunized mice. Infect. Immun. 67: 3674-3679.

Berd, D., 1998. Cancer vaccines: reborn or just recycled? Semin. Oncol. 25: 605-610.

Bermudes, D., Low, B., and Pawelek, J. 2000. Tumor-targeted *Salmonella*. Highly selective delivery vectors. Adv. Exp. Med. Biol. 465: 57-63.

Boehm, U., Klamp, T., Groot, M., and Howard, J.C., 1997. Cellular responses to interferon-gamma. Annu. Rev. Immunol. 15: 749-95.

Boon, T., Cerottini, J.C., Van den Eynde, B., van der Bruggen, P., and Van Pel, A. 1994. Tumor antigens recognized by T lymphocytes. Annu. Rev. Immunol. 12: 337-365.

Buchmeier, N.A., and Heffron, F. 1991. Inhibition of macrophage phagosome-lysosome fusion by *Salmonella typhimurium*. Infect. Immun. 59: 2232-2238.

Calmette, A.C., Guerin, C., and Weill-Halle, B. 1924. Essais de premunition par le BCG comtre l'infection tuberculeuse de l'homme et des animaux. B. Bull. Acad. Natl. Med. (Paris) 91: 787-796.

Camilli, A., Tilney, L.G., and Portnoy, D.A. 1993. Dual roles of *plcA* in *Listeria monocytogenes* pathogenesis. Mol. Microbiol. 8: 143-157.

Cella, M., Scheidegger, D., Palmer-Lehmann, K., Lane, P., Lanzavecchia, A., and Alber, G. 1996. Ligation of CD40 on dendritic cells triggers production of high levels of interleukin-12, and enhances T cell stimulatory capacity: T-T help via APC activation. J. Exp. Med. 184: 747-752.

Chang, H.L., Gillett, N., Figari, I., Lopez, A.R., Palladino, M.A., and Derynck, R. 1993. Increased transforming growth factor beta expression inhibits cell proliferation *in vitro*, yet increases tumorigenicity, and tumor growth of Meth A sarcoma cells. Cancer Res. 53: 4391-4398.

Chomez, P., De Backer, O., Bertrand, M. De Plaen, E., Boon, T., and Lucas, S. 2001. An overview of the MAGE gene family with the identification of all human members of the family. Cancer Res. 61: 5544-5551.

Choo, C.K., Rorke, E.A., and Eckert, R.L. 1994. Differentiation-independent constitutive expression of the human papillomavirus type 16 E6, and E7 oncogenes in the CaSki cervical tumour cell line. J. Gen. Virol. 75: 1139-1147.

Coley, W.B. 1893. The treatment of malignant tumors by repeated inoculations of erysipelas: with a report of ten original cases. Am. J. Med. Sci. 105: 487-511.

Coley, W.B. 1909. The treatment of inoperable sarcoma by bacterial toxins (the mixed toxins of the streptococcus of erysipelas, and the bacillus prodigiosus). Practitioner 83: 589-613.

Cooper, A.M., D'Souza, C., Frank, A.A., and Orme, I.M. 1997. The course of *Mycobacterium tuberculosis* infection in the lungs of mice lacking expression of either perforin- or granzymes-mediated cytolytic mechanisms. Infect. Immun. 65:1317-1320.

Creasey, A.A. , Reynolds, M.T., and Laird, W. 1986. Cures, and partial regression of murine, and human tumors by recombinant human tumor necrosis factor. Cancer Res. 46: 5687-5690.

Darji, A., Guzman, C.A., Gerstel, B., Wachholz, P., Timmis, K.N., Wehland, T., Chakraborty, T., and Weiss, S. 1997. Oral somatic transgene vaccination using attenuated *S. typhimurium.* Cell 91: 765-775.

Darji, A., Bruder, D., zur Lage, S., Gerstel, B., Chakraborty, T., Wehland, J., and Weiss, S. 1998. The role of the bacterial membrane protein ActA in immunity, and protection against *Listeria monocytogenes.* J. Immunol. 161: 2414-2420.

De Bruijn, M.L., Greenstone, H.L., Vermeulen, H., Melief, C.J., Lowy, D.R., Schiller, J.T., and Kast, W.M. 1998. L1-specific protection from tumor challenge elicited by HPV16 virus-like particles. Virology 250:371-376.

DiTirro, J., Rhoades, E.R., Roberts, A.D., Burke, J.M., Mukasa, A. Cooper, A.M., Frank, A.A., Born, W.K., and Orme, I.M. 1998. Disruption of the cellular inflammatory response to *Listeria monocytogenes* infection in mice with disruptions in targeted genes. Infect. Immun. 66: 2284-2289.

Dranoff, G., Jaffee, E., Lazenby, A., Golumbek, P., Levitsky, H., Brose, K., Jackson, V., Hamada, H., Pardoll, D., and Mulligan, R.C. 1993. Vaccination with irradiated tumor cells engineered to secrete murine granulocyte-macrophage colony-stimulating factor stimulates potent, specific, and long-lasting anti-tumor immunity. Proc. Natl. Acad. Sci. USA. 90: 3539-3543.

Eisenstein, T.K., Bushnell, B., Meissler, J.J., Dalal, N., Schafer, R., and Havas, H.F. 1995. Immunotherapy of a plasmacytoma with attenuated *Salmonella.* Med. Oncol. 12: 103-108.

Erb, K.J., Holloway, J.W., Sobeck, A., Moll, H., and Le Gros, G. 1998. Infection of mice with *Mycobacterium bovis* Bacillus Calmette-Guerin (BCG) suppresses allergen-induced airway eosinophilia. J. Exp. Med. 187: 561-569.

Everest, P., Allen, J., Papakonstantinopoulou, A., Mastroeni, P., Roberts, M., and Dougan, G. 1997. *Salmonella typhimurium* infections in mice deficient in interleukin-4 production: role of IL-4 in infection-associated pathology. J. Immunol. 159: 1820-1827.

Fidler, I.J. 1975. Biological behavior of malignant melanoma cells correlated to their survival *in vivo*. Cancer Res. 35: 218-224.

Flynn, J.L., Weiss, W.R., Norris, K.A., Seiffert, H.S., Kumar, S., and So, M. 1990. Generation of a cytotoxic T-lymphocyte response using a *Salmonella* antigen delivery system. Mol. Microbiol. 4: 2111-2118.

Flynn, J.L., Goldstein, M.M., Triebold, K.J., Koller, B., and Bloom, B.R. 1992. Major histocompatibility complex class I restricted T cells are required for resistance to *Mycobacterium tuberculosis* infection. Proc. Natl. Acad. Sci. USA. 89: 12013-12017.

Fuchs, E.J., and Matzinger, P. 1996. Is cancer dangerous to the immune system? Semin. Immunol. 8: 271-280.

Gaillard, J.L., Berche, P., Mounier, J., Richard, S., and Sansonetti, P. 1987. *In vitro* model of penetration, and intracellular growth of *Listeria monocytogenes* in the human enterocyte-like cell line Caco-2. Infect. Immun. 55: 2822-2829.

Gellin, B.G., and Broome, C.V. 1989. Listeriosis. JAMA 261: 1313-1320.

George, A. 1996. Generation of gamma interferon responses in murine Peyer's patches following oral immunization. Infect. Immun. 64: 4606-4611.

Germann, T., Gately, M.K., Schoenhaut, D.S., Lohoff, M., Mattner, F., Fischer, S., Jin, S.C., Schmitt, E., and Rude, E. 1993. Interleukin-12/T cell stimulating factor, a cytokine with multiple effects on T helper type 1 (Th1) but not on Th2 cells. Eur. J. Immunol. 23: 1762-1770.

Greenstone, H.L., Nieland, J.D., de Visser, K.E., De Bruijn, M.L., Kirnbauer, R., Roden, R.B., Lowy, D.R., Kast, W.M., and Schiller, J.T. 1998. Chimeric papillomavirus virus-like particles elicit antitumor immunity against the E7 oncoprotein in an HPV16 tumor model. Proc. Natl. Acad. Sci. USA. 95: 1800-1805.

Gunn, G.R., Zubair, A., Peters, C., Pan, Z.K., Wu, T.C., and Paterson, Y. 2001. Two *Listeria monocytogenes* vaccine vectors that express different molecular forms of HPV-16 E7 induce qualitatively different T cell immunity that correlates with their ability to induce regression of established tumors immortalized by HPV-16. J. Immunol. 167: 6471-6479.

Habal, N., Gupta, R.K., Bilchik, A.J., Yee, R., Leopoldo, Z., Ye, W., Elashoff, R.M., and Morton, D.L. 2001. CancerVax, an allogeneic tumor cell vaccine, induces specific humoral, and cellular immune responses in advanced colon cancer. Ann. Surg. Oncol. 8: 389-401.

Halbert, C.L., Demers, G.W., and Galloway, D.A. 1992. The E6, and E7 genes of human papillomavirus type 6 have weak immortalizing activity in human epithelial cells. J. Virol. 66: 2125-2134.

Haranaka, K., Satomi, N., and Sakurai, A. 1984. Antitumor activity of murine tumor necrosis factor (TNF) against transplanted murine tumors, and heterotransplanted human tumors in nude mice. Int. J. Cancer. 34: 263-267.

Harding, C.V., and Pfeifer, J.D. 1994. Antigen expressed by *Salmonella typhimurium* is processed for class I major histocompatibility complex presentation by macrophages but not infected epithelial cells. Immunol. 83: 670-674.

Harris, J.E., Ryan, L., Hoover, H.C. Jr., Stuart, R.K., Oken, M.M., Benson, A.B. 3rd, Mansour, E., Haller, D.G., Manola, J., and Hanna, M.G. Jr. 2000. Adjuvant active specific immunotherapy for stage II, and III colon cancer with an autologous tumor cell vaccine: Eastern Cooperative Oncology Group Study E5283. J. Clin. Oncol. 18: 148-157.

Harrison, J.A., Villarreal-Ramos, B., Mastroieni, P., Demarco de Hormaeche, R., and Hormaeche, C.E. 1997. Correlates of protection induced by live Aro⁻ *Salmonella typhimurium* vaccines in the murine typhoid model. Immunol. 90: 618-625.

Haywood, G.R., and McKhann, C.F. 1971. Antigenic specificities on murine sarcoma cells. Reciprocal relationship between normal transplantation antigens (H-2), and tumor-specific immunogenicity. J. Exp. Med. 133: 1171-1187.

Hess, J., Dietrich, G., Gentschev, I., Miko, D., Goebel, W., and Kaufmann, S.H.E. 1997. Protection against murine listeriosis by an attenuated recombinant *Salmonella typhimurium* vaccine strain that secretes the naturally somatic antigen superoxide dismutase. Infect. Immun. 65: 1286-1292.

Hone, D.M. Shata, M.T., Pascual, D.W., and Lewis, G.K. 1999. Mucosal Vaccination with *Salmonella* Vaccine Vectors. In: Intracellular Bacterial Vaccine Vectors: Immunology, Cell Biology, and Genetics, Y. Paterson ed. Wiley-Liss, A John Wiley & Sons, Inc. Publication. New York. p. 171-222.

Hsieh, C.S., Macatonia, S.E., Tripp, C.S., Wolf, S.F., O'Garra, A., and Murphy, K. M. 1993. Development of TH1 CD4+ T cells through IL-12 produced by *Listeria*-induced macrophages. Science 260: 547-549.

Huang, A.Y., Golumbek, P., Ahmadzadeh, M., Jaffee, E., Pardoll, D., and Levitsky, H. 1994. Role of bone marrow-derived cells in presenting MHC class I-restricted tumor antigens. Science 264: 961-965.

Hui, K., Grosveld, F., and Festenstein, H. 1984. Rejection of transplantable AKR leukemia cells following MHC DNA-mediated cell transformation. Nature 311: 750-752.

Ikonomidis, G., Paterson, Y., Kos, F.J., and Portnoy, D.A. 1994. Delivery of a viral antigen to the class I processing, and presentation pathway by *Listeria monocytogenes*. J. Exp. Med. 180: 2209-2218.

Ikonomidis, G., Portnoy, D.A., Gerhard, W., and Paterson, Y. 1997. Influenza-specific immunity induced by recombinant *Listeria monocytogenes* vaccines. Vaccine 15: 433-440.

Jensen, E.R., Selvakumar, R., Shen, H., Ahmed, R., Wettstein, F.O., Miller, J.F. 1997. Recombinant *Listeria monocytogenes* vaccination eliminates papillomavirus-induced tumors, and prevents papilloma formation from viral DNA. J. Virol. 71:8467-8474

June, C.H., Ledbetter, J.A., Linsley, P.S., and Thompson, C.B. 1990. Role of the CD28 receptor in T-cell activation. Immunol. Today 11: 211-216.

Kanda, T., Watanabe, S., and Yoshiike, K. 1988. Immortalization of primary rat cells by human papillomavirus type 16 subgenomic DNA fragments controlled by the SV40 promoter. Virology 165: 321-325.

Kocks, C., Gouin, E., Tabouret, M., Berche, P., Ohayon, H., and Cossart, P. 1992. *L. monocytogenes*-induced actin assembly requires the *actA* gene product, a surface protein. Cell 68: 521-531.

Krul, M.R., Tijhaar, E.G., Kleijne, J.A., Van Loon, A.M., Nievers, M.G., Schipper, H., Geerse, L., Can der Kolk, M., Steereberg, P.A., Mooi, F.R., and Den Otter, W. 1996. Induction of an antibody response in mice against human papillomavirus (HPV) type 16 after immunization with HPV recombinant *Salmonella* strains. Cancer Immunol. 43: 44-48.

Lamm, D.L. 1992. Long-term results of intravesical therapy for superficial bladder cancer. Urol. Clin. North America 19: 573-580.

Leong, S.P., Enders-Zohr, P., Zhou, Y.M., Stuntebeck, S., Habib, F.A., Allen, R.E. Jr., Sagebiel, R.W., Glassberg, A.B., Lowenberg, D.W., and Hayes, F.A. 1999. Recombinant human granulocyte macrophage-colony stimulating factor (rhGM-CSF), and autologous melanoma vaccine mediate tumor regression in patients with metastatic melanoma. J. Immunother. 22: 166-174.

Li, Q., Normolle, D.P., Sayre, D.M., Zeng, X., Sun, R., Jiang, G., Redman, B.D., and Chang, A.E. 2000. Immunological effects of BCG as an adjuvant in autologous tumor vaccines. Clin. Immunol. 94: 64-72.

Lin, K.Y., Guarnieri, F.G. Staveley-O'Carroll, K.F., Levitsky, H.I., August, J.T., Pardoll, D.M., and Wu, T.C. 1996. Treatment of established tumors with a novel vaccine that enhances major histocompatibility class II presentation of tumor antigen. Cancer Research 56: 21-26.

Londono, L.P., Chatfield, S., Tindle, Herd, K., Gao, X.M. Frazer, I., and Dougan, G. 1996. Immunization of mice using *Salmonella typhimurium* expressing human papillomavirus type 16 E7 epitopes inserted into hepatitis B virus core antigen. Vaccine 14: 545-552.

Lopez, S., Marco, A.J., Prats, N., and Czuprynski, C.J. 2000. Critical role of neutrophils in eliminating *Listeria monocytogenes* from the central nervous system during experimental murine listeriosis. Infect. Immun. 68: 4789-4791.

Lowy, D.R., and Schiller, J.T. 1999. Papillomaviruses: prophylactic vaccine prospects. Biochim. Biophys. Acta 1423: M1-8.

Luo, Y., Chen X., Downs, T.M., DeWolf, W.C., and O'Donnell, M.A., 1999. IFN-alpha 2B enhances Th1 cytokine responses in bladder cancer patients receiving *Mycobacterium bovis* bacillus Calmetter-Guerin immunotherapy. J. Immunol. 162: 2399-2405.

Luo, Y., Chen X., Han, R., and O'Donnell, M.A. 2001. Recombinant bacille Calmette-Guerin (BCG) expressing human interferon-alpha 2B demonstrates enhanced immunogenicity. Clin. Exp. Immunol. 123: 179-180.

Macatonia, S.E., Hosken, N.A., Litton, M., Vieira, P., Hsieh, C.S., Culpepper, J.A., Wysocka, M., Trinchieri, G., Murphy, K.M., and O'Garra, A. 1995. Dendritic cells produce IL-12, and direct the development of Th1 cells from naive CD4+ T cells. J. Immunol. 154: 5071-5079.

Mackaness, G.B. 1969. The influence of immunologically committed lymphoid cells on macrophage activity *in vivo*. J. Exp. Med. 129: 973-992.

Maheshwari, R.K., Srikantan, V., Bhartiya, D., Kleinman, H.K., and Grant, D.S. 1991. Differential effects of interferon gamma, and alpha on *in vitro* model of angiogenesis. J. Cell Physiol. 146: 164-169.

Manetti, R., Parronchi, P., Giudizi, M.G., Piccinni, M. P., Maggi, E., Trinchieri, G., and Romagnani, S. 1993. Natural killer cell stimulatory factor (interleukin 12 [IL-12]) induces T helper type 1 (Th1)-specific immune responses, and inhibits the development of IL-4-producing Th cells. J. Exp. Med. 177: 1199-1204.

Marquis, H., Bouwer, H.G., Hinrichs, D.J., and Portnoy, D.A. 1993. Intracytoplasmic growth, and virulence of *Listeria monocytogenes* auxotrophic mutants. Infect. Immun. 61: 3756-3760.

Mastrangelo, M.J., Maguire, H.C. Jr., Sato, T., Nathan, F.E., and Berd, D. 1996. Active specific immunization in the treatment of patients with melanoma. Semin. Oncol. 23: 773-781.

Mastroeni, P., Villarreal-Ramos, B., and Hormaeche, C.E. 1992. Role of T cells, TNF-α, and IFN-γ in recall of immunity to oral challenge with virulent *Salmonellae* in mice vaccinated with live attenuated *aro-Salmonella* vaccines. Microbial Pathogenesis. 13: 477-491

Mata, M., and Paterson, Y. 1999. Th1 T cell responses to HIV-1 Gag protein delivered by a *Listeria monocytogenes* vaccine are similar to those induced by endogenous listerial antigens. J. Immunol. 163: 1449-1456.

Mazzaccaro, R.J., Gedde, M., Jensen, E.R., van Santen, H.M., Ploegh, H.L., Rock, K.L., and Bloom, B.R. 1996. Major histocompatibility class I presentation of soluble antigen facilitated by *Mycobacterium tuberculosis* infection. Proc. Natl. Acad. Sci. USA. 93: 11786-11791.

Medina, E., Paglia, P., Rohde, M., Colombo, M.P., and Guzman, C.A. 2000. Modulation of host immune responses stimulated by *Salmonella* vaccine carrier strains by using different promoters to drive the expression of the recombinant antigen. Eur. J. Immunol. 30: 768-777.

Melero, I., Bach, N., and Chen, L. 1997. Costimulation, tolerance, and ignorance of cytolytic T lymphocytes in immune responses to tumor antigens. Life Sci. 60: 2035-2041.

Milstein, J.B., and Gibson, J.J. 1990. Quality control of BCG vaccines by the World Health Organization: a review of factors that may influence vaccine effectiveness, and safety. WHO/EPI/ge/89 89-93.

Mocci, S., Dalrymple, S.A., Nishinakamura, R., and Murray, R. 1997. The cytokine stew, and innate resistance to *L. monocytogenes*. Immunol. Rev. 158: 107-114.

Morales, A., and Nickel, J.C. 1992. Immunotherapy for superficial bladder cancer. A development, and clinical overview. Urol. Clin. North America 19: 549-556.

Murray, P.J., Aldovini, A., and Young, R.A. 1996. Manipulation, and potentiation of antimycobacterial immunity using recombinant BCG secreting murine cytokines. Proc. Natl. Acad. Sci. USA. 93: 934-939.

Mutis, T., Cornelisse, Y.E., and Ottenhoff, T.H. 1993. *Mycobacteria* induce CD4+ T cells that are cytotoxic, and display Th1-like cytokine secretion profile: heterogeneity in cytotoxic activity, and cytokine secretion levels. Eur. J. Immunol. 23: 2189-2195.

Nardelli-Haefliger, D., Roden, R.B., Benyacoub, J., Sahli, R., Kraechenbuhl, J.P., Schiller, J.T. Lachat, P., Potts, A., and De Grandi, P. 1997. Human papillomavirus type 16 virus like particles expressed in attenuated *Salmonella typhimurium* elicit mucosal, and systemic neutralizing antibodies in mice. Infect. Immun. 65: 3328-3336.

Niethammer, A.G., Xiang, R., Ruehlmann, J.M., Lode, H.N., Dolman, C.S., Gillies, S.D., and Reisfeld, R.A. 2001. Targeted interleukin 2 therapy enhances protective immunity induced by an autologous oral DNA vaccine against murine melanoma. Cancer Res. 61: 6178-6184.

Onizuka, S., Tawara, I., Shimizu, J., Sakaguchi, S., Fujita, T., and Nakayama, E. 1999. Tumor rejection by *in vivo* administration of anti-CD25 (interleukin-2 receptor alpha) monoclonal antibody. Cancer Res. 59: 3128-3133.

Overwijk, W.W., Lee, D.S., Surman, D.R., Irvine, K.R., Touloukian, C.E., Chan, C.C., Carroll, M.W., Moss, B., Rosenberg, S.A., and Restifo, N.P. 1999. Vaccination with a recombinant vaccinia virus encoding a "self" antigen induces autoimmune vitiligo, and tumor cell destruction in mice: requirement for CD4(+) T lymphocytes. Proc. Natl. Acad. Sci. USA. 96: 2982-2987.

Pace, J.L., Russell, S.W., LeBlanc, P.A., and Murasko, D.M. 1985. Comparative effects of various classes of mouse interferons on macrophage activation for tumor cell killing. J. Immunol. 134: 977-981.

Paglia, P., Arioli, I., Frahm, N., Chakraborty, T., Colombo, M.P., and Guznam, C.A. 1997. The defined attenuated *Listeria monocytogenes* mutant is an effective oral vaccine carrier to trigger a long-lasting immune response against a mouse fibrosarcoma. Eur. J. Immunol. 27: 1570-1575.

Paglia, P., Medina, E., Arioli, I., Guznam, C.A., and Colombo, M.P. 1998. Gene transfer in dendritic cells, induced by oral DNA vaccination with *Salmonella typhimurium,* results in protective immunity against a murine fibrosarcoma. Blood 92: 3172-3176

Pan, Z.K., Ikonomidis, G., Lazenby, A., Pardoll, D., and Paterson, Y. 1995a. A recombinant *Listeria monocytogenes* vaccine expressing a model tumour antigen protects mice against lethal tumour cell challenge, and causes regression of established tumours. Nat. Med. 1: 471-477.

Pan, Z.K., Ikonomidis, G., Pardoll, D., and Paterson, Y. 1995b. Regression of established tumors in mice mediated by the oral administration of a recombinant *Listeria monocytogenes* vaccine. Cancer Res. 55: 4776-4779.

Pan, Z.K., Weiskirch, L.M., and Paterson, Y. 1999. Regression of established B16F10 melanoma with a recombinant *Listeria monocytogenes* vaccine. Cancer Res. 59: 5264-5269.

Pardoll, D.M.1998. Cancer vaccines. Nat. Med. 4: 525-531.

Paterson, Y., and Ikonomidis, G. 1996. Recombinant *Listeria monocytogenes* cancer vaccines. Curr. Opin. Immunol. 8: 664-669.

Pawelek J.M., Low K.B., and Bermudes D. 1997. Tumor-targeted *Salmonella* as a novel anticancer vector. Cancer Res. 57:4537-4544.

Piccirillo, C.A., and Shavach, E.M. 2001. Cutting Edge: control of CD8(+) T cell activation by CD4(+)CD25(+) immunoregulatory cells. J. Immunol. 167: 1137-1140.

Portnoy, D.A., Chakraborty, T., Goebel, W., and Cossart, P. 1992. Molecular determinants of *Listeria monocytogenes* pathogenesis. Infect. Immun. 60: 1263-1267.

Ramarathinam, L., Shaban, R.A., Niesel, D.W., and Klimpel, G.R. 1991. Interferon gamma (IFN-γ) production of gut-associated lymphoid tissue, and spleen following oral *Salmonella typhimurium* challenge. Microbial Pathogenesis 11: 347-356.

Read, S., Malmstrom, V., and Powrie, F. 2000. Cytotoxic T lymphocyte-associated antigen 4 plays an essential role in the function of CD25(+)CD4(+) regulatory cells that control intestinal inflammation. J. Exp. Med. 192: 295-302.

Resnick, R.M., Cornelissen, M.T., Wright, D.K., Eichinger, G.H., Fox, H.S., ter Schegget, J., and Manos, M.M. 1990. Detection, and typing of human papillomavirus in archival cervical cancer specimens by DNA amplification with consensus primers. J. Natl. Cancer Inst. 82: 1477-1484.

Restifo, N.P., Esquivel, F., Asher, A.L., Stotter, H., Barth, R.J., Bennink, J.R., Mule, J.J. Yewdell, J.W., and Rosenberg, S.A. 1991. Defective presentation of endogenous antigens by a murine sarcoma. Implications for the failure of an anti-tumor immune response. J. Immunol. 147: 1453-1459.

Revaz, V., Benyacoub, J., Kast, W.M., Schiller, J.T., De Grandi, P., and Nardelli-Haefliger, D. 2001. Mucosal vaccination with a recombinant *Salmonella typhimurium* expressing human papillomavirus type 16 (HPV16) L1 virus-like particles (VLPs) or HPV16 VLPs purified from insect cells inhibits the growth of HPV16-expressing tumor cells in mice. Virology 279: 354-360.

Rosenberg, S.A. 1984. Immunotherapy of cancer by systemic administration of lymphoid cells plus interleukin-2. J. Biol. Response. Mod. 3: 501-511.

Rosenberg, S.A., Mule, J.J., Spiess, P.J., Reichert, C.M., and Schwarz, S.L. 1985. Regression of established pulmonary metastases, and subcutaneous tumor mediated by the systemic administration of high-dose recombinant interleukin 2. J. Exp. Med. 161: 1169-1188.

Sakaguchi, S., Sakaguchi, N., Asano, M., Itoh, M., and Toda, M. 1995. Immunologic self-tolerance maintained by activated T cells expressing IL-2 receptor alpha-chains (CD25). Breakdown of a single mechanism of self-tolerance causes various autoimmune diseases. J. Immunol. 155: 1151-1164.

Saltzman, D.A., Katsanis, E., Heise, C.P., Hasz, D.E., Vigdorovich, V., Kelly, S.M., Curtiss, R. 3rd, Leonard, A.S., and Anderson, P.M. 1997. Antitumor mechanisms of attenuated *Salmonella typhimurium* containing the gene for human interleukin-2: a novel antitumor agent? J. Pediatr. Surg. 32: 301-306.

Saltzman, D.A., Katsanis, E., Heise, C.P., Hasz, D.E., Vigdorovich, V., Kelly, S.M., Curtiss, R. 3rd, Leonard, A.S., and Anderson, P.M. 1996. Attenuated

Salmonella typhimurium containing interleukin-2 decreases MC-38 hepatic metastases: a novel anti-tumor agent. Cancer Biother. Radiopharm. 11: 145-153.

Sato, N., Nariuchi, H., Tsuruoka, N., Nishihara, T., Beitz, J.G., Calabresi, P., and Frackelton, A.R. 1990. Actions of TNF, and IFN-gamma on angiogenesis *in vitro*. J. Invest. Dermatol. 95: 85S-89S.

Schafer, R., Portnoy, D.A., Brassell, S.A., and Paterson, Y. 1992. Induction of a cellular immune response to a foreign antigen by a recombinant *Listeria monocytogenes* vaccine. J. Immunol. 149: 53-59.

Schreiber, H., Ward, P.L., Rowley, D.A., and Stauss, H.J. 1988. Unique tumor-specific antigens. Annu. Rev. Immunol. 6: 465-483.

Schwaab, T., Heaney, J.A., Schned, A.R., Harris, R.D., Cole, B.F., Noelle, R.J., Phillips, D.M., Stempkowski, L., and Ernstoff, M.S. 2000. A randomized phase II trial comparing two different sequence combinations of autologous vaccine, and human recombinant interferon gamma, and human recombinant interferon alpha2B therapy in patients with metastatic renal cell carcinoma: clinical outcome, and analysis of immunological parameters. J. Urol. 163: 1322-1327.

Shu, U, Kiniwa, M., Wu, C.Y., Maliszewski, C., Vezzio, N., Hakimi, J., Gately, M., and Delespesse, G. 1995. Activated T cells induce interleukin-12 production by monocytes via CD40-CD40 ligand interaction. Eur. J. Immunol. 25: 1125-1128.

Smith, G.A., Marquis, H., Jones, S., Johnston, N.C., Portnoy, D.A., and Goldfine, H. 1995. The two distinct phospholipases C of *Listeria monocytogenes* have overlapping roles in escape from a vacuole, and cell-to-cell spread. Infect. Immun. 63: 4231-4237.

Stevanovic, S., and Schild, H. 1999. Quantitative aspects of T cell activation—peptide generation, and editing by MHC class I molecules. Semin. Immunol. 11: 375-384.

Tepper, R.I., Coffman, R.L., and Leder, P. 1992. An eosinophil-dependent mechanism for the antitumor effect of interleukin-4. Science 257: 548-551.

Tilney, L.G., and Portnoy, D.A. 1989. Actin filaments, and the growth, movement, and spread of the intracellular bacterial parasite, *Listeria monocytogenes*. J. Cell Biol. 109: 1597-1608.

Torre-Amione, G., Beauchamp, R.D., Koeppen, H., Park, B.H., Schreiber, H., Moses, H. L., and Rowley, D. A. 1990. A highly immunogenic tumor transfected with a murine transforming growth factor type beta 1 cDNA escapes immune surveillance. Proc. Natl. Acad. Sci. USA. 87: 1486-1490.

Trinchieri, G., and Scott, P. 1999. Interleukin-12: basic principles, and clinical applications. Curr. Top. Microbiol. Immunol. 238: 57-78.

Trowsdale, J., Travers, P., Bodmer, W.F., and Patillo, R.A. 1980. Expression of HLA-A, -B, and -C, and beta 2-microglobulin antigens in human choriocarcinoma cell lines. J. Exp. Med. 152: 11s-17s.

Unanue, E.R. 1997. Studies in listeriosis show the strong symbiosis between the innate cellular system, and the T-cell response. Immunol. Rev. 158: 11-25.

Urashima, M., Suzuki, H., Yuza, Y., Akiyama, M. Ohno, N., and Eto, Y. 2000. An oral CD40 ligand gene therapy against lymphoma using attenuated *Salmonella typhimurium*. Blood 95: 1258-1263.

Urban, J.L., Burton, R.C., Holland, J.M., Kripke, M.L., and Schreiber, H. 1982. Mechanisms of syngeneic tumor rejection. Susceptibility of host-selected progressor variants to various immunological effector cells. J. Exp. Med. 155: 557-573.

Uyttenhove, C., Maryanski, J., and Boon, T. 1983. Escape of mouse mastocytoma P815 after nearly complete rejection is due to antigen-loss variants rather than immunosuppression. J. Exp. Med. 157: 1040-1052.

Van Den Brule, A.J., Walboomers, J.M., Du Maine, M., Kenemans, P., and Meijer, C.J. 1991. Difference in prevalence of human papillomavirus genotypes in cytomorphologically normal cervical smears is associated with a history of cervical intraepithelial neoplasia. Int. J. Cancer. 48: 404-408.

Vazquez-Boland, J.A., Kocks, C., Dramsi, S., Ohayon, H., Geoffroy, C., Mengaud, J., and Cossart, P. 1992. Nucleotide sequence of the lecithinase operon of *Listeria monocytogenes*, and possible role of lecithinase in cell-to-cell spread. Infect. Immun. 60: 219-230.

Verma, N.K., Ziegler, H.K., Wilson, M., Khan, M., Safley, S., Stocker, B.A., and Schoolnik, G.K. 1995. Delivery of class I, and class II MHC-restricted T cell epitopes of listeriolysin of *Listeria monocytogenes* by attenuated *Salmonella*. Vaccine 13: 142-150

Voest, E.E., Kenyon, B. M., O'Reilly, M. S., Truitt, G., D'Amato, R. J., and Folkman, J. 1995. Inhibition of angiogenesis *in vivo* by interleukin 12. J. Natl. Cancer Inst. 87: 581-586.

Wallich, R., Bulbuc, N., Hammerling, G. J., Katzav, S., Segal, S., and Feldman, M. 1985. Abrogation of metastatic properties of tumour cells by *de novo* expression of H-2K antigens following H-2 gene transfection. Nature 315: 301-305.

Watts, C. 1997. Capture, and processing of exogenous antigens for presentation on MHC molecules. Annu. Rev. Immunol. 15: 821-850.

Wiemann, B., and Starnes, C.O. 1994. Coley's toxins, tumor necrosis factor, and cancer research: a historical perspective. Pharmacol. Ther. 64: 529-564.

Winkelhake, J.L., Stampfl, S., and Zimmerman, R.J. 1987. Synergistic effects of combination therapy with human recombinant interleukin-2, and tumor necrosis factor in murine tumor models. Cancer Res. 47: 3948-3953.

Wood, G.W., Holladay, F.P., Turner, T., Wang, Y.Y., Chiga, M. 2000. A pilot study of autologous cancer cell vaccination, and cellular immunotherapy using anti-CD3 stimulated lymphocytes in patients with recurrent grade III/IV astrocytoma. J. Neurooncol. 48: 113-120.

Wortzel, R.D., Philipps, C., and Schreiber, H. 1983. Multiple tumour-specific antigens expressed on a single tumour cell. Nature 304: 165-167.

Xiang, R. Lode, H.N., Chao, T.H., Ruehlmann, J.M. Dolman, C.S., Rodriguez, F., Whitton, J.L., Overwijk, W.W., Restifo, N.P., and Reisfeld, R.A. 2000. An autologous oral DNA vaccine protects against murine melanoma. Proc. Natl. Acad. Sci. USA. 97: 5492-5497

Yang, J., and Mitsuyama, M. 1997. An essential role for endogenous interferon-gamma in the generation of protective T cells against *Mycobacterium bovis* BCG in mice. Immunol. 91: 529-535

Yip, D., Strickland, A.H., Karapetis, C.S., Hawkins, C.A., Harper, P.G. 2000. Immunomodulation therapy in colorectal carcinoma. Cancer Treat. Rev. 26:169-190.

York, I. A., and Rock, K. L. 1996. Antigen processing, and presentation by the class I major histocompatibility complex. Annu. Rev. Immunol. 14: 369-396.

Zheng, L.M., Luo, X., Li, Z., Le, T., Ittensohn, M., Trailsmith, M., Bermudes, D., Lin, S.L., and King, I.C. 2000. Tumor amplified protein expression therapy: *Salmonella* as a tumor-selective protein delivery vector. Oncol. Res. 12: 127-135.

Zoller, M., and Christ, O. 2001. Prophylactic tumor vaccination: comparison of effector mechanisms initiated by protein versus DNA vaccination. J. Immunol. 166: 3440-3450.

From: *Vaccine Delivery Strategies*
Edited by: Guido Dietrich and Werner Goebel

Chapter 15

Dendritic Cell-Based Vaccination against Tumors and Infectious Diseases

Christof Berberich, Wolfgang Strittmatter and Heidrun Moll

ABSTRACT

Recent insights into the pivotal functions of dendritic cells (DCs) for the initiation and regulation of immune responses have provided the basis to design DC-based cellular vaccines for immune interventions against tumors and infectious diseases. Data collected from pre-clinical and clinical studies document that DC-based vaccination protocols can induce high levels of protective immunity and may exhibit immunotherapeutical potential. Although some obstacles to this novel approach must still be overcome, the development of methods to generate large numbers of DCs from precursor cells has paved the way for their clinical applications.

INTRODUCTION

An efficient and durable immune response relies on the simultaneous action of antigen-presenting cells (APCs), CD4[+] helper T (Th) cells, CD8[+] cytotoxic T cells (CTLs) and antibody-secreting B cells. APCs play a pivotal role in this scenario as they are capable to bridge the innate, cellular and humoral arms of the immune system. Among the APCs, dendritic cells (DCs) represent a unique system of sensors of invading pathogens or tumor cells. Equipped with highly specialized functions for antigen presentation and interaction with naive T cells, DCs are able to initiate and regulate adaptive immune responses. DCs reside in peripheral tissues in an immature state to allow for efficient and constant uptake of invading pathogens or apoptotic cells. Exposure of DCs to inflammatory stimuli converts these cells from an antigen-capturing to an antigen-presenting mode which is defined as DC maturation (Banchereau and Steinman, 1998). The production of cytokines and upregulation of chemokine receptors during DC activation directs DC migration to the secondary lymph nodes for stimulation of both Th and CTL responses.

Capitalizing on the potent adjuvant properties of DCs, these cells have been tested as vaccine carriers for prophylactic and therapeutic vaccinations against several tumors or in models of infectious diseases for which conventional immunotherapies have failed or are still not available. This chapter focuses on recent findings regarding the instructive role of DCs in the development of immune responses and reviews the emerging literature on DC-based antitumor and anti-infective vaccination trials in experimental models and clinical studies.

CONTROL OF IMMUNITY BY DCS

Evidence for Different DC Subsets

How DCs are able to control such opposite functions like the stimulation of effector T cells for antimicrobial or tumor defense, on the one hand, and the suppression of self-reactive T cells for induction of peripheral tolerance, on the other hand, is one of the most intriguing issues of the DC immunobiology. The observation that the DC system comprises a network of different subpopulations, which are phenotypically and functionally heterogeneous, has provided a clue to this question. However, the functions of particular DC subsets do not appear to be fixed, but can be modified in response to signals from the microenvironment, thus permitting a high degree of flexibility during the development of the immune response (Lanzavecchia and Sallusto, 2001; Pulendran *et al.*, 2001). Based on the origin and localization of the cells and expression of the surface marker CD8α, two major DC subpopulations can be distinguished in mice: the lymphoid and the myeloid lineage (Maraskovsky *et al.*, 1996; Kelsall and Strober, 1996; Vremec and Shortman, 1997). Both subsets are derived from common CD34$^+$ stem cells in the bone marrow (Romani *et al.*, 1994). Lymphoid DCs are positive for the surface molecule CD8α and can be found in the T cell areas of secondary lymphoid organs and in the thymic cortex. The myeloid lineage has been proposed to consist of CD8α^- cells of the interstitial DC pathway and the Langerhans cell (LC)-derived DCs expressing only small, if any, amounts of CD8α. Myeloid DCs are preferentially localized in the marginal zones of the spleen, lymph nodes and Peyer's patches or, in the case of LCs, in epithelia. Similar to the murine DC system, two subsets of primary DCs were also identified in humans (Caux *et al.*, 1996; Kohrgruber *et al.*, 1999; Pulendran *et al.*, 2000). Myeloid DCs are positive for the surface markers CD11c and CD1a, in contrast to the lymphoid DCs which are CD11c$^-$, CD1a$^-$, but express high amounts of interleukin (IL)-3 receptor (Grouard *et al.*, 1997). Due to their plasma cell-like morphology characterized by large extensions of the endoplasmatic reticulum, lymphoid DCs have also been termed plasmacytoid DCs (Grouard *et al.*, 1997).

Mode of DC Function: DCs are Functionally Heterogeneous

A common feature of all DC subtypes is their capacity to respond to inflammatory signals derived from microbes (Reis e Sousa *et al.*, 1999a) or from necrotic cells (Gallucci *et al.*, 1999) with the activation of a specific maturation program. In addition, high levels of proinflammatory cytokines have also been described as potent activators of DC maturation (Josien *et al.*, 2000). Several Toll-like receptors expressed on the surface of DCs have been shown to be critically involved in the signal transduction of inflammatory stimuli into the nucleus leading to the transcriptional activation of specific gene targets (Takeuchi *et al.*, 1999). While immature DCs in body surface tissues are highly specialized for antigen uptake from the environment, they lose these properties during maturation, but up-regulate major histocompatibility (MHC) class II, costimulatory and adhesion molecules to allow for optimal antigen presentation (Cella *et al.*, 1997; Thery and Amigorena, 2001). Interestingly, in a process referred to as cross-presentation, DCs are capable to target exogenous antigens simultaneously to MHC class I and class II antigen-processing pathways for the induction of CD8$^+$ and CD4$^+$ T cell responses (Heath and Carbone, 2001). Activated DCs produce an array of various chemokines in a time-ordered fashion in order to regulate their own migratory capacities and the recruitment of effector cells such as macrophages or natural killer (NK) cells (Sallusto *et al.*, 1999). Of particular importance is the up-regulation of the chemokine receptor-7 (CCR7) which is essential to drive the migration of DCs to the lymphatics and then to the T cell areas (Förster *et al.*, 1999). The tight interaction of mature DCs with naive T cells leads to the formation of the so-called immunological synapse. Sustained T cell receptor signaling in this highly specialized area of contact between T cells and DCs triggers T cell proliferation and differentiation into effector T cells (Lanzavecchia and Sallusto, 2001).

DCs can integrate different stimuli and selectively prime Th1- and Th2-mediated immunity, respectively. The nature of DCs that induce the appropriate kind of Th response has been the subject of intense studies. Originally, it has been proposed that Th1 cells may be stimulated by DC1-like myeloid DCs, whereas lymphoid DCs preferentially induce Th2 responses (Maldonado-López *et al.*, 1999; Pulendran *et al.*, 1999). However, this rather simplistic concept has been challenged by recent data showing that both DC subpopulations are able to induce Th1 and Th2 responses, depending on the maturation stimulus and cytokine microenvironment (Cella *et al.*, 2000). Production of the Th1-biasing cytokine IL-12 in response to different inflammatory stimuli is considered the most critical factor that determines the balance between Th1 and Th2 effector cells. In addition to the nature of the inflammatory stimulus, the kinetics of activation and IL-12 production have also been shown to determine the quality of the immune response. Upon continuous exposure to pathogen-derived products, e.g. parasite antigen and bacterial lipopolysaccharide (LPS), or T cell-derived stimuli such as CD40 ligand, DCs produce IL-12 during a relatively narrow time window at the beginning of the maturation process, but down-regulate cytokine production at later stages and become even refractory to further stimulation (Reis e Sousa *et al.*, 1999b; Langenkamp *et al.*, 2000). For that reason, DCs that synthesize IL-12 have also been termed "active" DCs while "late" DCs have exhausted their capacity to produce this cytokine. Most notably, loss of IL-12 production in the exhausted phenotype switches DCs from a Th1- to a Th2-inducing mode (Langenkamp *et al.*, 2000). Exhaustion of the active, Th1-promoting DC phenotype may be important to down-regulate the inflammatory response and to protect from immunopathology. Together, these findings suggest that Th cell polarization by DCs is determined at several levels including the nature and kinetics of the maturation stimuli, expression of pattern recognition receptors, DC lineage differences, and the chemokine and cytokine microenvironment.

While only mature DCs are able to stimulate effector T cell responses, increasing experimental evidence points to an essential role of immature DCs in mediating tolerance by the induction of suppressive regulatory T cells (Tr). It has been hypothesized that immature DCs, in the absence of inflammatory stimuli, permanently phagocytose protein antigens from apoptotic cells and migrate at low rates to draining lymph nodes. However, these spontaneously migrating immature DCs do not induce effector T cells, but prime Tr cells (Jonuleit *et al.*, 2000). Tr cells are poorly proliferative after stimulation and produce predominantly IL-10 which may directly act on activated Th1 cells by inhibiting proliferation and cytokine production (Jonuleit *et al.*, 2000; Dhodapkar *et al.*, 2001). The phenotype and function of Tr may be maintained in the periphery through constant interactions with autoantigen-presenting DCs. Consequently, the eradication of Tr has been shown to result in the development of autoimmune diseases (Sakaguchi *et al.*, 1995; Garza *et al.*, 2000). Therefore, the induction of tolerance versus immunity appears to be largely determined by the ratio of tolerogenic immature to immunogenic mature DC.

Our increasing knowledge of the mechanisms by which DCs can induce different T cell responses has opened new perspectives for the therapeutic manipulation of the immune system using DC-based vaccination strategies. While immature DCs may be useful in patients with autoimmune diseases, activated, but not exhausted, mature DCs must be used for the induction of potent T cell responses against tumors or infectious agents (Figure 1).

DC-Based Immunotherapy Of Cancer

DC-Based Vaccines in Experimental Tumor Models

The unique capacity of DCs to initiate and regulate immune responses has focused the attention of many investigators on the potential utilization of these cells for therapeutic immune interventions. After disillusions with the performance of tumor antigens as immunotherapeutics, the concept of DC-based vaccinations emerged first in the field of tumor research. In murine tumor models, a large body of experimental data has demonstrated that DCs are able to induce potent antigen-specific antitumor responses and may protect mice against a lethal challenge with tumor cells (Grabbe *et al.*, 1991;

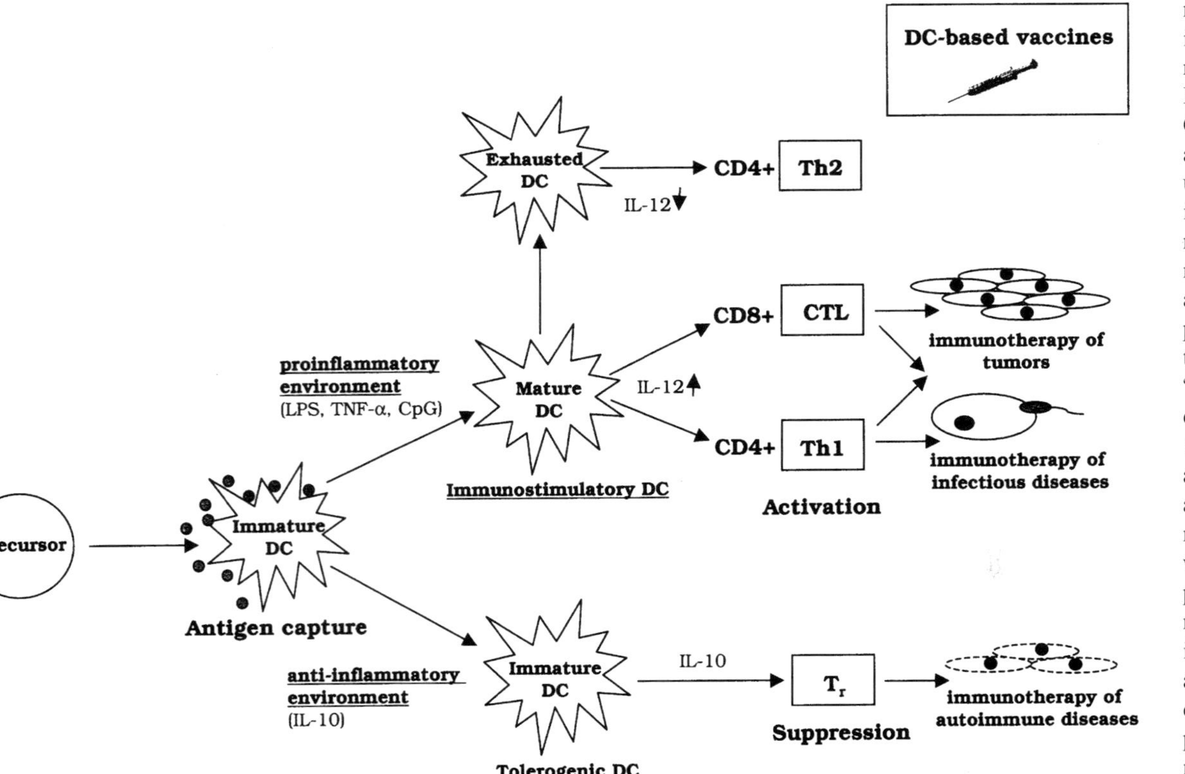

Figure 1. The type of immune response induced by DC-based immunization depends on the maturation status of DCs. Immature DCs originating from $CD34^+$ bone marrow stem cells are highly specialized for antigen uptake. In response to inflammatory stimuli, DCs mature and up-regulate molecules involved in T cell activation. Stimulated DCs produce IL-12 within a narrow time-window, but this activity is "exhausted" upon continuous exposure to the stimuli. Only IL-12-producing "active" DCs are able to induce efficient antitumor and anti-infective T cell responses (CTL and Th1), whereas "exhausted" DCs preferentially prime Th2 responses. In the absence of inflammatory signals, or in an anti-inflammatory cytokine environment, DC maturation is prevented. Immature DCs can mediate tolerance by the induction of Tr cells.

Mayordomo *et al.*, 1995; Celluzzi *et al.*, 1996; Paglia *et al.*, 1996; Porgador *et al.*, 1996). In some cases, even therapeutic efficacy of DC-based vaccines was reported, leading to the regression of an established tumor (Mayordomo *et al.*, 1996; Celluzzi and Falo, 1998). Most of these studies were based on the isolation of DCs from bone marrow, followed by *in vitro* loading of DCs with tumor antigen or peptides thereof and injection of the antigen-presenting cells into naive recipients. However, the use of "conventional" peptide pulsing has serious limitations for application in humans. The restriction given by the patient's HLA (human leukocyte antigen) class I haplotype would require a vaccination strategy with peptides tailored to the individual patient. The problem may be overcome by pulsing DCs with a broader panel of HLA-binding tumor antigen-derived peptides. Thus, the use of whole recombinant protein, instead of peptides, for vaccination seems the most obvious way to resolve problems related to HLA restriction. Other approaches are based on transfection with tumor tissue-derived RNA (Boczkowski *et al.*, 1996), loading with whole tumor cell extracts (Fields *et al.*, 1998), fusion with tumor cells (Gong *et al.*, 1997) or transduction with viral vectors (Specht *et al.*, 1997; Song *et al.*, 1997) and deserve further attention. In the future, these approaches may lead to promotor-specific DNA vaccination which would permit *in vivo* targeting of DCs.

It is important to understand that the immunostimulatory potential of DCs is not only dependent on the kind of antigen used, but that the optimization of a DC-based antitumor vaccination strategy primarily depends on the ability to direct the immune reaction to a durable CTL response. In this respect, it is notable that genetically modified DCs expressing both MHC class I and class II epitopes have been shown to be much more potent inducers of antitumor immunity than "conventionally" antigen-pulsed DCs that had been loaded *ex vivo* with a MHC class I-binding peptide (Schnell *et al.*, 2000). Hence, an important conclusion from this study is that vaccination with both tumor-specific CTL and Th cell epitopes is required for the generation of a potent antitumor response. Tumor antigen engineering with short immunodominant Th cell epitopes, originating from tetanus toxoid or diphtheria toxoid, is an attractive approach to increase the immunogenicity of the corresponding tumor proteins or peptides to be used for vaccination (Dalum *et al.*, 1997).

When using viral vectors for antigen delivery to DCs, immunomodulatory properties of viruses, which may hamper the generation of potent T cell responses, must be taken into account. These include viral immune evasion mechanisms that affect DC maturation and migration or induce the selective down-regulation of molecules that are essential for efficient antigen presentation (Klagge and Schneider-Schaulies, 1999; Tortorella *et al.*, 2000). In order to minimize these inhibitory effects, the most frequently used viral vectors for DC transduction are derived from vaccinia virus, adenovirus, herpes simplex virus and retrovirus (Jenne *et al.*, 2001).

Of particular interest is the observation that the use of growth and differentiation factors of DCs, such as GM-CSF, may greatly enhance the efficacy of DC-based vaccines. Indeed, DCs that had been transiently transfected with the GM-CSF gene showed increased efficacy to induce primary immune response *in vivo* (Curiel-Lewandrowski *et al.*, 1999). A similar effect could also be demonstrated when inflammatory stimuli such as LPS, TNF-α or CD40 ligand were present in the culture media during DC preparation and antigen pulsing. (Mackey *et al.*, 1998; Brunner *et al.*, 2000).

Clinical Trials Employing DC-Based Vaccination Protocols

The possibility to generate large amounts of mature DCs from peripheral blood monocytes (Romani *et al.*, 1996) or from proliferating CD34$^+$ precursor cells (Arrighi *et al.*, 1999) has provided the basis to test DC-based vaccination protocols in the immunotherapy of cancer patients. Currently, these clinical trials are still in phases I or II. Melanoma antigens were among the earliest characterized types of human tumor-associated antigens. Therefore, most clinical trials so far have been performed in advanced stage IV melanoma patients (Nestle *et al.*, 1998; Thurner *et al.*, 1999) for whom conventional chemotherapy had failed. Recently, the effect of DC-based immunotherapy has also been tested for other tumors such as renal cell cancer (Kugler *et al.*, 2000), prostate carcinoma (Tjoa *et al.*, 1999) or fibrosarcoma (Geiger *et al.*, 2000). These trials showed that vaccinations with autologous DCs are well tolerated and induce specific anticancer responses. In some cases, tumor regression and even complete remissions after repeated treatments have been reported. Interestingly, the route of DC administration did not appear to influence the efficacy of the immune response. However, it must be emphasized that these trials have been performed with relatively small cohorts of heavily pretreated patients and longer follow-up times of the patients' responses are not representative. While these observations are quite promising, clinical studies in patients with other tumors, by contrast, have been rather disappointing (Gjertsen *et al.*, 1996; Morse *et al.*, 1999). This demonstrates that many key questions regarding this approach must still be answered, including such essential points like the method of antigen delivery to DCs, the quality and number of DCs as well as the route and schedule of DC administration. Another critical issue refers to the risk of autoimmune reactions. Although indications of autoimmunity have not been reported from clinical trials performed so far, recent data obtained in a mouse model point to the possibility that strong responses to antigens shared between tumor and host cells may induce fatal autoimmune disease (Ludewig *et al.*, 2000). These results argue against the use of crude tumor lysates and support the notion that the search for tumor-restricted antigens, or antigens not co-expressed in vital organs, is still a major challenge for a broader application of DC-based protocols in the treatment of cancer.

DC-BASED VACCINATION AGAINST INFECTIOUS DISEASES

Interaction of Microbial Pathogens with DCs

Consistent with their function as sentinels of the immune system, DCs recognize signals derived from invading microorganisms such as LPS (De Smedt *et al.*, 1996), CpG motifs-containing bacterial DNA (Sparwasser *et al.*, 1998) or parasite antigens (Moll *et al.*, 1993; Reis e Sousa *et al.*, 1997). Toll-like receptors including TLR4 (Poltorak *et al.*, 1998) and TLR9 (Hemmi *et al.*, 2000) have been implicated in this signaling. DCs are particularly frequent in peripheral tissues, such as the skin or lung, where microbial pathogens gain access to their host. Numerous viruses, bacteria, fungi and protozoan parasites have been shown to infect DCs (Moll and Berberich, 2001). However, in contrast to macrophages, the functions of DCs are not aimed at avid ingestion and clearance of invading microorganisms, but at alerting the immune system. Indeed, the observation that the number and fate of intracellular microbes in DCs may be distinct from that in other cell types (García-del Portillo *et al.*, 2000) supports the notion that DCs are host cells with highly specialized functions. Pathogen-DC interactions influence DC functions at several levels. Bacteria and protozoan parasites up-regulate the expression of MHC and costimulatory molecules allowing for more efficient antigen presentation (Flohé *et al.*, 1997; Yrlid *et al.*, 2001). Microbial molecules elicit the production of IL-12 by DCs which triggers the development of a Th1 response (Reis e Sousa *et al.*, 1997, Gorak *et al.*, 1998; Flohé *et al.*, 1998). Dependent on the expression of specific pattern recognition receptors, DCs are able to discriminate even between different developmental stages of the same pathogen or between viable and inactivated forms of a parasite in terms of the type of immune response elicited. In a recent report, d'Ostiani *et al.* (2000) provided evidence that only phagocytosis of yeast forms of *Candida albicans* activated DCs for IL-12 production and priming of a protective Th1 response, while ingestion of fungal hyphae induced an IL-4-biased Th2 response. Infection by live tachyzoites of *Toxoplasma gondii* has been reported to be a much stronger stimulus for DC maturation than the phagocytosis of soluble antigens or heat-killed preparations (Subauste and Wessendarp, 2000). However, by impairing DC maturation and antigen presentation to T cells, other pathogens have evolved efficient mechanisms of immune evasion (Urban *et al.*, 1999; Van Overtvelt *et al.*, 1999; Engelmayer *et al.*, 1999). Taken together, a major conclusion from these findings is that the nature of pathogen-DC interactions largely determines the quality of the immune response elicited.

DCs as Cellular Vaccines Against Infectious Diseases

In contrast to the field of tumor therapy, the exploration of DC-based immune interventions in infectious disease settings has just begun. The first preclinical study in an animal model of a bacterial infection was reported in 1997 (Mbow *et al.*, 1997). DCs are now being examined as adjuvant and vaccine delivery system in a wide spectrum of infectious diseases caused by various viral, bacterial, fungal and parasitic pathogens. Most notably, despite the enormous heterogeneity of the pathogens tested, microbial antigen-pulsed DCs are remarkably efficient in inducing both humoral and T cell-mediated responses which often result in complete protection against disease. For example, DC-based vaccinations were shown to elicit protective immunity against bacterial infections caused by *Borrelia burgdorferi* (Mbow *et al.*, 1997), *Chlamydia trachomatis* (Su *et al.*, 1998) and *Mycobacterium tuberculosis* (Demangel *et al.*, 1999), against viral infections caused by lymphocytic choriomeningitis virus (Ludewig *et al.*, 1998), influenza virus (López *et al.*, 2000) or genital herpes simplex virus (Schon *et al.*, 2001) and against fungal and parasitic infections caused by *Candida albicans* (d'Ostiani *et al.*, 2000), *Toxoplasma gondii* (Bourguin *et al.*, 1998), *Leishmania major* (Flohé *et al.*, 1998) and *Leishmania donovani* (Ahuja *et al.*, 1999). A number of immunological parameters that are associated with the induction of protection by DC-based immunization approaches were studied. In the model of experimental murine leishmaniasis, it was found that DC-mediated protection was long-lasting, i.e. it was maintained after subsequent challenges with the parasites and correlated with the development of a Th1-type cytokine profile (Flohé *et al.*, 1998). A single treatment with *ex vivo* antigen-pulsed DCs was sufficient to induce maximal effects. Furthermore, the homing pattern of adoptively transferred DCs seems to be important because the effectiveness of DC-based vaccination against *L. major* was dependent on the route of immunization (Flohé *et al.*, 1998). In an attempt to further increase the efficacy of DC-based protocols for anti-infective therapy, DCs were genetically engineered to overexpress the Th1-inducing cytokine IL-12 (Ahuja *et al.*, 1999) or to down-regulate the expression of IL-10 which is known to exert a negative effect on the development of Th1 responses (Igietseme *et al.*, 2000). In both cases, the use of genetically modulated DCs for *ex vivo* antigen pulsing has proven to increase the magnitude of a protective immune response. Notably, treatment of an already established *L. donovani* infection with IL-12-transduced, soluble antigen-pulsed DCs could reduce the parasite burden by one to two orders of magnitude (Ahuja *et al.*, 1999), suggesting that DCs engineered in this manner may be a valuable tool for the therapy of chronic infectious diseases.

In summary, DC-based anti-infective vaccines and immunotherapies represent a novel, yet growing field. The results from murine infectious disease models hold the promise that these vaccination strategies may also be clinically applicable for the prevention and control of severe intracellular infections. In this context, the observation that human CTL strongly proliferated after exposure to DCs pulsed with a HLA-binding peptide derived from a 19 kDa lipoprotein of *M. tuberculosis* (Mohagheghpour *et al.*, 1998) is very encouraging. Although it is currently not feasible to use *ex vivo* antigen-loaded autologous DCs in large-scale settings for prophylactic vaccinations, the development of DC-based immune interventions may be useful for the treatment of patients in whom conventional anti-infective therapies have failed or to cure infections against which no other treatment options are yet available.

CONCLUSIONS

Over the last years, considerable insights have been gained into the mechanisms by which DCs induce and regulate the fate of immune responses to microbial pathogens, tumor cells or self antigens. The possibility to generate sufficient numbers of these potent APCs *in vitro* from precursor cells has opened new perspectives for the immunotherapy of tumors and infectious diseases. Although the data from the experimental disease models and the first clinical trials using DC-based immune interventions are highly encouraging, better vaccine formulations and the development of standardized clinical protocols are required to consider this method a realistic option among the routine methods of treatment. Major issues that have to be addressed include (a) selection of tumor-associated and microbial antigens that are suitable for DC targeting, (b) engineering of immunogenic recombinant proteins and/or vectors that induce a MHC class I and/or class II-driven immune response and (c) the identification of genes and proteins that are selectively expressed during DC differentiation or in distinct functional states of DCs and may represent targets for enhancement of the efficacy of DC-based vaccine.

REFERENCES

Ahuja, S.S., Reddick, R.L., Sato, N., Montalbo, E., Kostecki, V., Zhao, W., Dolan, M.J., Melby, P.C., and Ahuja, S.K. 1999. Dendritic cell (DC)-based anti-infective strategies: DCs engineered to secrete IL-12 are a potent vaccine in a murine model of an intracellular infection. J. Immunol. 163: 3890-3897.

Arrighi, J.F., Hauser, C., Chapuis, B., Zubler, R.H., and Kindler, V. 1999. Long-term culture of human CD34$^+$ progenitors with FLT3-ligand, thrombopoietin, and stem cell factor induces extensive amplification of a CD34$^-$ CD14$^-$ and a CD34$^-$ CD14$^+$ dendritic cell precursor. Blood 93: 2244-2252.

Banchereau, J., and Steinman, R.M. 1998. Dendritic cells and the control of immunity. Nature 392: 245-252.

Boczkowski, D., Nair, S.K., Snyder, D., and Gilboa, E. 1996. Dendritic cells pulsed with RNA are potent antigen-presenting cells *in vitro* and *in vivo*. J. Exp. Med. 184: 465-472.

Bourguin, I., Moser, M., Buzoni-Gatel, D., Tielemans, F., Bout, D., Urbain, J., and Leo, O. 1998. Murine dendritic cells pulsed *in vitro* with *Toxoplasma gondii* antigens induce protective immunity *in vivo*. Infect. Immun. 66: 4867-4874.

Brunner, C., Seiderer, J., Schlamp, A., Bidlingmaier, M., Eigler, A., Haimerl, W., Lehr, H.A., Krieg, A.M., Hartmann, G., and Endres, S. 2000. Enhanced dendritic cell maturation by TNF-α or cytidine-phosphate-guanosine DNA drives T cell activation *in vitro* and therapeutic anti-tumor immune responses *in vivo*. J. Immunol. 165: 6278-6286.

Caux, C., Vanbervliet, B., Massacrier, C., Dezutter-Dambuyant, C., de Saint-Vis, B., Jacquet, C., Yoneda, K., Imamura, S., Schmitt, D., and Banchereau, J. 1996. CD34$^+$ hematopoietic progenitors from human cord blood differentiate along two independent dendritic cell pathways in response to GM-CSF + TNFα. J. Exp. Med. 184: 695-706.

Cella, M., Engering, A., Pinet, V., Pieters, J., and Lanzavecchia, A. 1997. Inflammatory stimuli induce accumulation of MHC class II complexes on dendritic cells. Nature 388: 782-787.

Cella, M., Facchetti, F., Lanzavecchia, A., and Colonna, M. 2000. Plasmacytoid dendritic cells activated by influenza virus and CD40L drive a potent Th1 polarization. Nature Immunol. 1: 305-310.

Celluzzi, C.M., Mayordomo, J.I., Storkus, W.J., Lotze, M.T., and Falo, L.D.Jr. 1996. Peptide-pulsed dendritic cells induce antigen-specific CTL-mediated protective tumor immunity. J. Exp. Med. 183: 283-287.

Celluzzi, C.M., and Falo, L.D.Jr. 1998. Physical interaction between dendritic cells and tumor cells results in an immunogen that induces protective and therapeutic tumor rejection. J. Immunol. 160: 3081-3085.

Curiel-Lewandrowski, C., Mahnke, K., Labeur, M., Roters, B., Schmidt, W., Granstein, R.D., Luger, T.A., Schwarz, T., and Grabbe, S. 1999. Transfection of immature murine bone marrow-derived dendritic cells with the granulocyte-macrophage colony-stimulating factor gene potently enhances their *in vivo* antigen-presenting capacity. J. Immunol. 163: 174-183.

Dalum, I., Jensen, M.R., Gregorius, K., Thomasen, C.M., Elsner, H.I., and Mouritsen, S. 1997. Induction of cross-reactive antibodies against a self protein by immunization with a modified self protein containing a foreign T helper epitope. Mol. Immunol. 34: 1113-1120.

Demangel, C., Bean, A.G., Martin, E., Feng, C.G., Kamath, A.T., and Britton, W.J. 1999. Protection against aerosol *Mycobacterium tuberculosis* infection using *Mycobacterium bovis* Bacillus Calmette Guérin-infected dendritic cells. Eur. J. Immunol. 29: 1972-1979.

De Smedt, T., Pajak, B., Muraille, E., Lespagnard, L., Heinen, E., De Baetselier, P., Urbain, J., Leo, O., and Moser, M. 1996. Regulation of dendritic cell numbers and maturation by lipopolysaccharide *in vivo*. J. Exp. Med. 184: 1413-1424.

Dhodapkar, M.V., Steinman, R.M., Krasovsky, J., Munz, C., and Bhardwaj, N. 2001. Antigen-specific inhibition of effector T cell function in humans after injection of immature dendritic cells. J. Exp. Med. 193: 233-238.

d'Ostiani, C.F., Del Sero, G., Bacci, A., Montagnoli, C., Spreca, A., Mencacci, A., Ricciardi-Castagnoli, P., and Romani, L. 2000. Dendritic cells discriminate between yeasts and hyphae of the fungus *Candida albicans*. Implications for initiation of T helper cell immunity *in vitro* and *in vivo*. J. Exp. Med. 191: 1661-1674.

Engelmayer, J., Larsson, M., Subklewe, M., Chahroudi, A., Cox, W.I., Steinman, R.M., and Bhardwaj, N. 1999. Vaccinia virus inhibits the maturation of human dendritic cells: a novel mechanism of immune evasion. J. Immunol. 163: 6762-6768.

Fields, R.C., Shimizu, K., and Mule, J.J. 1998. Murine dendritic cells pulsed with whole tumor lysates mediate potent antitumor immune responses *in vitro* and *in vivo*. Proc. Natl. Acad. Sci. USA. 95: 9482-9487.

Flohé, S., Lang, T., and Moll, H. 1997. Synthesis, stability, and subcellular distribution of major histocompatibility complex class II molecules in Langerhans cells infected with *Leishmania major*. Infect. Immun. 65: 3444-3450.

Flohé, S.B., Bauer, C., Flohé, S., and Moll, H. 1998. Antigen-pulsed epidermal Langerhans cells protect susceptible mice from infection with the intracellular parasite *Leishmania major*. Eur. J. Immunol. 28: 3800-3811.

Förster, R., Schubel, A., Breitfeld, D., Kremmer, E., Renner-Müller, I., Wolf, E., and Lipp, M. 1999. CCR7 coordinates the primary immune response by establishing functional microenvironments in secondary lymphoid organs. Cell 99: 23-33.

Gallucci, S., Lolkema, M., and Matzinger, P. 1999. Natural adjuvants: endogenous activators of dendritic cells. Nature Med. 5:1249-1255.

García-del Portillo, F., Jungnitz, H., Rohde, M., and Guzman, C.A. 2000. Interaction of *Salmonella enterica* serotype typhimurium with dendritic cells is defined by targeting to compartments lacking lysosomal membrane glycoproteins. Infect. Immun. 68: 2985-2991.

Garza, K.M., Chan, S.M., Suri, R., Nguyen, L.T., Odermatt, B., Schoenberger, S.P., and Ohashi, P.S. 2000. Role of antigen-presenting cells in mediating tolerance and autoimmunity. J. Exp. Med. 191: 2021-2027.

Geiger, J., Hutchinson, R., Hohenkirk, L., McKenna, E., Chang, A., and Mule, J. 2000. Treatment of solid tumours in children with tumour-lysate-pulsed dendritic cells. Lancet 356: 1163-1165.

Gjertsen, M.K., Bakka, A., Breivik, J., Saeterdal, I., Gedde-Dahl, T., Stokke, K.T., Solheim, B.G., Egge, T.S., Soreide, O., Thorsby, E., and Gaudernack, G. 1996. *Ex vivo* ras peptide vaccination in patients with advanced pancreatic cancer: results of a phase I/II study. Int. J. Cancer 65: 450-453.

Gong, J., Chen, D., Kashiwaba, M., and Kufe, D. 1997. Induction of antitumor activity by immunization with fusions of dendritic and carcinoma cells. Nature Med. 3: 558-561.

Gorak, P.M., Engwerda, C.R., and Kaye, P.M. 1998. Dendritic cells, but not macrophages, produce IL-12 immediately following *Leishmania donovani* infection. Eur. J. Immunol. 28: 687-695.

Grabbe, S., Bruvers, S., Gallo, R.L., Knisely, T.L., Nazareno, R., and Granstein, R.D. 1991. Tumor antigen presentation by murine epidermal cells. J. Immunol. 146: 3656-3661.

Grouard, G., Rissoan, M.C., Filgueira, L., Durand, I., Banchereau, J., and Liu, Y.J. 1997. The enigmatic plasmacytoid T cells develop into dendritic cells with interleukin (IL)-3 and CD40 ligand. J. Exp. Med. 185: 1101-1111.

Heath, W.R., and Carbone, F.R. 2001. Cross-presentation, dendritic cells, tolerance and immunity. Annu. Rev. Immunol. 19: 47-64.

Hemmi, H., Takeuchi, O., Kawai, T., Kaisho, T., Sato, S., Sanjo, H., Matsumoto, M., Hoshino, K., Wagner, H., Takeda, K., and Akira, S. 2000. A Toll-like receptor recognizes bacterial DNA. Nature 408: 740-745.

Igietseme, J.U., Ananaba, G.A., Bolier, J., Bowers, S., Moore, T., Belay, T., Eko, F.O., Lyn, D., and Black, C.M. 2000. Suppression of endogenous IL-10 gene expression in dendritic cells enhances antigen presentation for specific Th1 induction: potential for cellular vaccine development. J. Immunol. 164: 4212-4219.

Jenne, L., Schuler, G., and Steinkasserer, A. 2001. Viral vectors for dendritic cell-based immunotherapy. Trends Immunol. 22: 102-107.

Jonuleit, H., Schmitt, E., Schuler, G., Knop, J., and Enk, A.H. 2000. Induction of interleukin 10-producing, nonproliferating CD4$^+$ T cells with regulatory properties by repetitive stimulation with allogeneic immature human dendritic cells. J. Exp. Med. 192: 1213-1222.

Josien, R., Li, H.L., Ingulli, E., Sarma, S., Wong, B.R., Vologodskaia, M., Steinman, R.M., and Choi, Y. 2000. TRANCE, a tumor necrosis factor family member, enhances the longevity and adjuvant properties of dendritic cells *in vivo*. J. Exp. Med. 19: 495-502.

Kelsall, B.L., and Strober, W. 1996. Distinct populations of dendritic cells are present in the subepithelial dome and T cell regions of the murine Peyer's patch. J. Exp. Med. 183: 237-247.

Klagge, I.M., and Schneider-Schaulies, S. 1999. Virus interactions with dendritic cells. J. Gen. Virol. 80: 823-833.

Kohrgruber, N., Halanek, N., Groger, M., Winter, D., Rappersberger, K., Schmitt-Egenolf, M., Stingl, G., and Maurer, D. 1999. Survival, maturation, and function of CD11c$^-$ and CD11c$^+$ peripheral blood dendritic cells are differentially regulated by cytokines. J. Immunol. 163: 3250-3259.

Kugler, A., Stuhler, G., Walden, P., Zoller, G., Zobywalski, A., Brossart, P., Trefzer, U., Ullrich, S., Müller, C.A., Becker, V., Gross, A.J., Hemmerlein, B., Kanz, L., Müller, G.A., and Ringert, R.H. 2000. Regression of human metastatic renal cell carcinoma after vaccination with tumor cell-dendritic cell hybrids. Nature Med. 6: 332-336.

Langenkamp, A., Messi, M., Lanzavecchia, A., and Sallusto, F. 2000. Kinetics of dendritic cell activation: impact on priming of Th1, Th2 and nonpolarized T cells. Nature Immunol. 1: 311-316.

Lanzavecchia, A., and Sallusto, F. 2001. The instructive role of dendritic cells on T cell responses: lineages, plasticity and kinetics. Curr. Opin. Immunol. 13: 291-298.

López, C.B,, Fernandez-Sesma, A., Czelusniak, S.M., Schulman, J.L., and Moran, T.M. 2000. A mouse model for immunization with *ex vivo* virus-infected dendritic cells. Cell. Immunol. 206: 107-115.

Ludewig, B., Ehl, S., Karrer, U., Odermatt, B., Hengartner, H., and Zinkernagel, R.M. 1998. Dendritic cells efficiently induce protective antiviral immunity. J. Virol. 72: 3812-3818.

Ludewig, B., Ochsenbein, A.F., Odermatt, B., Paulin, D., Hengartner, H., and Zinkernagel, R.M. 2000. Immunotherapy with dendritic cells directed against tumor antigens shared with normal host cells results in severe autoimmune disease. J. Exp. Med. 191: 795-804.

Mackey, M.F., Gunn, J.R., Maliszewsky, C., Kikutani, H., Noelle, R.J., and Barth, R.J., Jr. 1998. Dendritic cells require maturation via CD40 to generate protective antitumor immunity. J. Immunol. 161: 2094-2098.

Maldonado-López, R., De Smedt, T., Michel, P., Godfroid, J., Pajak, B., Heirman, C., Thielemans, K., Leo, O., Urbain, J., and Moser, M. 1999. $CD8\alpha^+$ and $CD8\alpha^-$ subclasses of dendritic cells direct the development of distinct T helper cells *in vivo*. J. Exp. Med. 189: 587-592.

Maraskovsky, E., Brasel, K., Teepe, M., Roux, E.R., Lyman, S.D., Shortman, K., and McKenna, H.J. 1996. Dramatic increase in the numbers of functionally mature dendritic cells in Flt3 ligand-treated mice: multiple dendritic cell subpopulations identified. J. Exp. Med. 184: 1953-1962.

Mayordomo, J.I., Zorina, T., Storkus, W.J., Zitvogel, L., Celluzzi, C., Falo, L.D., Melief, C.J., Ildstad, S.T., Kast, W.M., Deleo, A.B., and Lotze, M.T. 1995. Bone marrow-derived dendritic cells pulsed with synthetic tumour peptides elicit protective and therapeutic antitumour immunity. Nature Med. 1: 1297-1302.

Mayordomo, J.I., Loftus, D.J., Sakamoto, H., De Cesare, C.M., Appasamy, P.M., Lotze, M.T., Storkus, W.J., Appella, E., and DeLeo, A.B. 1996. Therapy of murine tumors with p53 wild-type and mutant sequence peptide-based vaccines. J. Exp. Med. 183: 1357-1365.

Mbow, M.L., Zeidner, N., Panella, N., Titus, R.G., and Piesman, J. 1997. *Borrelia burgdorferi*-pulsed dendritic cells induce a protective immune response against tick-transmitted spirochetes. Infect. Immun. 65: 3386-3390.

Mohagheghpour, N., Gammon, D., Kawamura, L.M., van Vollenhoven, A., Benike, C.J., and Engleman, E.G. 1998. CTL response to *Mycobacterium tuberculosis*: identification of an immunogenic epitope in the 19-kDa lipoprotein. J. Immunol. 161: 2400-2406.

Moll, H., Fuchs, H., Blank, C., and Röllinghoff, M. 1993. Langerhans cells transport *Leishmania major* from the infected skin to the draining lymph node for presentation to antigen-specific T cells. Eur. J. Immunol. 23: 1595-1601.

Moll, H., and Berberich, C. 2001. Dendritic cells as vectors for vaccination against infectious diseases. Int. J. Med. Microbiol 291: 323-329.

Morse, M.A., Deng, Y., Coleman, D., Hull, S., Kitrell-Fisher, E., Nair, S., Schlom, J., Ryback, M.E., and Lyerly, H.K. 1999. A Phase I study of active immunotherapy with carcinoembryonic antigen peptide (CAP-1)-pulsed, autologous human cultured dendritic cells in patients with metastatic malignancies expressing carcinoembryonic antigen. Clin. Cancer Res. 5: 1331-1338.

Nestle, F.O., Alijagic, S., Gilliet, M., Sun, Y., Grabbe, S., Dummer, R., Burg, G., and Schadendorf, D. 1998. Vaccination of melanoma patients with peptide- or tumor lysate-pulsed dendritic cells. Nature Med. 4: 328-332.

Paglia, P., Chiodoni, C., Rodolfo, M., and Colombo, M.P. 1996. Murine dendritic cells loaded *in vitro* with soluble protein prime cytotoxic T lymphocytes against tumor antigen *in vivo*. J. Exp. Med. 183: 317-322.

Poltorak, A., He, X., Smirnova, I., Liu, M.Y., Huffel, C.V., Du, X., Birdwell, D., Alejos, E., Silva, M., Galanos, C., Freudenberg, M., Ricciardi-Castagnoli, P., Layton, B., and Beutler, B. 1998. Defective LPS signaling in C3H/HeJ and C57BL/10ScCr mice: mutations in Tlr4 gene. Science 282: 2085-2088.

Porgador, A., Snyder, D., and Gilboa, E. 1996. Induction of antitumor immunity using bone marrow-generated dendritic cells. J. Immunol. 156: 2918-2926.

Pulendran, B., Smith, J.L., Caspary, G., Brasel, K., Pettit, D., Maraskovsky, E., and Maliszewski, C.R. 1999. Distinct dendritic cell subsets differentially regulate the class of immune response *in vivo*. Proc. Natl. Acad. Sci. USA. 96: 1036-1041.

Pulendran, B., Banchereau, J., Burkeholder, S., Kraus, E., Guinet, E., Chalouni, C., Caron, D., Maliszewski, C., Davoust, J., Fay, J., and Palucka, K. 2000. Flt3-ligand and granulocyte colony-stimulating factor mobilize distinct human dendritic cell subsets *in vivo*. J. Immunol. 165: 566-572.

Pulendran, B., Banchereau, J., Maraskovsky, E., and Maliszewski, C. 2001. Modulating the immune response with dendritic cells and their growth factors. Trends Immunol. 22: 41-47.

Reis e Sousa, C., Hieny, S., Scharton-Kersten, T., Jankovic, D., Charest, H., Germain, R.N., Sher, A. 1997. *In vivo* microbial stimulation induces rapid CD40 ligand-independent production of interleukin 12 by dendritic cells and their redistribution to T cell areas. J. Exp. Med. 186: 1819-1829.

Reis e Sousa, C., Sher, A., and Kaye, P. 1999a. The role of dendritic cells in the induction and regulation of immunity to microbial infection. Curr. Opin. Immunol. 11: 392-399.

Reis e Sousa, C., Yap, G., Schulz, O., Rogers, N., Schito, M., Aliberti, J., Hieny, S., and Sher, A. 1999b. Paralysis of dendritic cell IL-12 production by microbial products prevents infection-induced immunopathology. Immunity 11: 637-647.

Romani, N., Gruner, S., Brang, D., Kämpgen, E., Lenz, A., Trockenbacher, B., Konwalinka, G., Fritsch, P.O., Steinman, R.M., and Schuler, G. 1994. Proliferating dendritic cell progenitors in human blood. J. Exp. Med. 180: 83-93.

Romani, N., Reider, D., Heuer, M., Ebner, S., Kämpgen, E., Eibl, B., Niederwieser, D., and Schuler, G. 1996. Generation of mature dendritic cells from human blood. An improved method with special regard to clinical applicability. J. Immunol. Methods 196: 137-151.

Sakaguchi, S., Sakaguchi, N., Asano, M., Itoh, M., and Toda, M. 1995. Immunologic self-tolerance maintained by activated T cells expressing IL-2 receptor α-chains (CD25). Breakdown of a single mechanism of self-tolerance causes various autoimmune diseases. J. Immunol. 155: 1151-1164.

Sallusto, F., Palermo, B., Lenig, D., Miettinen, M., Matikainen, S., Julkunen, I., Förster, R., Burgstahler, R., Lipp, M., and Lanzavecchia, A. 1999. Distinct patterns and kinetics of chemokine production regulate dendritic cell function. Eur. J. Immunol. 29: 1617-1625.

Schnell, S., Young, J.W., Houghton, A.N., and Sadelain, M. 2000. Retrovirally transduced mouse dendritic cells require CD4[+] T cell help to elicit antitumor immunity: implications for the clinical use of dendritic cells. J. Immunol. 164: 1243-1250.

Schon, E., Harandi, A.M., Nordstrom, I., Holmgren, J., and Eriksson, K. 2001. Dendritic cell vaccination protects mice against lethality caused by genital herpes simplex virus type 2 infection. J. Reprod. Immunol. 50: 87-104.

Song, W., Kong, H.L., Carpenter, H., Torii, H., Granstein, R., Rafii, S., Moore, M.A., and Crystal, R.G. 1997. Dendritic cells genetically modified with an adenovirus vector encoding the cDNA for a model antigen induce protective and therapeutic antitumor immunity. J. Exp. Med. 186: 1247-1256.

Sparwasser, T., Koch, E.S., Vabulas, R.M., Heeg, K., Lipford, G.B., Ellwart, J.W., and Wagner, H. 1998. Bacterial DNA and immunostimulatory CpG oligonucleotides trigger maturation and activation of murine dendritic cells. Eur. J. Immunol. 28: 2045-2054.

Specht, J.M., Wang, G., Do, M.T., Lam, J.S., Royal, R.E., Reeves, M.E., Rosenberg, S.A., and Hwu, P. 1997. Dendritic cells retrovirally transduced with a model antigen gene are therapeutically effective against established pulmonary metastases. J. Exp. Med. 186: 1213-1221.

Su, H., Messer, R., Whitmire, W., Fischer, E., Portis, J.C., Caldwell, H.D. 1998. Vaccination against chlamydial genital tract infection after immunization with dendritic cells pulsed *ex vivo* with nonviable *Chlamydiae*. J. Exp. Med. 188: 809-818.

Subauste, C.S., and Wessendarp, M. 2000. Human dendritic cells discriminate between viable and killed *Toxoplasma gondii* tachyzoites: dendritic cell activation after infection with viable parasites results in CD28 and CD40 ligand signaling that controls IL-12-dependent and -independent T cell production of IFN-γ. J. Immunol. 165:1498-1505.

Takeuchi, O., Hoshino, K., Kawai, T., Sanjo, H., Takada, H., Ogawa, T., Takeda, K., and Akira, S. 1999. Differential roles of TLR2 and TLR4 in recognition of gram-negative and gram-positive bacterial cell wall components. Immunity 11: 443-451.

Thery, C., and Amigorena, S. 2001. The cell biology of antigen presentation in dendritic cells. Curr. Opin. Immunol. 13: 45-51.

Thurner, B., Haendle, I., Röder, C., Dieckmann, D., Keikavoussi, P., Jonuleit, H., Bender, A., Maczek, C., Schreiner, D., von den Driesch, P., Bröcker, E.B., Steinman, R.M., Enk, A., Kämpgen, E., and Schuler, G. 1999. Vaccination with mage-3A1 peptide-pulsed mature, monocyte-derived dendritic cells expands specific cytotoxic T cells and induces regression of some metastases in advanced stage IV melanoma. J. Exp. Med. 190: 1669-1678.

Tjoa, B.A., Simmons, S.J., Elgamal, A., Rogers, M., Ragde, H., Kenny, G.M., Troychak, M.J., Boynton, A.L., and Murphy, G.P. 1999. Follow-up evaluation of a phase II prostate cancer vaccine trial. Prostate 40: 125-129.

Tortorella, D., Gewurz, B.E., Furman, M.H., Schust, D.J., and Ploegh, H.L. 2000. Viral subversion of the immune system. Annu. Rev. Immunol. 18: 861-926.

Urban, B.C., Ferguson, D.J., Pain, A., Willcox, N., Plebanski, M., Austyn, J.M., and Roberts, D.J. 1999. *Plasmodium falciparum*-infected erythrocytes modulate the maturation of dendritic cells. Nature 400: 73-77.

Van Overtvelt, L., Vanderheyde, N., Verhasselt, V., Ismaili, J., De Vos, L., Goldman, M., Willems, F., and Vray, B. 1999. *Trypanosoma cruzi* infects human dendritic cells and prevents their maturation: inhibition of cytokines, HLA-DR, and costimulatory molecules. Infect. Immun. 67: 4033-4040.

Vremec, D., and Shortman, K. 1997. Dendritic cell subtypes in mouse lymphoid organs: cross-correlation of surface markers, changes with incubation, and differences among thymus, spleen, and lymph nodes. J. Immunol. 159: 565-573.

Yrlid, U., Svensson, M., Hakansson, A., Chambers, B.J., Ljunggren, H.G., and Wick, M.J. 2001. *In vivo* activation of dendritic cells and T cells during *Salmonella enterica* serovar typhimurium infection. Infect. Immun. 69: 5726-5735.

From: *Vaccine Delivery Strategies*
Edited by: Guido Dietrich and Werner Goebel

Chapter 16

Edible Vaccines

Jie Yu, James E. Carter and
William H.R. Langridge

ABSTRACT

Advances in plant molecular biology over the past two decades have resulted in the expression of foreign genes in an increasing variety of plant species. Transgenic plants expressing recombinant proteins are becoming more effective production systems for vaccines. Inoculation with edible plants producing pathogen and self proteins has shown promising results for protective immunization against infectious diseases and induction of immune tolerance against autoimmune diseases. Ease of administration and the reduced cost of vaccine production provided by recombinant plant technology may soon enable a global immunization program.

INTRODUCTION

The concept of vaccination originated in the late 18th century, when the English physician Edward Jenner inoculated an 8-year-old boy, James Phipps with cowpox virus isolated from a milkmaid. This first parenteral vaccination enabled the patient to develop a protective resistance to smallpox. After more than two hundred years, parenteral vaccination has become one of the most cost–effective medical intervention methods available for control and eradication of disease epidemics worldwide. However, implementation of a global vaccination program in developing nations has been impossible due to a combination of poverty and political unrest resulting in inadequate health care, and the prohibitive cost of vaccine administration.

To rectify this situation, basic changes are required in the way vaccines are produced, distributed and administered to make them more effective, less expensive, easier to administer and more widely available. In 1990, the World Health Organization (WHO) launched the Children's Vaccine Initiative establishing goals for the development of vaccines that are safe, inexpensive, easily (orally) administered and widely accessible (Mitchell *et al.*, 1993). The establishment of these goals and the advent of modern methods of molecular genetics ultimately led to the idea of oral vaccine production in transgenic food plants (Mason *et al.*, 1992).

TRANSGENIC PLANTS AS VACCINE PRODUCTION AND DELIVERY SYSTEMS

Traditional methods of plant breeding were practiced for hundreds of years with great success in improving observable plant characteristics (traits) and agricultural properties, such as larger yields, improved protein content, resistance to insect and fungal attack and resistance to virus and bacterial disease. However, the classical plant breeding approach is slow and imprecise due to the transfer of all the traits of the donor organism to the recipient, which can considerably alter the expression of the desired genes. However, in the past decade, the development of new molecular biology methods, especially recombinant DNA techniques, has contributed substantially to shortening the time required to identify and clone specific genes encoding desirable traits and has made plant systems particularly valuable for production of recombinant proteins with nutritional and therapeutic value (Schell, 1987; Mason and Arntzen, 1995; Arntzen *et al.*, 1997, and 1998; Mor *et al.*, 1998). Genetic engineering technology has also been applied to the production of proteins with pharmaceutical value including antibodies and antigenic proteins for use as vaccines (Figure 1).

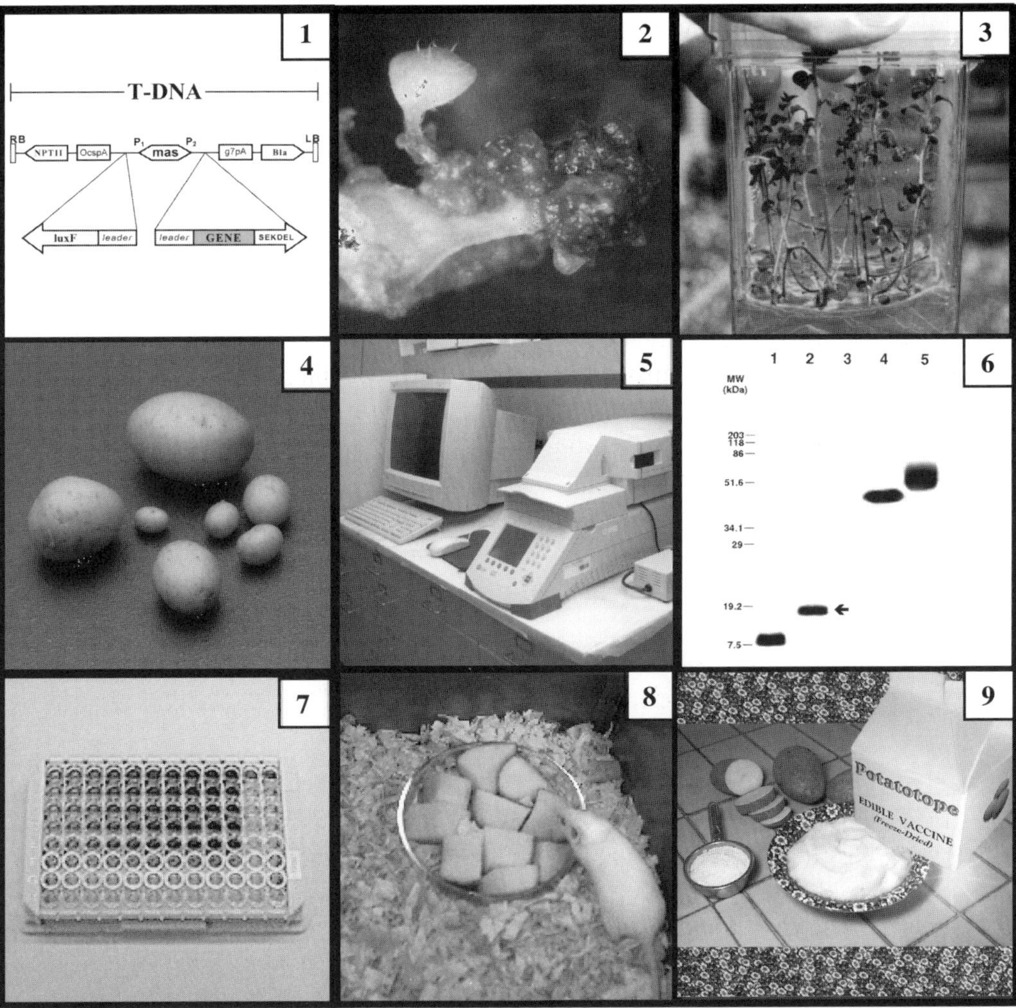

Figure 1. Graphic representation of major stages involved in developing an edible vaccine in transformed plants. 1) Plant expression vectors containing genes encoding antigens or autoantigens are inserted into host plant tissues via *A. tumefaciens* mediated stable transformation methods. 2) From three to six weeks after transformation, shoots emerge from callus growing on transformed stem tissues. 3) Transformed shoots are propagated to form roots in ten to twelve weeks (potato plants shown). 4) Transgenic tubers are harvested from mature plants approximately six months after transformation. 5) PCR analysis of genomic DNA isolated from transformed plants confirms the presence of vaccine genes. 6) Immunoblot confirmation of vaccine proteins in potatoes. 7) ELISA quantification of vaccine protein levels synthesized in transformed plants. 8) Animal pre-clinical trials for determination of plant-produced vaccine protective efficacy. 9) Following successful human clinical trials, plant vaccine product will likely be distributed in freeze-dried form to ensure consistency in dosage and to increase shelf-life.

ADVANTAGES OF PLANT-BASED VACCINES

One of the greatest advantages of plant genetic engineering is that entire plants can be regenerated from individual transformed cells (Streatfield *et al.*, 2001). When a plant is wounded, plant growth factors (hormones), trigger rapid cell regeneration called a "callus" to grow over the surface of the wound. If individual cells or a piece of this embryonic callus tissue is removed and placed in a culture medium containing the appropriate nutrients and plant growth hormones, the callus cells will continue to grow and differentiate into shoots and roots and ultimately a complete flowering plant will be produced. If rapid regeneration of plants from callus tissue is combined with gene transfer into cells of the callus, transgenic plants can be conveniently grown from individual transformed cells to produce stable breeding lines, with normal morphology, which can be propagated by conventional horticultural techniques and stored and distributed as seeds or vegetative proteins (tubers). Plant produced proteins are inexpensive to synthesize. Unlike bacterial or animal cells, plant cultivation does not require special media or equipment. Since plants photosynthesize, they require only water, CO_2, soil and sunlight for growth and development (Moffat, 1995). Another obvious benefit of transgenic plants as vaccine production systems is their potential for scaled-up production (Mor *et al.*, 1998), in which large amounts of recombinant protein can be produced at minimal cost. For example, the plant biotech company Agracetus has developed a transformed strain of corn that can produce 1.5 kg of pharmaceutical quality antibodies per acre. A cost-effectiveness analysis carried out by the Scripps Research Institute showed that the "plantibodies" could be produced at approximately one U.S. dollar per gram (Ma and Vine, 1999).

To develop a protective recombinant subunit vaccine, the immunogenicity of the antigen must be maintained . This depends on retention of the correct amino acid sequence, structure, protein folding and post-translational modifications. Since plants are eukaryotic systems, there are significant advantages over bacterial or viral expression systems with respect to post-translational modification of proteins synthesized in plants. Small antigen epitopes, large structural proteins, and even complex virus capsid-like particles can be expressed and assembled in plants with the assistance of ER-resident chaperones homologous to those in mammalian cells. Targeting recombinant proteins to the ER, storage vacuoles and the Golgi apparatus can be achieved using either native or plant leader sequences (Hijarrubia *et al.*, 1997). For example, by co-expression of antibody heavy and light chains, a full-length antibody, functionally identical to its mammalian counterpart, can be synthesized and assembled in plants (Hiatt *et al.*, 1989). Expression of the rabies virus glycoprotein in trangenic tomatoes demonstrated the ability of plant cells to carry out post-translational glycosylation essential for the biological function of proteins of animal origin (McGarvey *et al.*, 1995). However, the plant glycosylation pattern differs to a small degree from mammals in the composition of complex glycans. In plant proteins, complex glycans tend to be smaller than mammalian glycans and differ in terminal sugar residues. However, with respect to the recombinant proteins expressed so far, this difference has not led to detectable losses of structure or biological function.

Additional advantages of the plant production system include biological safety and ease of purification. Plant viruses are not known to infect humans. In addition, vaccines produced in plants eliminate contamination with animal viruses. If tissue specific promoters are used, the vaccine antigens can be exclusively expressed in storage organs such as seeds, fruits or tubers (Arakawa *et al.*, 1997; McGarvey *et al.*, 1995; Wenzler *et al.*, 1989). Extraction and purification from plant tissues is relatively simple. The idea of an edible plant vaccine is also very tempting from the perspective of simplicity. Vaccines produced in transgenic plants can be harvested by conventional agricultural machinery and administered to patients simply by eating the leaves, fruit, tubers or seeds that contain the appropriate amounts of vaccine antigen required for immune protection (Arntzen, 1997). To date there are more than 30 antigens isolated from infectious pathogens and autoantigens from autoimmune diseases that have been synthesized in a variety of edible plants (Table 1).

Although plants are attractive systems for vaccine production, they have certain limitations. Many groups of plants are polyploid. Thus plants regenerated from single cells may not be genetically homogeneous, which may cause variation in yield of the recombinant protein. An additional potential problem is that many important crop plants such as maize, rice and wheat belong to the class monocotyledonae which was proved to be difficult to transform with *Agrobacterium* based *in vivo* DNA vectoring systems. For this group of plants, DNA coated metal particle bombardment of plant tissue has so far proven to be the most effective method of transformation, as protoplast regeneration has not proven to be easy to accomplish in these species.

Table 1. Diseases currently targeted by plant-based vaccines.

Disease/Pathogen	Plant used	Method*	Reference
B-cell lymphoma	Tobacco	V/A	McCormick *et al.*, 1999
Bovine pneumonia pasteurellosis	White clover	S	Lee *et al.*, 2001
Canine parvovirus	Tobacco	V	Fernandez-Fernandez *et al.*, 1998
	Arabidopsis	S	Gil *et al.*, 2001
Cholera (*Vibrio cholerae*)	Potato	S	Arakawa *et al.*, 1997
	Tobacco	C	Daniell *et al.*, 2001
Cholera, *E. coli*, and rotavirus (diarrhea)	Potato	S	Yu *et al.*, 2001
Colon cancer	Tobacco	A	Verch *et al.*, 1998
Colon, breast, and other epithelial tumors	Tobacco	A	Vaquero *et al.*, 1999
	Rice, Wheat	A	Stoger *et al.*, 2000
Dental caries (*Streptococcus mutans*)	Tobacco	A	Ma *et al.*, 1998
Diabetes, type 1A (autoimmune)	Tobacco, Potato	S	Ma *et al.*, 1997
	Potato	S	Arakawa *et al.*, 1998b, and 1999
Enterotoxigenic *E. coli*	Tobacco	S	Haq *et al.*, 1995
	Potato	S	Haq *et al.*, 1995
	Potato	S	Tacket *et al.*, 1998
	Potato	S	Mason *et al.*, 1998
	Potato	S	Lauterslager *et al.*, 2001
	Corn	S	Streatfield *et al.*, 2001
Foot-and-mouth disease virus	Cowpea	V	Usha *et al.*, 1993
	Arabidopsis	S	Carrillo *et al.*, 1998
	Alfalfa	S	Wigdorovitz *et al.*, 1999a
	Tobacco	V	Wigdorovitz *et al.*, 1999b
Genital herpes (herpes simplex virus-2)	Soybean	A	Zeitlin *et al.*, 1998
Hepatitis B virus	Tobacco	S	Mason *et al.*, 1992
	Tobacco	S	Thanavala *et al.*, 1995
	Lupine	S	Kapusta *et al.*, 1999
	Lettuce	S	Kapusta *et al.*, 1999
	Potato	S	Richter *et al.*, 2000
Hepatitis C virus	Tobacco	V	Nemchinov *et al.*, 2000
Human cytomegalovirus	Tobacco	S	Tackaberry *et al.*, 1999
Human immunodeficiency virus	Cowpea	V	Porta *et al.*, 1994
	Tobacco	V	Sugiyama *et al.*, 1995
	Cowpea	V	McLain *et al.*, 1996
	Tobacco	V	Yusibov *et al.*, 1997
	Tobacco	V	Joelson *et al.*, 1997

Table 1 continued

Human rhinovirus 14	Cowpea	V	Porta *et al.*, 1994
Influenza virus	Tobacco	V	Sugiyama *et al.*, 1995
Malaria	Tobacco	V	Turpen *et al.*, 1995
Measles virus	Tobacco	S	Huang *et al.*, 2001
Mink enteritis virus	Cowpea	V	Dalsgaard *et al.*, 1997
Murine hepatitis virus	Tobacco	V	Koo *et al.*, 1999
Norwalk virus (diarrhea)	Tobacco	S	Mason *et al.*, 1996
	Potato	S	Tacket *et al.*, 2000
Pseudomonas aeruginosa	Cowpea	V	Brennan *et al.*, 1999a
Rabbit hemorrhagic disease virus	Potato	S	Castanon *et al.*, 1999
	Tobacco	V	Fernandez-Fernandez *et al.*, 2001
Rabies virus	Tomato	S	McGarvey *et al.*, 1995
	Tobacco	V	Yusibov *et al.*, 1997
	Tobacco, Spinach	V	Modelska *et al.*, 1998
Respiratory syncytial virus	Apple leaf	S	Sandhu *et al.*, 1999
	Tomato	S	Sandhu *et al.*, 2000
	Tobacco	V	Belanger *et al.*, 2000
Staphylococcus aureus	Cowpea, Tobacco	V	Brennan *et al.*, 1999b
Swine-transmissible gastroenteritis virus	*Arabidopsis*	S	Gomez *et al.*, 1998
	Potato	S	Gomez *et al.*, 2000
	Tobacco	S	Tuboly *et al.*, 2000
	Corn	S	Streatfield *et al.*, 2001

*S = stable (nuclear) transformation, V = engineered plant virus, A = plant-produced antibodies, C = chloroplast transformation.

PRODUCTION OF ANTIBODIES IN TRANSGENIC PLANTS FOR PASSIVE IMMUNIZATION

The first demonstration of recombinant antibody expression in transgenic plants was reported by Hiatt *et al.* (1989). The gamma and kappa immunoglobulin chains were expressed in separate tobacco plants. Cross pollination of the two plants generated progeny expressing both heavy and light chains, which self assembled into functional antibodies. A number of strategies have been applied to improve antibody yields. Addition of a leader sequence increased antibody accumulation to 1.3% of total soluble plant protein (TSP). Fusion of the endoplasmic-reticulum retention signal KDEL to the C-terminus of the antibody fragment has increased single chain Fv protein yield to 4% - 6.8% of total soluble protein (Schouten *et al.*,1996). Targeted aggregation of antibodies in the apoplasm (extracellular space) and in plant storage tissues such as tubers, fruits, and seeds has considerably improved the quantity and long-term storage of therapeutic proteins (Fiedler and Conrad, 1995; Conrad and Fiedler, 1998). The most complex recombinant antibody synthesized in plants to date is the secretory immunoglobulin "Guy's 13" (Ma *et al.*, 1995). A series of sexual crosses between four different transgenic *Nicotiana tabacum* plants expressing four individual components of secretory immunoglobulin (a murine joining chain, a rabbit secretory protein component, a light chain and a hybrid IgA-G antibody heavy chain), resulted in a transformed plant that expressed all four peptide chains simultaneously. The four components of the secretory immunoglobulin assembled into a functional high molecular weight (470 kDa) secretory IgA that specifically recognized the streptococcal adhesion molecule (SAI/II) of *Streptococcus mutans*, which is the major cause of dental caries. The dimeric sIgA-G expression levels in the plant reached 5-8% of the total plant protein and the secretory antibody was shown to prevent oral colonization by *S. mutans* in human trials (Ma *et al.*, 1998). Production of a functional complex secretory antibody in plants demonstrated the amazing capability that plants have to synthesize and assemble complex protein molecules for passive immunotherapy. With a known DNA sequence encoding the variable region, virtually any recombinant antibody can now be synthesized in transgenic plants. A humanized monoclonal antibody against herpes simplex virus (HSV) glycoprotein B was produced in transgenic soybean (Zeitlin *et al.*, 1998). The plant derived antibody was stable in human semen and cervical mucus, and its efficacy for prevention of HSV-2 infection in the mouse was similar to the same antibody expressed in mammalian cell-culture (Zeitlin *et al.*, 1998).

PLANT PRODUCED VACCINES FOR IMMUNIZATION AGAINST INFECTIOUS DISEASES

The mammalian mucosal immune system is an integrated network of antigen presenting cells (APC's), T helper lymphocytes and antibody producing B lymphocytes. Induction of the mucosal immune response can result in protective immunity in both the peripheral compartment (blood and lymph) and at mucosal membrane sites (Freytag and Clements, 1999). When one considers that most infectious agents come in contact with the host at mucosal surfaces, oral vaccination becomes the most attractive approach for protective immunization. Induction of mucosal immune responses by oral vaccines may not only protect the host from morbidity and mortality due to infection, but may possibly prevent infection altogether (Brandtzaeg, 1995; Czerkinsky *et al.*, 1995). A number of strategies have been pursued to develop plants as vaccine production and delivery systems. One productive approach employs *Agrobacterium tumefaciens* mediated stable transformation. In this method, the T-DNA region of an *A. tumefaciens* Ti plasmid that contains genes encoding recombinant proteins is transferred into plant cells and becomes stably integrated into the plant genome. Selectable markers such as neomycin phosphotransferase II (NPTII) and dihydrofolate reductase are included for selection of transformed plants. The integrated genes are passed on to subsequent generations with expression levels ranging generally from 0.01% to 0.4% of TSP. The second method uses genetically modified plant viruses for the expression of antigen epitopes in plants. Such plant viruses can replicate to high levels in infected plant tissues. Within weeks the recombinant protein expression levels can reach up to 2.0% of total plant soluble protein. This method is labor intensive as virus infection kills the host plant which makes virus reinfection necessary for each vaccine harvest. The viral products can not be easily used directly for vaccination. However, in comparison with bacterial or mammalian systems, relatively simple vaccine purification procedures are required. Recent success in chloroplast engineering makes this organelle an ideal compartment for expression of viral and bacterial antigens. Large numbers (thousands) of copies of foreign genes can be introduced into single plant cells by chloroplast transformation methods. Thus, this transformation method can generate exceptionally high levels of foreign proteins, up to 46% of total soluble protein have been recorded (Bogorad, 2000). The introduction of foreign genes without using antibiotic selection makes the chloroplast an attractive system for edible vaccine production.

Transient Plant Virus Mediated Expression

There are generally two approaches in which modified plant viruses have been used for synthesis and accumulation of recombinant proteins in plants. In the first case, the foreign genes are transcribed from viral promoters, which produce soluble antigen proteins during virus infection. The second method involves modification of viral capsid proteins to carry vaccine epitopes. Due to the expression of multiple copies of antigen epitopes on the surface of a virus particle, this method has been the most widely used (Beachy *et al.*, 1996; Yu *et al.*, 2000).

Tobacco Mosaic Virus (TMV)

TMV is a rod shaped RNA plant virus. The virus particle is composed of approximately 2100 copies of well characterized TMV coat protein (CP) surrounding a helical genomic RNA molecule. Selected B cell epitopes of malaria were either fused to the C terminus or inserted into the surface loop region of the TMV coat protein (Turpen *et al.*, 1995). A leaky stop codon was used to produce both wild type and modified coat protein. Infection of tobacco plants with the chimeric virus generated wild type TMV CP and the fusion protein at a ratio of approximately 20:1. The malaria epitopes were recognized by anti-malarial antibodies in ELISA and Western blot assay (Turpen *et al.*, 1995). Epitopes from human immunodeficiency virus (HIV) glycoprotein and *H. influenzae* haemagglutinin have also been fused to the C-terminus of the TMV CP (Sugiyama *et al.*, 1995). Virus particles purified from infected plants reacted with antiserum specific for each epitope. The results suggested the presence of foreign peptides on the viral surface. To generate contraceptives, TMV CP has been engineered for expression of murine ZP3 protein, a primary binding site for sperm during fertilization (Fitchen *et al*, 1995). Modified virus particles isolated from infected plant tissues were used for mouse immunization and anti-ZP3 antibodies were detected in immunized mice. Although there was some evidence of anti-ZP3 antibodies bound to the zona pellucida, no impact on the fertility of the treated mice has yet been demonstrated.

Cowpea Mosaic Virus (CPMV)

CPMV is an RNA genome virus containing approximately 60 copies of large and small protein subunits. Structural studies of the small coat protein revealed several loop regions on the virus surface that may not be directly involved in intersubunit interactions. Epitopes from protein VP1 of foot and mouth disease virus (FMDV) were inserted into the loop region of the small coat protein between amino acids 18 and 19 (Usha *et al.*, 1993; Porta *et al.*, 1994). RNA transcripts from modified clones were able to replicate in cowpea protoplasts. FMDV specific antiserum was able to recognize the virus particles. Immunosorbent electron microscopy detected assembly of the chimeric virus particle in cowpea leaf tissues. However, serial passage of the virus showed rapid loss of the FMDV sequences inserted in CPMV. A redesigned chimeric protein has led to genetically more stable chimeric CPMVs. Peptides from VP1 of human rhinovirus and from gp41 of HIV-1 were inserted into the small protein between amino acids 22 and 23 and stably expressed (McLain *et al.*, 1996). In both cases, the chimeric virus particles possessed the antigenic properties of the inserted sequences and in case of the human rhinovirus (HRV)-14 peptide, the inserted epitope was able to elicit an antibody response in rabbits. The CPMV expression system has been adopted for development of an animal vaccine. A linear epitope from the VP2 capsid protein of mink enteritis virus (MEV) was introduced into CPMV. Recombinant virus particles harvested from black eyed bean were subsequently used for subcutaneous injection in mink (Dalsgaard *et al.*, 1997). A significant reduction in virus shed and relief of clinical disease symptoms were found following challenge with virulent MEV. This was the first demonstration that plant virus based vaccines can protect animals from infectious disease.

Other Plant Viruses

Other plant viruses like alfalfa mosaic virus (AMV), plum pox virus (PPV), potato virus X (PVX) and tomato bushy-stunt virus (TBSV) have also been explored for vaccine production (Joelson *et al.*, 1997; Brennan *et al.*, 1999b; Fernandez-Fernandez *et al.*, 2001). Antigenic peptides from rabies virus and HIV were expressed on AMV coat proteins (Yusibov *et al.*, 1997). The plant produced peptides were purified and used for mouse immunization. Both antigens elicited specific virus neutralizing antibodies in immunized mice. In another experiment, 50 µg of plant derived rabies virus peptides in the form of recombinant virus particles were injected into mice intraperitoneally for three separate immunizations (Modelska *et al.*, 1998). Fourteen days after the last immunization, the mice were challenged with a lethal dose of rabies virus. Forty percent of immunized mice survived and never developed clinical signs of the disease. Oral administration (by gastric intubation or feeding) of plant produced rabies virus antigens stimulated significant serum

IgG and IgA titers in mice and provided partial protection against infection with an attenuated rabies virus strain. Interestingly, mice fed virus infected spinach leaves (25 µg of antigen per dose) stimulated higher levels of immune response than when the virus was administered by gastric intubation (250 µg per dose). The higher levels of immune response indicated that feeding of the pathogen enhanced delivery of virus particles to the mucosal immune system.

Respiratory syncytial virus (RSV) is the primary cause of respiratory infection in infants. Peptides from the G protein of RSV were fused to the N terminus of the AMV coat protein and expressed in *Nicotiana tabacum* cv (Belanger *et al.*, 2000). The recombinant AMV viruses were passaged five consecutive times in new plants without loss of the coat protein insert. The high replication rate of AMV generated 50 µg of RSV peptide per gram of fresh plant tissue comparable to foreign protein expression levels reported for cow pea mosaic virus. Intraperitioneal administration of plant derived RSV peptides (1.0 mg/ dose) three times protected mice against challenge infection. However, despite the high yield of the virus expression system, there remains a size limitation of the antigenic peptide that can be inserted into the virus coat protein. In most cases the inserted peptides are less than 40 amino acids. From a clinical vaccine perspective, a single linear antigen epitope may not provide complete protection against an infectious disease.

A. *tumefaciens* Mediated Stable Transformation

The first reported vaccine candidate expressed in transgenic plants was the cell surface adhesin protein (spa A) from *streptococcus mutans*, a major bacterial cause of tooth decay (Curtiss and Cardineau, 1990). The *spaA* gene was introduced into tobacco by *Agrobacterium*-mediated transformation methods. The protein was expressed at levels of up to 0.02% of total leaf protein. Oral immunization with this plant-synthesized vaccine stimulated the production of protective secretory IgA in saliva. The 185 kD size of SpaA protein demonstrated the ability of the plant genome to accommodate large foreign gene inserts, a distinct advantage for vaccine efficacy.

Hepatitis B virus (HBV) is the major cause of acute and chronic hepatitis in humans. The HBV surface antigen (HbsAg) was the first viral antigen to be produced in transgenic plants (Mason *et al.*, 1992). The expression level of HbsAg in tobacco plants was about 0.01% of TSP. The recombinant HbsAg assembled into subviral particles of 22 nm in diameter similar to those found in the sera of human patients (Thanavala *et al.*, 1995). Intraperitioneal immunization of mice (0.5ug/dose) induced anti-HbsAg antibodies. The primed T cells from immunized mice could be stimulated by a yeast derived HbsAg in a T cell proliferation assay (Richter *et al.*, 2000). The results demonstrated that both B and T cell epitopes of plant produced HbsAg are preserved. One drawback is that transgenic tobacco leaves can not be fed directly to animals. The HbsAg was later expressed in potato plants. Various strategies have been explored to enhance antigen expression in the plant, including addition of 5' and 3' flanking elements, different promoters and protein targeting within plant cells. The highest antigen expression level was 0.25 % of total soluble protein (Richter *et al.*, 2000). Oral immunization with raw potatoes (5.5ug/dose) plus 10 μg of cholera toxin added as adjuvant stimulated a serum antibody response. A booster dose of 0.5 μg yeast derived HbsAg resulted in an immediate high level secondary antibody response. This study opens the way for the development of oral vaccines for non-enteric human pathogenic HBV. Transgenic lupin and lettuce plants expressing HbsAg have also been generated (Kapusta *et al.*, 1999). A one time feeding of 5 g lupin callus (5.5 *ng*/g HbsAg) induced an HbsAg specific IgG response. Encouraged by the results of animal studies, human volunteers were immunized twice orally with HbsAg expressing transgenic lettuce leaves containing approximately 22 to 30 μg of HbsAg per dose (Kapusta *et al.*, 1999). Two of three volunteers developed serum IgG antibodies against HbsAg at levels considered protective, suggesting that humans may be orally immunized against HBV with edible plant vaccines. However, more human volunteers must be added in future trials to draw statistically significant conclusions.

Enterotoxigenic *E.coli* (ETEC) is considered to be one of the most common causes of traveler's diarrhea. ETEC possesses two major pathogenic traits: colonization of the small intestine and production of enterotoxins. The binding subunit of heat-labile ETEC enterotoxin (LTB) was expressed in transgenic potato and tabacco plants at a level of 0.01% of total soluble protein (Haq *et al.*, 1995). Codon optimization of the LTB gene in plants significantly increased the expression level to 0.15% of total soluble protein. Oral administration of the plant derived LTB in mice induced both serum IgG and mucosal IgA which neutralized the enterotoxin in a cell protection assay (Mason *et al.*, 1998). This plant vaccine project advanced to human clinical trials. Raw potato tubers (50 g to 100 g) containing 0.5 mg to 1 mg recombinant LTB were consumed by 14 volunteers on day 0, 7, and 21. Both systemic and mucosal immune responses to LTB were detected in volunteers (Tacket *et al.*, 1998). This work demonstrated for the first time that an edible vaccine against a bacterial antigen produced in transgenic plants could generate an immune response in humans.

Cholera is an acute diarrheal disease that has caused recurrent lethal pandemics largely in the developing world. The cholera toxin (CT) isolated from *Vibrio cholerae* is one of the most potent immunogens ever found. CT is a hetero-hexameric protein in which a single toxic A subunit is associated with a ring-like B pentamer formed by the association of five identical B monomers. The toxic A subunit is readily cleaved by exogenous proteases to form A1 and A2 peptide fragments, linked via a single disulphide bond (Hol *et al.*, 1995). The A1 subunit catalyses ADP-ribosylation of a Gs protein, which leads to an elevation in cyclic AMP (cAMP) levels in the cell (Stavric *et al.*, 1978). Increased cAMP levels cause continuous activation of protein kinases which phosphorylate membrane porins which in turn results in chloride ion efflux causing a concomitant osmotic movement of water into the gut lumen and characteristic profuse watery diarrhea. The A2 peptide fragment is a helical adaptor peptide whose major function is to interact with the B subunit and link the A1 subunit with the B subunit pentamer (Zhang *et al.*, 1995). The CTB pentamers bind to G_{M1} ganglioside sugars presented on mammalian cell surfaces, including the cell surface of intestinal epithelial cells (Merrit *et al.*, 1994). To develop a plant based cholera vaccine, potatoes were engineered to produce the cholera toxin B subunit (CTB) (Arakawa *et al.*, 1997). An ER retention signal was fused to the C-terminus of the CTB protein to facilitate accumulation of CTB in plant cells. Expression levels in potato tubers reached 0.3% of total soluble protein. Like the native CTB, the plant synthesized CTB formed a G_{M1} ganglioside binding pentameric structure. Mice fed 3 g of transgenic potato tubers (30 ug CTB), generated significant levels of serum and mucosal antibodies against CTB (Arakawa *et al.*, 1998a). Following intraileal injection with CT, the immunized mice showed up to a 60% reduction in fluid accumulation in the small intestine. Of additional importance, the authors showed that the immune response could be significantly boosted by a single oral dose two months later indicating the presence of memory B cells.

Previous experiments showed that CT and CTB are not only immunogenic, they (especially CT), also possess significant mucosal adjuvanticity, being able to enhance the immunogenicity of relatively poor mucosal antigens when mixed or conjugated with the antigens (Jackson *et al.*, 1993; Holmgren *et al.*, 1994; Hajishengallis *et al.*, 1995; Czerkinsky *et al.*, 1996). Yu and Langridge reported the expression of a cholera toxin fusion protein with a rotavirus antigen and an ETEC antigen in transgenic potatoes (Yu *et al.*,

2000). A 22 amino acid epitope from rotavirus enterotoxin NSP4 was fused to the C terminus of CTB and an ETEC fimbrial antigen CFA/I was fused to the N terminus of the cholera toxin A2 subunit. The chimeric antigens were synthesized in potato tuber tissues and assembled into cholera holotoxin-like structures that retained enterocyte binding affinity. Mice fed 3 g (about 30 μg vaccine) transgenic tuber tissue generated both serum and mucosal antibodies against all three antigens. A strong Th1 response with elevated levels of interleukin 2 and interferon γ was detected in immunized mice. Passively immunized mouse pups showed a significant reduction in diarrhea symptoms against rotavirus challenge (Yu and Langridge, 2001). The results of this work address two important issues in plant-based oral vaccine development. The use of CTB as a carrier molecule for targeting multiple antigens to the mucosal immune system lowered the amount of antigen protein required for oral administration, which helps to circumvent problems associated with the presently low expression levels of foreign antigen proteins in transgenic plants. Secondly, the expression of multiple antigens in a single plant has opened the way for designing multicomponent plant vaccines for simultaneous protection against several infectious diseases or multivalent vaccines including several antigens against a single pathogen.

Norwalk virus is a major cause of acute viral gastroenteritis in humans. The virus particle is constructed of a single capsid protein. Norwalk virus capsid protein (NVCP) expressed in tobacco and potato plants formed 38 nm virus-like particles (Mason *et al.*, 1996). Mice given NVCP extracts from tobacco leaves by gavage developed serum IgG and secretory IgA that recognized Norwalk virus particles. Four of 20 human volunteers who ingested 150 g potato (215-751 mg NVCP) developed specific serum IgG, and 6 of 20 volunteers developed specific IgA, even though the antibody response was modest (Tacket *et al.*, 2000).

The VP1 protein of FMDV was also expressed in *Arabidopsis thaliana* and alfalfa transgenic plants by means of *A. tumefaciens* mediated transformation (Carrillo *et al.*, 1998; Wigdorovitz *et al.*, 1999a). In comparison with the CPMV plant virus transfer system previously described, the whole intact VP1 gene was introduced into plants. The authors also demonstrated protection in immunized mice against virulent FMDV infection. This experiment extends the importance of plant vaccines into veterinary vaccination programs in addition to human applications.

Chloroplast Engineering

A. tumefaciens mediated nuclear transformation has been widely used for stable plant expression of foreign antigens for vaccine purposes. However, most monocotyledonous plants, are outside the host range of *A. tumefaciens*, and are difficult to transform by this *in vivo* method. Recent successes in chloroplast genome engineering have provided an alternative for increased foreign gene expression in plants (Bogorad, 2000). Certain characteristics of the chloroplast make it an ideal compartment for vaccine production. The simplicity of the plastid genome, only 120-150 genes per chromosome, makes it relatively easy to manipulate. The high copy numbers of each gene can generate extremely high levels of foreign protein, up to 46% of total soluble protein have been observed (De Cosa *et al.*, 2001). Many genes are organized in operons, thus, multiple genes can be transcribed together from one DNA insert. The insertion of foreign genes is site specific by homologous recombination comparing random insertion mediated by *A. tumefaciens*. Furthermore, chloroplasts can be used for production of gene products that are toxic in the cytoplasm. For environmental safety concerns, chloroplast engineering can be a friendly method. No antibiotic resistant marker genes are essential for selection of transformants. Chloroplast genes are not present in pollen. Thus, spreading of a foreign gene to plants in the environment would not be possible.

Up to the present, most efforts in chloroplast engineering have been focused on improving agricultural traits such as herbicide resistance, pathogen resistance and drought tolerance (De Cosa *et al.*, 2001). The expression of CTB in tobacco chloroplasts was the first report of chloroplast transformation to develop edible plant vaccines (Daniell *et al.*, 2001). The CTB protein level accumulated to approximately 4.1% of total soluble leaf protein. Chloroplast derived CTB was found to assemble into oligomers capable of binding the G_{M1} ganglioside receptors. This report has demonstrated the potential of the chloroplast system for vaccine production. Since the chloroplast is more like a prokaryotic system, it is ideal for the expression of antigens of bacterial origin. One potential negative feature may be that the chloroplast may not be suitable for expression of antigens of higher eukaryotic human, viral or animal origin, which could require more complicated post-translational processing machinery which does not exist within the chloroplast.

EDIBLE VACCINE AGAINST AUTOIMMUNE DISEASES

Th1 lymphocyte mediated autoimmune diseases such as multiple sclerosis, rheumatoid arthritis, and Type 1 diabetes mellitus (IDDM), currently affect 30-42 million people worldwide with increasing numbers annually. In normal persons, autoreactive T cells are generally downregulated or eliminated. However, predisposed genetic backgrounds and environmental factors may trigger activation of autoreactive T cells, causing tissue-specific or systemic damage (Luppi *et al.*, 1995; Weiner *et al.*, 2000). Insulin dependent diabetes mellitus is one of the best studied autoimmune diseases (Jean-Francois and Lucienne, 2001). Previous work has demonstrated that oral administration of disease specific autoantigens such as insulin and glutamic acid decarboxylase (GAD), could prevent or delay the onset of autoimmune diabetes symptoms in prediabetic non-obese diabetic (NOD) mice (Blanas *et al.*, 1996; Whitacre *et al.*, 1996; Bergerot *et al.*, 1997; Weiner, 1997). In 1997, GAD was expressed in transgenic tabacco at levels reaching approximately 0.4% TSP (Ma *et al.*, 1997). Approximately 1.0-1.5 mg of plant derived GAD was fed daily to prediabetic NOD mice. After 4 weeks of feeding, a significant suppression of diabetes symptoms was detected. However, the therapeutic potential of autoantigen therapy was limited by the substantial amounts of plant produced antoantigens required to induce a state of oral tolerance. To expedite targeting of autoantigens to the immune system, GAD and proinsulin were fused to the CTB molecule (Arakawa *et al.*, 1998b;1999). The chimeric CTB fusion proteins were produced in potatoes at a level of 0.1% of total soluble protein (Arakawa *et al.*, 1998b; 1999). The CTB-INS and CTB-GAD fusion proteins were able to assemble into pentamers, which retained G_{M1} ganglioside binding affinity and antigenicity of insulin and GAD. NOD mice fed 3 g of transgenic potato tuber containing 30 µg of autoantigens once a week for 5 weeks showed a substantial reduction in pancreatic islet inflammation (insulitis), and a substantial delay of clinical diabetes (hyperglycemia) onset. This experiment indicated that the dose of autoantigens required to induce tolerance could be reduced from 1 mg daily for 7 months to 30 µg once per week for 5 weeks for an equivalent therapeutic result and underscored the value of the CTB carrier system and the feasibility of plant derived edible vaccines for prevention of Th1 lymphocyte mediated autoimmune diseases.

One of the most attractive aspects of plant based immunization is the apparent simplicity of immunization against both infectious and autoimmune diseases. The most obvious outward difference between plant mediated immunization against infectious disease and the generation of plant based protection against the autoimmune disease development is the fusion of the carrier protein with either antigenic protein for protection against infectious disease or fusion of the carrier with an autoantigen to provide immunotolerance against autoimmune disease development. From an immunological perspective, mucosal immunization with an antigen appears to stimulate a dominant Th1 cell response resulting in induction of cytotoxic macrophages and cytotoxic lymphocytes which secrete inflammatory cytokines (IL-2 and IFN-γ thereby generating an inflammatory response. Alternatively, immunization with small amounts of autoantigens delivered by food plants stimulate an immunotolerizing 'bystander suppression' response in which autoantigen activated Th2 lymphocytes migrate to the site of inflammation and secrete cytokines including IL-4, IL-10 and TGF-β, which suppress cytotoxic macrophages and lymphocytes from secreting inflammatory cytokines.

SAFETY OF GENETICALLY MODIFIED (GM) PLANTS AND PLANT-BASED VACCINES

Various products from bio-engineered organisms have been acknowledged in the scientific community and licensed for commercial use. However, due to a lack of adequate safety information, the concept of genetically modified (GM) plants has stirred confusion and fear in the public sector (Stewart *et al.*, 2000). Ongoing protests in Europe continue to remind scientists of the importance of the establishment of safety criteria to evaluate the potential risk of the application of GM plant products. Some of the safety aspects which apply to plant vaccines which must be addressed include: the horizontal transfer of foreign genes from GM crops to wild relatives, the possibility of development of food allergies from edible plant vaccines, the toxicity of vaccine gene products to humans, and additional environmental concerns. A recent report indicates that pollen from *Bacillus thuringiensis* (Bt) toxin producing corn could kill Monarch butterfly caterpillars, which suggested a potential risk of GM plants for altering the environment in potentially unfavorable ways (Losey *et al.*, 1999). However, critics indicate that Bt bacteria, which are themselves widely used as pesticidal sprays, could also harm a variety of desirable butterflies. In 1996, a study reported that people allergic to Brazil nuts would also be allergic to GM soybeans that express a Brazil nut protein (Nordlee *et al.*, 1996). Since the experimentation was performed in a laboratory environment, unlike the release of traditionally bred killer bees into the environment, further experimentation was discontinued. Again critics say that foods such as peanuts and Brazil nuts themselves pose much higher risk of allergies than GM plants. In fact GM plants or transgenic plant vaccines are more genetically defined and thus much safer than conventional plant products obtained by conventional crossing methods. The question of food allergy of plant vaccines can be tested directly during clinical trials or by analyzing the sequence of the foreign proteins to see if they resemble known food allergens. Multiple mutations or deletions could limit the host range of the genetically modified plant viruses or prevent *in vivo* recombination to form virulent strains (Danner, 1997). In comparison with conventional injection of killed or live attenuated bacterial or viral vaccines, edible plant vaccines appear to be much safer and more palatable than their injectable counterparts. The lack of public education concerning the safety and benefits of GM plants has contributed significantly to the current negative responses. Clearly, the scientific community has a responsibility for maintaining open communication about the risk assessment and risk management necessary to help build public confidence in bio-engineered plant vaccines.

PLANT VACCINES' FUTURE PERSPECTIVES

The predicted increase in the world population from 6 billion to 8-9 billion by 2050 will require development of novel methods for simple, easy to prepare and disseminate protection against infectious and autoimmune diseases. Plants, harvesters of light energy, are one of the most inexpensive sources of protein and therefore, potentially also one of the cheapest sources of recombinant proteins. The potential for production scale-up makes plants possibly the most cost-effective source of vaccines yet developed (Arntzen, 1997, 1998; Richter and Kipp, 1999). However, certain basic questions must be addressed. A substantial obstacle to effective plant-based vaccines remains the low level of accumulation of foreign antigens in plant tissues. This issue becomes even more problematic for less immunogenic antigens. Manipulation of antigen encoding genes at both the transcriptional and translational levels may increase the expression levels of recombinant protein in the plant. Such strategies include addition of transcriptional and translational enhancer sequences, addition of targeted leader peptides, addition of ER retention signals (Schouten *et al.*, 1996), application of constitutively active promoters, adjustment of the codon usage to favor plant gene expression, and removal of RNA splice sites and intron sequences (Mor *et al.*, 1998; Ma *et al.*, 1999). However, there may be further limitations to how much foreign protein can be synthesized or accumulated in stably transformed plant cells without sacrificing biomass.

Alternative solutions to increased production of antigen proteins in plants which can improve the utilization of the plant product by man or animals include improved targeting of antigen molecules to enterocytes or to lymphocytes of the mucosal immune system, which could significantly reduce the amount of plant-produced antigen protein presently needed for successful oral immunization (Arakawa *et al.*, 1998). An accumulating body of evidence indicates that the cholera toxin B subunit is an effective carrier molecule for targeting antigens specifically to receptors located in the intestinal epithelial cell membrane. The inclusion of HIV transactivation sequences (Tat) peptides (Barka *et al.*, 2000), another source of a general enterocyte targeting molecule, is currently under active investigation in our laboratory. Cholera toxin A subunits that have been genetically altered to eliminate toxicity while maintaining strong adjuvant activity may also be employed to increase the mucosal immune response. The addition of plant secretion signals to the antigen proteins could permit recombinant proteins produced by the plant to be continuously secreted into liquid culture media, never reaching toxic levels that might compromise the health of the plant production system.

Simple purification methods may permit the harvest of large amounts of recombinant proteins accumulated in liquid culture media. Under sterile environmental conditions of optimal temperature and light, trangenic plants can produce foreign proteins approaching 24 hours a day. Increased expression levels of antigen protein in the plant could reduce the dose of plant vaccine delivered for immunization. This source of antigen variability might be reduced by minimal processing of the plant material, for example, freeze drying followed by grinding and mixing the dried tissues to create uniform batches of plant-based antigen.

Foreign proteins are frequently subjected to post-translational modifications in plant cells following synthesis (McGarvey *et al.*, 1995). Post-translational processes such as correct protein folding, glycosylation, and proteolysis may greatly affect antigen stability and immunogenicity. While post-translational modification in plants is similar to that found in animal cells, small but critical variations may occur. Therefore, continued efforts to study the structure and function of plant-produced antigen proteins must be emphasized.

In addition, the issue of biological safety of plant delivered vaccines must continue to be addressed in great detail. Regulations for the use of trangenic plant tissues for vaccine purposes must be established before human clinical trials can be initiated. Finally, the environmental impact of growing transgenic plants in the field must be assessed to settle issues of public safety. Thus, considerable research into basic molecular mechanisms of the immune response and targeting of antigen and autoantigen molecules is required as well as continuous dissemination of education of citizens concerning immunologic safety issues such as immunotolerization, effective dosage for immunization and frequency of vaccine administration must be accomplished before children can simply be protected against diseases by drinking a glass of tomato juice or eating a slice of transgenic banana.

REFERENCES

Arakawa, T., Chong, D.K., and Langridge, W.H. 1998a. Efficacy of a food plant-based oral cholera toxin B subunit vaccine. Nat. Biotechnol. 16: 292-297.

Arakawa, T., Chong, D.K., Merritt, J.L., and Langridge, W.H. 1997. Expression of cholera toxin B subunit oligomers in transgenic potato plants. Transgenic Res. 6: 403-413.

Arakawa, T., Chong, D.K.X., Yu, J., Hough, J., Engen, P.C., Elliott, J.F., and Langridge, W.H.R. 1999. Suppression of autoimmune diabetes by a plant-delivered cholera toxin B subunit-human glutamate decarboxylase fusion protein. Transgenics 3: 51-60.

Arakawa, T., Yu, J., Chong, D.K., Hough, J., Engen, P.C., and Langridge, W.H. 1998b. A plant-based cholera toxin B subunit-insulin fusion protein protects against the development of autoimmune diabetes. Nat. Biotechnol. 16: 934-938.

Arntzen, C.J. 1997. High-tech herbal medicine: Plant-based vaccines. Nat. Biotech. 15: 221-222.

Arntzen, C.J. 1998. Pharmaceutical foodstuffs—oral immunization with transgenic plants. Nat. Med. Vaccine Supplement 4: 502-503.

Barka, T., Gresik, E.W., and van Der, N.H. 2000. Transduction of TAT-HA-beta-galactosidase fusion protein into salivary gland-derived cells and organ cultures of the developing gland, and into rat submandibular gland in vivo. J. Histochem. Cytochem. 48: 1453-1460.

Beachy, R.N., Fitchen, J.H., and Hein, M.B. 1996. Use of plant viruses for delivery of vaccine epitopes. Ann. N.Y. Acad. Sci. 792: 43-49.

Belanger, H., Fleysh, N., Cox, S., Bartman, G., Deka, D., Trudel, M., Koprowski, H., and Yusibov, V. 2000. Human respiratory syncytial virus vaccine antigen produced in plants. FASEB J. 14: 2323-2328.

Bergerot, I., Ploix, C., Petersen, J., Moulin, V., Rask, C., Fabien, N., Lindblad, M., Mayer, A., Czerkinsky, C., Holmgren, J., and Thivolet, C. 1997. A cholera toxoid-insulin conjugate as an oral vaccine against spontaneous autoimmune diabetes. Proc. Natl. Acad. Sci. USA. 94: 4610-4614.

Blanas, E., Carbone, F.R., Allison, J., Miller, J.F., and Heath, W.R. 1996. Induction of autoimmune diabetes by oral administration of autoantigen. Science 274: 1707-1709.

Bogorad, L. 2000. Engineering chloroplasts: An alternative site for foreign genes, proteins, reactions and products. Trends Biotechnol. 18: 257-263.

Brandtzaeg, P. 1995. Basic mechanisms of mucosal immunity. A major adaptive defense system. Immunologists 3: 89-96.

Brennan, F.R., Gilleland, L.B., Staczek, J., Bendig, M.M., Hamilton, W.D., and Gilleland, H.E., Jr. 1999a. A chimaeric plant virus vaccine protects mice against a bacterial infection. Microbiology 145: 2061-2067.

Brennan, F.R., Jones, T.D., Longstaff, M., Chapman, S., Bellaby, T., Smith, H., Xu, F., Hamilton, W.D., and Flock, J.I. 1999b. Immunogenicity of peptides derived from a fibronectin-binding protein of *S. aureus* expressed on two different plant viruses. Vaccine 17: 1846-1857.

Carrillo, C., Wigdorovitz, A., Oliveros, J.C., Zamorano, P.I., Sadir, A.M., Gomez, N., Salinas, J., Escribano, J.M., and Borca, M.V. 1998. Protective immune response to foot-and-mouth disease virus with VP1 expressed in transgenic plants. J. Virol. 72: 1688-1690.

Castanon, S., Marin, M.S., Martin-Alonso, J.M., Boga, J.A., Casais, R., Humara, J.M., Ordas, R.J., and Parra, F. 1999. Immunization with potato plants expressing VP60 protein protects against rabbit hemorrhagic disease virus. J. Virol. 73: 4452-4455.

Conrad, U. and Fiedler, U. 1998. Compartment-specific accumulation of recombinant immunoglobulins in plant cells: An essential tool for antibody production and immunomodulation of physiological functions and pathogen activity. Plant Mol. Biol. 38: 101-109.

Curtiss, R., and Cardineau, G.A. 1990. World Intellectual Property Organization PCT/US89/03799.

Czerkinsky, C., Quiding, M., Eriksson, K., Nordstrom, I., Lakew, M., Weneras, C., Kilander, A., Bjorck, S., Svennerholm, A.M., Butcher, E., *et al.* 1995. Induction of specific immunity at mucosal surfaces: Prospects for vaccine development. Adv. Exp. Med. Biol. 371B: 1409-1416.

Czerkinsky, C., Sun, J.B., Lebens, M., Li, B.L., Rask, C., Lindblad, M., and Holmgren, J. 1996. Cholera toxin B subunit as transmucosal carrier-delivery and immunomodulating system for induction of anti infectious and antipathological immunity. Ann. NY. Acad. Sci. 778: 185-193.

Dalsgaard, K., Uttenthal, A., Jones, T.D., Xu, F., Merryweather, A., Hamilton, W.D., Langeveld, J.P., Boshuizen, R.S., Kamstrup, S., Lomonossoff, G.P., Porta, C., Vela, C., Casal, J.I., Meloen, R.H., and Rodgers, P.B. 1997. Plant-derived vaccine protects target animals against a viral disease. Nat. Biotechnol. 15: 248-252.

Daniell, H., Lee, S.B., Panchal, T., and Wiebe, P.O. 2001. Expression of the native cholera toxin B subunit gene and assembly as functional oligomers in transgenic tobacco chloroplasts. J. Mol. Biol. 311: 1001-1009.

Danner, K. 1997. Acceptability of bio-engineered vaccines. Comp. Immunol. Microbiol. Infect. Dis. 20: 3-12.

De Cosa, B., Moar, W., Lee, S.B., Miller, M., and Daniell, H. 2001. Overexpression of the Bt cry2Aa2 operon in chloroplasts leads to formation of insecticidal crystals. Nat. Biotechnol. 19: 71-74.

Fernandez-Fernandez, M.R., Martinez-Torrecuadrada, J.L., Casal, J.I., and Garcia, J.A. 1998. Development of an antigen presentation system based on plum pox potyvirus. FEBS Lett. 427: 229-235.

Fernandez-Fernandez, M.R., Mourino, M., Rivera, J., Rodriguez, F., Plana-Duran, J., and Garcia, J.A. 2001. Protection of rabbits against rabbit hemorrhagic disease virus by immunization with the VP60 protein expressed in plants with a potyvirus-based vector. Virology 280: 283-291.

Fiedler, U. and Conrad, U. 1995. High-level production and long-term storage of engineered antibodies in transgenic tobacco seeds. Biotechnology 13: 1090-1093.

Fitchen, J., Beachy, R.N., and Hein, M.B. 1995. Plant virus expressing hybrid coat protein with added murine epitope elicits autoantibody response. Vaccine 13: 1051-1057.

Freytag, L.C. and Clements, J.D. 1999. Bacterial toxins as mucosal adjuvants. Curr. Top. Microbiol. Immunol. 236: 215-236.

Gil, F., Brun, A., Wigdorovitz, A., Catala, R., Martinez-Torrecuadrada, J.L., Casal, I., Salinas, J., Borca, M.V., and Escribano, J.M. 2001. High-yield expression of a viral peptide vaccine in transgenic plants. FEBS Lett. 488: 13-17.

Gomez, N., Carrillo, C., Salinas, J., Parra, F., Borca, M.V., and Escribano, J.M. 1998. Expression of immunogenic glycoprotein S polypeptides from transmissible gastroenteritis coronavirus in transgenic plants. Virology 249: 352-358.

Gomez, N., Wigdorovitz, A., Castanon, S., Gil, F., Ordas, R., Borca, M.V., and Escribano, J.M. 2000. Oral immunogenicity of the plant derived spike protein from swine-transmissible gastroenteritis coronavirus. Arch. Virol. 145: 1725-1732.

Hajishengallis, G., Hollingshead, S.K., Koga, T., and Russell, M.W. 1995. Mucosal immunization with a bacterial protein antigen genetically coupled to cholera toxin A2/B subunits. J. Immunol. 154: 4322-4332.

Haq, T.A., Mason, H.S., Clements, J.D., and Arntzen, C.J. 1995. Oral immunization with a recombinant bacterial antigen produced in transgenic plants. Science 268: 714-716.

Hiatt, A., Cafferkey, R., and Bowdish, K. 1989. Production of antibodies in transgenic plants. Nature 342: 76-78.

Hijarrubia, M.J., Casqueiro, J., Gutierrez, S., Fernandez, F.J., and Martin, J.F. 1997. Characterization of the *bip* gene of *Aspergillus awamori* encoding a protein with an HDEL retention signal homologous to the mammalian BiP involved in polypeptide secretion. Curr. Genet. 32: 139-146.

Hol, W.G.J., Sixma, T.K., and Meritt, E.A. 1995. Structure and function of *E. coli* heat-labile enterotoxin and cholera toxin B pentamer. In: Handbook of Natural Toxins. J. Moss, B. Iglewski, M. Vaughan, A.T. Tu, ed. Dekker, New York. p. 185-223.

Holmgren, J., Czerkinsky, C., Lycke, N., and Svennerholm, A.M. 1994. Strategies for the induction of immune responses at mucosal surfaces making use of cholera toxin B subunit as immunogen, carrier, and adjuvant. Am. J. Trop. Med. Hyg. 50: 42-54.

Huang, Z., Dry, I., Webster, D., Strugnell, R., and Wesselingh, S. 2001. Plant-derived measles virus hemagglutinin protein induces neutralizing antibodies in mice. Vaccine 19: 2163-2171.

Jackson, R.J., Fujihashi, K., Xu-Amano, J., Kiyono, H., Elson, C.O., and McGhee, J.R. 1993. Optimizing oral vaccines: Induction of systemic and mucosal B-cell and antibody responses to tetanus toxoid by use of cholera toxin as an adjuvant. Infect. Immun. 61: 4272-4279.

Jean-Francois, B., and Lucienne, C. 2001. Tolerance to islet autoantigens in type 1 diabetes. Annu. Rev. Immunol. 19: 131-161.

Joelson, T., Akerblom, L., Oxelfelt, P., Strandberg, B., Tomenius, K., and Morris, T.J. 1997. Presentation of a foreign peptide on the surface of tomato bushy stunt virus. J. Gen. Virol. 78: 1213-1217.

Kapusta, J., Modelska, A., Figlerowicz, M., Pniewski, T., Letellier, M., Lisowa, O., Yusibov, V., Koprowski, H., Plucienniczak, A., and Legocki, A.B. 1999. A plant-derived edible vaccine against hepatitis B virus. FASEB J. 13: 1796-1799.

Koo, M., Bendahmane, M., Lettieri, G.A., Paoletti, A.D., Lane, T.E., Fitchen, J.H., Buchmeier, M.J., and Beachy, R.N. 1999. Protective immunity against murine hepatitis virus (MHV) induced by intranasal or subcutaneous administration of hybrids of tobacco mosaic virus that carries an MHV epitope. Proc. Natl. Acad. Sci. USA. 96: 7774-7779.

Lauterslager, T.G., Florack, D.E., van der Wal, T.J., Molthoff, J.W., Langeveld, J.P., Bosch, D., Boersma, W.J., and Hilgers, L.A. 2001. Oral immunisation of naive and primed animals with transgenic potato tubers expressing LT-B. Vaccine 19: 2749-2755.

Lee, R.W., Strommer, J., Hodgins, D., Shewen, P.E., Niu, Y., and Lo, R.Y. 2001. Towards development of an edible vaccine against bovine pneumonic pasteurellosis using transgenic white clover expressing a *Mannheimia haemolytica* A1 leukotoxin 50 fusion protein. Infect. Immun. 69: 5786-5793.

Losey, J.E., Rayor, L.S., and Carter, M.E. 1999. Transgenic pollen harms monarch larvae. Nature 399: 214.

Luppi, P., Rossiello, M.R., Faas, S., and Trucco, M. 1995. Genetic background and environment contribute synergistically to the onset of autoimmune diseases. J. Mol. Med. 73: 381-393.

Ma, J.K., Hiatt, A., Hein, M., Vine, N.D., Wang, F., Stabila, P., van Dolleweerd, C., Mostov, K., and Lehner, T. 1995. Generation and assembly of secretory antibodies in plants. Science 268: 716-719.

Ma, J.K., Hikmat, B.Y., Wycoff, K., Vine, N.D., Chargelegue, D., Yu, L., Hein, M.B., and Lehner, T. 1998. Characterization of a recombinant plant monoclonal secretory antibody and preventive immunotherapy in humans. Nat. Med. 4: 601-606.

Ma, J.K. and Vine, N.D. 1999. Plant expression systems for the production of vaccines. Curr. Top. Microbiol. Immunol. 236: 275-292.

Ma, S.W., Zhao, D.L., Yin, Z.Q., Mukherjee, R., Singh, B., Qin, H.Y., Stiller, C.R., and Jevnikar, A.M. 1997. Transgenic plants expressing autoantigens fed to mice to induce oral immune tolerance. Nat. Med. 3: 793-796.

Mason, H.S. and Arntzen, C.J. 1995. Transgenic plants as vaccine production systems. Trends Biotechnol. 13: 388-392.

Mason, H.S., Ball, J.M., Shi, J.J., Jiang, X., Estes, M.K., and Arntzen, C.J. 1996. Expression of Norwalk virus capsid protein in transgenic tobacco and potato and its oral immunogenicity in mice. Proc. Natl. Acad. Sci. USA. 93: 5335-5340.

Mason, H.S., Haq, T.A., Clements, J.D., and Arntzen, C.J. 1998. Edible vaccine protects mice against *Escherichia coli* heat-labile enterotoxin (LT): Potatoes expressing a synthetic LT-B gene. Vaccine 16: 1336-1343.

Mason, H.S., Lam, D.M., and Arntzen, C.J. 1992. Expression of hepatitis B surface antigen in transgenic plants. Proc. Natl. Acad. Sci. USA. 89: 11745-11749.

McCormick, A.A., Kumagai, M.H., Hanley, K., Turpen, T.H., Hakim, I., Grill, L.K., Tuse, D., Levy, S., and Levy, R. 1999. Rapid production of specific vaccines for lymphoma by expression of the tumor-derived single-chain Fv epitopes in tobacco plants. Proc. Natl. Acad. Sci. USA. 96: 703-708.

McGarvey, P.B., Hammond, J., Dienelt, M.M., Hooper, D.C., Fu, Z.F., Dietzschold, B., Koprowski, H., and Michaels, F.H. 1995. Expression of the rabies virus glycoprotein in transgenic tomatoes. Biotechnology 13: 1484-1487.

McLain, L., Durrani, Z., Wisniewski, L.A., Porta, C., Lomonossoff, G.P., and Dimmock, N.J. 1996. Stimulation of neutralizing antibodies to human immunodeficiency virus type 1 in three strains of mice immunized with a 22 amino acid peptide of gp41 expressed on the surface of a plant virus. Vaccine 14: 799-810.

Merrit, E.A., Sarfaty, S., Akker, F.V.D. L'Hoir, C., Martial, J.A., and Hol, W.G.J. 1994. Crystal structure of cholera toxin B-pentamer bound to recptor GM1 pentasaccharide. Protein Sci. 3: 166-175.

Mitchell, V.S., Philipose, N.M., and Sanford J.P. 1993. The children's vaccine initiative. National Academy Press. 36: 57-59.

Modelska, A., Dietzschold, B., Sleysh, N., Fu, Z.F., Steplewski, K., Hooper, D.C., Koprowski, H., and Yusibov, V. 1998. Immunization against rabies with plant-derived antigen. Proc. Natl. Acad. Sci. USA. 95: 2481-2485.

Moffat, A.S. 1995. Exploring transgenic plants as a new vaccine source. Science 268: 658-660.

Mor, T.S., Gomez-Lim, M.A., and Palmer, K.E. 1998. Perspective: Edible vaccines—A concept coming of age. Trends Microbiol. 6: 449-453.

Nemchinov, L.G., Liang, T.J., Rifaat, M.M., Mazyad, H.M., Hadidi, A., and Keith, J.M. 2000. Development of a plant-derived subunit vaccine candidate against hepatitis C virus. Arch. Virol. 145: 2557-2573.

Nordlee, J.A., Taylor, S.L., Townsend, J.A., Thomas, L.A., and Bush, R.K. 1996. Identification of a Brazil-nut allergen in transgenic soybeans. N. Engl. J. Med. 334: 688-692.

Porta, C., Spall, V.E., Loveland, J., Johnson, J.E., Barker, P.J., and Lomonossoff, G.P. 1994. Development of cowpea mosaic virus as a high-yielding system for the presentation of foreign peptides. Virology 202: 949-955.

Richter, L. and Kipp, P.B. 1999. Transgenic plants as edible vaccines. Curr. Top. Microbiol. Immunol. 240: 159-176.

Richter, L.J., Thanavala, Y., Arntzen, C.J., and Mason, H.S. 2000. Production of hepatitis B surface antigen in transgenic plants for oral immunization. Nat. Biotechnol. 18: 1167-1171.

Sandhu, J.S., Krasnyanski, S.F., Domier, L.L., Korban, S.S., Osadjan, M.D., and Buetow, D.E. 2000. Oral immunization of mice with transgenic tomato fruit expressing respiratory syncytial virus-F protein induces a systemic immune response. Transgenic Res. 9: 127-135.

Sandhu, J.S., Osadjan, M.D., Krasnyanski, S.F., Domier, L.L., Korban, S.S., and Buetow, D.E. 1999. Enhanced expression of the human respiratory syncytial virus-F gene in apple leaf protoplasts. Plant Cell Rep. 18: 394-397.

Schell, J.S.T. 1987. Transgenic plants as tools to study the molecular organizaiton of plant genes. Science 237: 1176-1183.

Schouten, A., Roosien, J., van Engelen, F.A., de Jong, G.A., Borst-Vrenssen, A.W., Zilverentant, J.F., Bosch, D., Stiekema, W.J., Gommers, F.J., Schots, A., and Bakker, J. 1996. The C-terminal KDEL sequence increases the expression level of a single-chain antibody designed to be targeted to both the cytosol and the secretory pathway in transgenic tobacco. Plant Mol. Biol. 30: 781-793.

Stavric, S., Speirs, J.I., Konowalchuk, J., and Jeffrey, D. 1978. Stimulation of cyclic AMP secretion in Vero cells by enterotoxins of *Escherichia coli* and *Vibrio cholerae*. Infect. Immun. 21: 514-517.

Stewart, C.N., Jr., Richards, H.A. 4th., and Halfhill, M.D. 2000. Transgenic plants and biosafety: Science, misconceptions and public perceptions. Biotechniques 29: 832-843.

Stoger, E., Vaquero, C., Torres, E., Sack, M., Nicholson, L., Drossard, J., Williams, S., Keen, D., Perrin, Y., Christou, P., and Fischer, R. 2000. Cereal crops as viable production and storage systems for pharmaceutical scFv antibodies. Plant Mol. Biol. 42: 583-590.

Streatfield, S.J., Jilka, J.M., Hood, E.E., Turner, D.D., Bailey, M.R., Mayor, J.M., Woodard, S.L., Beifuss, K.K., Horn, M.E., Delaney, D.E., Tizard, I.R., and Howard, J.A. 2001. Plant-based vaccines: Unique advantages. Vaccine 19: 2742-2748.

Sugiyama, Y., Hamamoto, H., Takemoto, S., Watanabe, Y., and Okada, Y. 1995. Systemic production of foreign peptides on the particle surface of tobacco mosaic virus. FEBS Lett. 359: 247-250.

Tackaberry, E.S., Dudani, A.K., Prior, F., Tocchi, M., Sardana, R., Altosaar, I., and Ganz, P.R. 1999. Development of biopharmaceuticals in plant expression systems: Cloning, expression and immunological reactivity of human cytomegalovirus glycoprotein B (UL55) in seeds of transgenic tobacco. Vaccine 17: 3020-3029.

Tacket, C.O., Mason, H.S., Losonsky, G., Clements, J.D., Levine, M.M., and Arntzen, C.J. 1998. Immunogenicity in humans of a recombinant bacterial antigen delivered in a transgenic potato. Nat. Med. 4: 607-609.

Tacket, C.O., Mason, H.S., Losonsky, G., Estes, M.K., Levine, M.M., and Arntzen, C.J. 2000. Human immune responses to a novel norwalk virus vaccine delivered in transgenic potatoes. J. Infect. Dis. 182: 302-305.

Thanavala, Y., Yang, Y.F., Lyons, P., Mason, H.S., and Arntzen, C. 1995. Immunogenicity of transgenic plant-derived hepatitis B surface antigen. Proc. Natl. Acad. Sci. USA. 92: 3358-3361.

Tuboly, T., Yu, W., Bailey, A., Degrandis, S., Du, S., Erickson, L., and Nagy, E. 2000. Immunogenicity of porcine transmissible gastroenteritis virus spike protein expressed in plants. Vaccine 18: 2023-2028.

Turpen, T.H., Reinl, S.J., Charoenvit, Y., Hoffman, S.L., Fallarme, V., and Grill, L.K. 1995. Malarial epitopes expressed on the surface of recombinant tobacco mosaic virus. Biotechnology 13: 53-57.

Usha, R., Rohll, J.B., Spall, V.E., Shanks, M., Maule, A.J., Johnson, J.E., and Lomonossoff, G.P. 1993. Expression of an animal virus antigenic site on the surface of a plant virus particle. Virology 197: 366-374.

Vaquero, C., Sack, M., Chandler, J., Drossard, J., Schuster, F., Monecke, M., Schillberg, S., and Fischer, R. 1999. Transient expression of a tumor-specific single-chain fragment and a chimeric antibody in tobacco leaves. Proc. Natl. Acad. Sci. USA. 96: 11128-11133.

Verch, T., Yusibov, V., and Koprowski, H. 1998. Expression and assembly of a full-length monoclonal antibody in plants using a plant virus vector. J. Immunol. Methods. 220: 69-75.

Weiner, H. L. 1997. Oral tolerance: Immune mechanisms and treatment of autoimmune diseases. Immunol. Today. 18: 335-343.

Weiner, H. L. 2000. Oral tolerance, an active immunologic process mediated by multiple mechanisms. J. Clin. Invest. 106: 935-937.

Wenzler, H.C., Mignery, G.A., Fisher, L.M., Park, W.D. 1989. Analysis of a chimaeric class I patatin-GUS gene fusion in transgenic potato plants: High level expression in tubers and sucrose-inducible expression in cultured leaf and stem explants. Plant Mol. Biol. 12: 41-50.

Whitacre, C.C., Gienapp, I.E., Meyer, A., Cox, K.L., and Javed, N. 1996. Treatment of autoimmune disease by oral tolerance to autoantigens. Clin. Immunol. Immunopathol. 80: S31-S39.

Wigdorovitz, A., Carrillo, C., Dus Santos, M.J., Trono, K., Peralta, A., Gomez, M.C., Rios, R.D., Franzone, P.M., Sadir, A.M., Escribano, J.M., and Borca, M.V. 1999a. Induction of a protective antibody response to foot and mouth disease virus in mice following oral or parenteral immunization with alfalfa transgenic plants expressing the viral structural protein VP1. Virology 255: 347-353.

Wigdorovitz, A., Perez Filgueira, D.M., Robertson, N., Carrillo, C., Sadir, A.M., Morris, T.J., and Borca, M.V. 1999b. Protection of mice against challenge with foot and mouth disease virus (FMDV) by immunization with foliar extracts from plants infected with recombinant tobacco mosaic virus expressing the FMDV structural protein VP1. Virology 264: 85-91.

Yu, J., Arakawa, T., and Langridge, W.H.R. 2000. Assembly of cholera toxin-antigen fusion proteins in transgenic potato. Transgenics 40: 1-10.

Yu, J., and Langridge, W.H.R. 2001. A plant-based multicomponent vaccine protects mice from enteric diseases. Nat. Biotechnol. 19: 548-552.

Yusibov, V., Modelska, A., Steplewski, K., Agadjanyan, M., Weiner, D., Hooper, D.C., and Koprowski, H. 1997. Antigens produced in plants by infection with chimeric plant viruses immunize against rabies virus and HIV-1. Proc. Natl. Acad. Sci. USA. 94: 5784-5788.

Zeitlin, L., Olmsted, S.S., Moench, T.R., Co, M.S., Martinell, B.J., Paradkar, V.M., Russell, D.R., Queen, C., Cone, R.A., and Whaley, K.J. 1998. A humanized monoclonal antibody produced in transgenic plants for immunoprotection of the vagina against genital herpes. Nat. Biotechnol. 16: 1361-1364.

Zhang, R.G., Scott, D.L., Westbrook, M.L., Nance, S., Spangler, B.D., Shipley, G.G., and Westbrook, E.M. 1995. The three-dimensional crystal structure of cholera toxin. J. Mol. Biol. 251: 563-573.

Index

F

Foreign antigen
  Expression in attenuated bacteria 193-199
  Factors affecting immunogenicity 194-198
Foreign gene stabilization 196-197
Fragment C 189
Freund's aduvant 26, 58

G

Gene *E* 165, 167
  Expression control 168-170
Gene transfer
  Applications 292-294
  Bacteria-mediated 290
Gene therapy 293-294
Gene gun 108
Genetically modified (GM) plant 386 *See Also* Transgenic Plants
Gut-associates lymphoid tissue (GALT) 186, 187

H

Haemophilus influenzae 2
  Capsular polysaccharide 2-4
  Type b vaccine 4, 12-13
    Coupling to carrier proteins 6
Heat shock protein 112-117
Heat-labile enterotoxin (HLT, LT) 29, 58, 62,63
  Activity 30-31
  Detoxified LT 32-36
  Mutations in the B subunit 31
  Recombinant A subunit 31-32
  Structure 29-30
Helicobacter pylori 194, 200
Helper T cell (Th), 23, 59
Hemagglutinin (HA) 91
Hepatitis 147
Hepatitis B virus (HBV) 108, 114
Herpes simplex virus 2 (HSV-2) 147
HlyA 213-215
  Secretion system 215-221
HlyB 213-215, 217
HlyD 213-215, 217
Hsp70 115, 116
Hsp73 111-115
Hsp90 115
Human immunodeficiency virus (HIV) 147, 247, 255, 270-271, 275

Human Papilloma virus (HPV) 256
Human active CpG sequence 142, 143

I

Immune response
  Extended bacterial ghost system 179-180
  Infection 22-23
  To tumor antigen 318-320
  To TCI 63
  Skin 57-63
Immunization
  Transcutaneous 53-73
  Using plant-based vaccines 377-386
Immunopotentiating reconstituted influenza virosomes 91-95 *See Also* IRIV
Immunostimulation 22-23
  Adjuvants 24-25
Immunotherapy of cancer
Influenza 58, 59, 140
  Protein 270, 275
  Nucleoprotein (NP)
  Vaccine 58, 62, 94
  Virosomes 91-95
Intracellular pathogen
Intranasal
Invasion
IRIV
  Vaccine 94-95
Iscoms 27

K

Klebsiella pneumoniae 167

L

lacZ 168,
Langerhans cell (LC) 55-57, 64, 66
Leishmania 255
  Leishmania donovanii 358
  Leishmania major 255
Lettuce 374, 375
Lipopolysaccharide (LPS) LPS 1
Liposomes 27, 83-85, 87-89
Listeria monocytogenes 212, 213, 215, 218, 232, 235, 263, 290
  Adjuvant effect 278-279
  Antigen delivery 269-273
  As a Colney's toxin 329-330
  Attenuation 267-269